Ourselves Unborn

Ourselves Unborn

A History of the Fetus in
Modern America

Sara Dubow

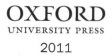

OXFORD
UNIVERSITY PRESS
2011

OXFORD
UNIVERSITY PRESS

Oxford University Press, Inc., publishes works that further
Oxford University's objective of excellence
in research, scholarship, and education.

Oxford   New York
Auckland   Cape Town   Dar es Salaam   Hong Kong   Karachi
Kuala Lumpur   Madrid   Melbourne   Mexico City   Nairobi
New Delhi   Shanghai   Taipei   Toronto

With offices in
Argentina   Austria   Brazil   Chile   Czech Republic   France   Greece
Guatemala   Hungary   Italy   Japan   Poland   Portugal   Singapore
South Korea   Switzerland   Thailand   Turkey   Ukraine   Vietnam

Published by Oxford University Press, Inc.
198 Madison Avenue, New York, New York 10016

www.oup.com

Oxford is a registered trademark of Oxford University Press

Library of Congress Cataloging-in-Publication Data
Dubow, Sara.
Ourselves unborn : a history of the fetus in modern America / Sara Dubow.
p. ; cm.
Includes bibliographical references and index.
ISBN 978-0-19-532343-6
1. Fetus—United States—History—20th century.   2. Fetus—Legal status,
laws, etc.—United States.   3. Obstetrics—United States—History—20th
century.   4. Perinatology—United States—History—20th century.
I. Title. [DNLM: 1. Fetus—United States.   2. Beginning of Human Life—United
States.   3. Civil Rights—history—United States.   4. History, 19th Century—United
States.   5. History, 20th Century—United States.   6. History, 21st Century—United
States.   7. Personhood—United States.   8. Public Policy—United States.
9. Social Environment—United States. WQ 210 D8180a 2011]
RG600.D83 2011
362.198'32—dc22   2010014000

Contents

Acknowledgments   vii

Introduction: Fetal Stories   1

Chapter 1: Discovering Fetal Life, 1870s–1920s   10

Chapter 2: Interpreting Fetal Bodies, 1930s–1970s   38

Chapter 3: Defining Fetal Personhood, 1973–1976   67

Chapter 4: Defending Fetal Rights, 1970s–1990s   112

Chapter 5: Debating Fetal Pain, 1984–2007   153

Epilogue: Fetal Meanings   184

Notes   191

Bibliography   239

Index   297

Acknowledgments

It is a tremendous pleasure to thank those who have supported me since I began this project in a graduate seminar at Rutgers University, developed it into a dissertation, and finally turned it into this book. Rutgers University provided me with exceptionally rich intellectual and personal resources. Alice Kessler-Harris is an extraordinary advisor, whose advice, wisdom, and friendship have profoundly shaped my thinking, writing, and teaching. Norma Basch, Jim Livingston, and Margaret Marsh were the ideal dissertation committee, and their dedication and engagement consistently inspired and motivated me. For demonstrating the integrity and generosity that characterize the Rutgers history department, I would also like to thank my professors and fellow graduate students Mia Bay, Jennifer Brier, Kim Brodkin, Paul Clemens, Gary Darden, John Dizgun, Dee Garrison, James Goodman, Matthew Guterl, Jennifer Jones, Dan Katz, Melissa Klapper, Peter Lau, Jan Lewis, David Oshinsky, Teresa Poor, Joan Scott, Charles Upchurch, and Deborah Gray White. I would like to especially acknowledge the friendship and support I received from Sarah Gordon, Justin Hart, and Jennifer Tammi, each of whom read different iterations of these chapters many times, made graduate school a sustaining and enriching experience, and has been a source of camaraderie and encouragement for the past fifteen years. I was also extremely fortunate in having excellent teachers and role models as an undergraduate at Williams College and a graduate student at the University of Massachusetts at Amherst. In particular, I would like to thank Charles Dew, Bruce Laurie, Carl Nightingale, Kathy Peiss, and Jim Wood.

I completed my dissertation and began revising my manuscript while I was teaching at the Brearley School, Hunter College High School, and Hunter College. I learned a great deal from my thoughtful colleagues and students, and am particularly grateful for all the advice and encouragement I received from Irving Kagan, Betty Kleinfeld, Susan Meeker, Jack Salzman, and Barbara Welter. I completed the book at Williams College, and I want to thank my colleagues in the history department for their friendship and support, and my students for inspiring me to become a better historian and better teacher. I also want to thank my student Denise Duquette for her outstanding work as my research assistant.

Rutgers University provided generous fellowship assistance, and I am also grateful for support from the Littleton-Griswold Grant for Research in U.S. Legal History, the Margaret Storrs Grierson Fellowship at the Sophia Smith Collection, the Schlesinger Library Research Support Grant, the Fellowship from the Franklin & Eleanor Roosevelt Faculty Seminar on Public Policy at Hunter College, and a PSC-CUNY Research Grant.

I have been very lucky to work with Oxford University Press and my editor Susan Ferber. Throughout the process, she has been incredibly attentive, balancing her support and encouragement with probing questions. My two anonymous readers provided me with useful and thoughtful critiques that have made this a better book.

My deepest thanks go to my friends and family. They have all listened to much talk about the fetus and have been my biggest supporters. Kate Delacorte, Nancy Diehl, Ellen Drought, Tim Hildreth, Adam Learman, Lisa Leinau, Adam Leven, Maggie Levy, Jeff Low, Andhra Lutz, Steve Martin, Ruth Potee, Joe Scavetta, Deirdre Williamson, Andrew Winston, and Traci and Joel Wolfe have helped me in countless ways. Through example and encouragement, my parents have inspired all of their children to live lives full of love and learning. I thank them, along with my grandmother, brothers, sister, in-laws, nephews, and nieces for their interest and belief in my work, and for their love and support. Finally, I want to thank Rick Berger, whose love, friendship, and encouragement has been invaluable.

Ourselves Unborn

INTRODUCTION
FETAL STORIES

The fetus is a familiar, contested, and provocative presence in American culture and politics. Ultrasound images used by activists at antiabortion protests, or produced in fetal photo studios where expectant parents can buy greeting cards and other keepsakes, illustrate the proliferation and power of the fetal image in contemporary society. Although ultrasound technology has made a particular image of the fetus extremely recognizable, that image represents only one moment on the historical continuum of encounters with the unborn. The meanings ascribed to the fetus in those encounters are neither inevitable nor self-evident. Rather, the fetus has long been a screen onto which society projects its deepest held assumptions and anxieties. *Ourselves Unborn: The Fetus in Modern America* examines how, from the late nineteenth to the early twenty-first century, Americans have articulated those assumptions and anxieties through arguments about the social value, legal identity, and political status of the human fetus.

Some recent examples illustrate how the fetus is currently imagined as part of the body politic, a citizen recognized and protected by the state. In October 2002, the United States Department of Health and Human Services added human embryos to the list of "human subjects" whose welfare must be taken into account by the Advisory Committee on Human Research Protections.[1] The next month, in revising the State Child Health Insurance Program (S-CHIP), HHS redefined the term *child* to begin at the moment of conception, making fetuses eligible for state-sponsored health insurance.[2] In April 2004, Congress signed into law the Unborn Victims of Violence Act, making the death of a pregnant woman and her zygote, embryo, or fetus in the execution of a federal crime punishable as two separate criminal violations. And in May 2004, a U.S. district judge in Missouri temporarily prohibited the deportation of a pregnant Mexican woman because "[i]f this child is an American citizen, we can't send his mother back until he is born."[3]

The policies regarding stem cell research and health insurance, the making of the killing of an unborn child a federal crime, and the immigration decision illustrate how the state constructs fetal citizens through bureaucratic technologies such as statutory policies, state and federal laws, and judicial rulings.[4] Although none of these four examples are about abortion per se, they, and the idea of fetal citizenship itself, are products of and participants in the politics of abortion that began in 1973. For nearly forty years, the *Roe v. Wade* decision has intersected with political exigencies, social tensions, religious beliefs, and technological developments to generate a series of conflicts about the meaning and status of the fetus.[5]

Some examples of these conflicts involved the so-called epidemic of "crack babies," the increasingly violent culture wars over abortion, and the eruption of a series of so-called maternal-fetal conflicts in the 1980s and 1990s. Pictures of pregnant women addicted to crack or of crack babies, and antiabortion billboards featuring aborted fetuses were part of the cultural landscape. Also part of that landscape was the escalating violence of the antiabortion movement, most horrifyingly illustrated by the bombings of abortion clinics and the assassinations of abortion providers, including, between 1993 and 1998, four physicians, two clinic employees, a security guard, and a clinic escort. In 2009, Dr. George Tiller, an abortion provider and one of the few physicians willing to perform late-term abortions, was assassinated.[6] Between 1977 and the end of September 1998, more than 3,385 bombings, arsons, blockades, episodes of vandalism, stalkings, assaults, and other acts of violence took place at clinics throughout the country.[7] The hysteria about crack babies dissipated, and the violence of the antiabortion movement was curtailed by the 1994 passage of the Freedom of Access to Clinics Entrances Act (FACE), which made it a federal crime to use force, the threat of force, or physical obstruction to prevent individuals from obtaining or providing reproductive health-care services. Nonetheless, the fetus remains a public presence.

The political culture of the 1980s and 1990s increasingly saw the interests and rights of pregnant women as separate from the interests and rights of the fetus. Courts were asked to resolve a series of perceived conflicts between women and fetuses: Could women be required to undergo sterilization procedures in order to work in certain environments? Could pregnant women be required to undergo caesarean sections without their consent? Could pregnant women be charged with child abuse or neglect if they were taking drugs? One of many examples of this phenomenon was the case of Cornelia Whitner, who had been arrested and charged with child neglect after delivering a baby with traces of cocaine in his system. In 1997, the South Carolina Supreme Court upheld her conviction. Among the countless political battles surrounding the meaning and status of the fetus since *Roe v. Wade*—battles that have included the construction of fetal citizenship, the "crack baby epidemic," and the violence of the antiabortion movement—these so-called maternal-fetal conflicts constituted just another episode in the history of public efforts to ascribe meanings to and monitor women's behavior on behalf of the fetus.

In the year following Whitner's arrest, Eric Rudolph bombed an abortion clinic in Birmingham, Alabama, and James Kopp murdered Dr. Bernard Slepian, an obstetrician and abortion provider in Buffalo, New York. At the same time, public health billboards featuring sonogram images of fetuses with messages like "Smoking will seriously damage the health of your unborn child. For their sake stop today!" proliferated in the public landscape. Stores like "A Peek in the Pod" opened, where for $295 expectant parents can buy a "keepsake package of prenatal memories" that includes a thirty-minute ultrasound session recorded on DVD, a computer screensaver, and photo frames.[8]

Ourselves Unborn: Fetal Meanings in Modern America historicizes the public fetus of the 1980s and 1990s in a larger context, contending that the meanings ascribed to the fetus from the late nineteenth century through the early twenty-first century have had more to do with social values and political circumstances than with biology or theology. Therefore, in order to understand the particular resonance of fetal discourses at particular historical moments, we need to read them against those social values and political circumstances. A fetus in 1870 is not the same thing as a fetus in 1930, which is not the same thing as a fetus in 1970, which is not the same thing as a fetus in 2010. Although multiple and competing fetuses have always coexisted, particular historical circumstances have generated and valorized different stories about the fetus. This book is about the relationship between those stories and those circumstances. By telling and interpreting stories about the origins, development, and significance of the fetus, people—individually and collectively—have expressed their assumptions and anxieties about personhood, family, motherhood, and national identity. By asking questions such as: How do people come to understand what embryos and fetuses are and what they mean? Why and how did people begin to make an emotional and political investment in the fetus? How do particular stories become politically and culturally significant? *Ourselves Unborn* examines the causes and consequences of the American obsession with the unborn.

The answers to those questions reveal deep patterns of change and continuity. In the late nineteenth century, fetal life was recognized and acknowledged only at the moment of "quickening" in the fourth or fifth month of pregnancy; by the late twentieth century, ultrasound exams could detect fetal life from the earliest days of conception.[9] In the late nineteenth century, embryologists and obstetricians were only beginning to understand the mechanisms of fertilization and development, and could neither observe nor intervene in that process; by the late twentieth century, reproductive endocrinologists could manage and manipulate fertility, and fetologists could diagnose and treat the fetus *in utero*.[10]

In the late nineteenth century, the fetus was not regulated, or even recognized, by law; a century later, the fetus was governed by a wide array of tort, criminal, property, and abortion laws.[11] In the late nineteenth century, almost no one knew what a fetus actually looked like; today, most people can easily identify sonogram images as a fetus.[12] Despite these quite remarkable developments, the meanings ascribed to the fetus are also marked by more subtle continuities and recurrent questions. Some of those questions—the ones about how fetal life develops—are embryological; some of them—the ones about what fetal life means—are philosophical; and some of them—the ones about whether fetal life should be protected—are political and ethical.

Fetal stories are constructed through a combination of theological, governmental, and medical technologies, as well as through everyday cultural practices. Since the late nineteenth century, these technologies and practices have intersected with larger conversations about the authority of science and religion, the relationship between individuals and society, and the meaning of individuality and personhood. By examining those intersections, the history of fetal meanings offers a new perspective on debates and assumptions at the center of the twentieth-century American history. The fetal stories of *Ourselves Unborn* are specifically American stories. Certainly, other cultures have rich histories in which individuals and the state ascribe particular meanings to the fetus and other historians have written those histories.[13] This book looks at the ways in which fetal stories are refracted through the prisms of the peculiarly American history of race, gender, ethnicity, and class; the relationships among religion, science, and politics; and the debates about individualism and democracy.

Ourselves Unborn builds on and engages with a rich literature on the various meanings and constructions of the fetus in Western culture and American history. Legal scholars and political scientists have traced a history of the fetus that identifies precedent-setting cases as significant turning points.[14] These works typically begin with the 1884 decision *Dietrich v. Northampton,* which established the legal precedent that a fetus has "no separate existence" from the mother and therefore cannot sue to obtain damages for injuries sustained *in utero.* The *Dietrich* precedent held for over sixty years, until 1946, when the *Bonbrest v. Katz* decision legitimized limited fetal rights by upholding a plaintiff's claims for damages for injuries incurred prenatally. The next significant turning point is the 1973 *Roe* decision that ruled that a fetus is not a person under the terms of the Fourteenth Amendment, but that the state has an interest in protecting the life of the fetus after viability. The legal history of the fetus generally ends with three landmark cases between 1990 and 2001: the 1990 case *In re A.C.,* in which the District of Columbia Court of Appeals ruled that physicians must honor the wishes of a competent woman regarding a cesarean section; the 1991 decision in *UAW v. Johnson Controls*, in which the Supreme Court declared that policies that bar women from specific jobs out of fear that these jobs might harm embryos or fetuses were a form of sexual discrimination that violates Title VII of the Civil Rights Act of 1964; and the 2001 decision in *Ferguson v. The City of Charleston*, in which the U.S. Supreme Court found unconstitutional a public South Carolina hospital's policy of surreptitiously testing pregnant women for drugs.[15] Within those parameters, legal scholars trace the patchwork of state laws having to do with fetal homicide, fetal abuse, and fetal neglect.

Medical historians begin their story much earlier, frequently with Aristotle's theories of human reproduction.[16] But the fetus's modern medical history in the United States generally begins in the 1880s, at Johns Hopkins University, with embryologist Franklin Mall's project to collect human embryos. The next turning point might be the 1930s and 1940s, with Arthur Hertig and John Rock's efforts to photograph specimens of early fertilized human ova between one and seventeen days of development, and Rock's 1944 success in fertilizing a human egg in a test tube.[17] Other important steps in this medical narrative include Dr. Ian Donald's development in the late 1950s of ultrasound technology for obstetrical purposes; the growing use of amniocentesis in the late 1960s; and Dr. William Liley's research and practice of intrauterine transfusions in the late 1960s and 1970s, which inaugurated the practice of fetal medicine, or fetology.[18]

Providing a different perspective on these medical and legal developments, feminist scholars have worked to expose the political and ideological motives behind the transformation of the maternal-fetal relationship from one experienced and defined by the pregnant woman to one interpreted and regulated by laws and physicians. Others have worked to reclaim that relationship from its overmedicalized and highly politicized position. Historians of abortion and reproductive rights begin with the premise that abortion has always been practiced, and trace its largely unregulated history until the mid-nineteenth century, when Dr. Horatio Storer started the antiabortion movement that succeeded in criminalizing abortion in almost every state by the early twentieth century.[19] This physician-led antiabortion movement has been seen as part of a larger effort to professionalize medicine, led by medical-school trained physicians who wanted to end midwives' control over reproduction, and endorsed by a society that wanted to control the behavior of women. Storer and his followers focused primarily on the ways in which abortion posed serious dangers to women, but also introduced the concept of fetal life into abortion politics. This body of scholarship focuses on the ways that abortion politics are a window into ideas about women and their appropriate role in society.

Religious scholars approach the history of the fetus from a variety of angles, based on the particular doctrines of Catholicism, Judaism, Buddhism, and Hinduism. This perspective illustrates a great variation. In Judaism, the fetus is a person only once the head has emerged from the birth canal and the first breath has been taken.[20] In Islam, the fetus becomes a person at 120 days of gestation.[21] Hindus believe that life is without a clear beginning or a clear end—conception and death are not the boundaries of life.[22] The Roman Catholic Church's position has changed over the past two thousand years from teaching that personhood occurs at 40 days after conception for a boy and 80 days for a girl, to teaching that personhood begins at conception.[23] Religious scholars also study how these doctrinal teachings are practiced in people's lives and in different cultural contexts, showing a tremendous gap between theory and practice.[24] A third perspective focuses on the intersections of religion and politics, either using religion to justify a particular position on abortion or stem cell research, for example, or showing how different groups have mobilized religious authority to make political claims.[25]

Cultural critics have analyzed the ways in which modes of visualization have enabled the identification of a fetus as a "person" separate from the mother, and constructed the fetus as a "citizen" with rights subject to the protection of the state.[26] Anthropologists have written about how women's experiences of pregnancy and childbirth have been altered by new technologies.[27] Working from a variety of disciplines and perspectives, these scholars have provocatively analyzed the social and political causes and consequences of contemporary fetal politics. But in overemphasizing the causal role of technology, much of this literature foreshortens the history of those politics and understates the significance of the fetus in American history. Although it is true that ultrasound technology has familiarized a particular visual image of the fetus, that image is only one moment along the historical continuum of Americans' encounters with the fetal body.

Cumulatively, this scholarship offers important insights into the varied meanings that have been ascribed to the fetus, and the ways in which those meanings have been constructed and deployed in modern America. However, it can also obscure the ways in which these different narratives—legal, political, medical, religious, anthropological, sociological, cultural—intersect and interact with one another. Understanding the history of fetal meanings in modern America involves tracing the relationships among these different narratives, and relating them to the larger context of social, political, and economic changes. This historical project required creating a kind of archive of the fetus, one that includes medical textbooks and journals, educational literature and "popular" science books, museum exhibitions and mass media, case law and legal journals, and legislation and legislative debates. Historicizing the fetus requires amassing and making sense of stories told by embryologists and physicians, museum curators and self-help literature, politicians and lawyers, religious leaders and social activists, and by women themselves. In revealing how people have come to understand what embryos and fetuses are, these stories highlight the causes and consequences of the cultural, emotional, and political investments that have been made in the fetus in modern America. That archive and those stories are the basis for *Ourselves Unborn.*

Organized loosely chronologically, the book does not move comprehensively through time, but, instead, examines particular themes and episodes as representative and illuminative of a particular era. Chapter 1, "Discovering Fetal Life, 1870s–1920s," focuses on the period during which embryology became a modern science, obstetrics became a profession, abortion became a crime, birth control became a movement, eugenics became a cause, and prenatal care became a policy. This chapter examines the ways in which the fetus was imagined in each of these shifts. Tracing the formulation of the idea that the fetus had a "right to be well-born," this chapter argues that fetal meanings in these years were shaped by anxieties about and responses to the ways in which the emerging industrial order was challenging traditional values and assumptions. This Progressive Era fetus was used to respond to the tremendous changes of these years, to express anxieties or excitement about industrialization, immigration, urbanization, feminism, modernity, and America's place in the world. The wide range of responses to those changes produced a protean fetus that meant different things to different people and that is used to endorse and comment upon a wide range of ideas and policies.

Chapter 2, "Interpreting Fetal Bodies, 1930s–1970s," analyzes the public encounters with the fetus through the dissection, display, and depiction of fetal bodies. Since the late nineteenth century, embryologists had been making wax models of human embryos and fetuses, and pathologists had been collecting real human embryos and fetuses to study.[28] As these collections expanded in the early twentieth century, ordinary Americans were increasingly exposed to fetal bodies through exhibits at fairs and museums, specimens in laboratories and classrooms, and photographs in textbooks and popular literature. This chapter analyzes how, during World War II and the early years of the Cold War, the corporeal fetal body that people encountered in public spaces became deployed as a symbol that paradoxically embodied both the strength and the vulnerability of the American individual and of American democracy in those perilous times. It then looks at how medical, political, and social changes wrought by 1960s liberalism generated a radically new abortion policies and politics that remade the fetus.

Chapter 3, "Defining Fetal Personhood, 1973–1976," focuses on two related episodes in Boston. The first episode is a series of local hearings on fetal research performed in Boston hospitals. The chapter examines the ways in which abortion politics transformed the longstanding and uncontroversial practice of fetal research into a politically and socially divisive issue. It then looks closely at the trial of Dr. Kenneth Edelin, an African-American obstetrician at Boston City Hospital. The fetal research hearings led investigators to BCH, where they heard reports of a purportedly questionable abortion performed by Edelin. The district attorney decided to pursue the issue. For performing a legal abortion on a seventeen-year-old girl, Edelin was charged with manslaughter. After a trial that consumed the city's attention for months, Edelin was convicted in February 1975. Both these events—the fetal research hearings and the Edelin trial—took place in a city riven by tensions over gender, race, class, and religion, tensions exacerbated by the contemporaneous busing crisis. The Edelin case and the fetal research controversy illustrate how fetal meanings in the 1970s emerged from those divisions transforming Boston and the nation.

The proliferation of rights-based movements for equality in the 1960s and 1970s provided the seductive language and compelling logic of "fetal rights" as a strategy of resistance. Chapter 4, "Defending Fetal Rights, 1970s–1990s," analyzes the context, intentions, and consequences of that strategy. Beginning in the 1970s, court-mandated medical interventions began invoking fetal rights while overriding women's civil rights as patients. At the same time, corporate-sponsored fetal protection policies began invoking fetal rights while overriding women's equal protection rights as workers. Beginning in the 1980s, states began prosecuting women for crimes of fetal abuse. This chapter analyzes the proliferation of claims on behalf of fetal rights that came at the cost of women's constitutional and legal rights. It situates this fetal rights discourse in the context of the growth of the New Right, and the backlash to the legalization of abortion, feminism, changing gender roles, and the welfare policies of the Great Society.

Chapter 5, "Debating Fetal Pain, 1984–2007," analyzes how fetal pain has been defined and debated in medical literature, in litigation, in legislative debates, and in public discourse. It begins in 1984, when Bernard Nathanson released *The Silent Scream,* a film in which he videotaped and narrated an abortion procedure performed on a twelve-week-old fetus, and ends in 2007, when the Supreme Court upheld the 2003 Partial Birth Abortion Ban Act in *Gonzales v. Carhart* and *Gonzales v. Planned Parenthood Federation of America, Inc., et. al.*[29] Debates about fetal pain and partial birth abortion emerged during the Reagan era, at the height of the religious right's influence and the "family values" movement; they are best understood in that context. This chapter argues these debates—shaped by conflicting visions of motherhood and gender roles, by politicized struggles over the relative authority of scientific evidence and religious values, and by arguments about the role of government in people's lives—ultimately became a referendum on liberalism.

Ourselves Unborn makes clear that competing fetal stories and contested fetal meanings have occupied an important place in the public sphere and collective imagination of the United States throughout the modern era. Illustrating how fetuses came to symbolize "ourselves unborn," this book also argues that stories about fetuses express individual and collective beliefs about individuality, motherhood, and American society. The fetus is sometimes a window into anxieties about race, gender, and motherhood; sometimes a projection of our beliefs about the relative authority of religion, science, or personal experience; and sometimes a proxy for seemingly unrelated issues like immigration, the Cold War, feminism, or liberalism. Analyzing the changing and contested meanings ascribed to the fetus from the late nineteenth century through the early twenty-first century offers a new perspective on those anxieties, beliefs, and issues, and explains why the fetus is such a powerful symbol in American culture and politics.

CHAPTER 1

DISCOVERING FETAL LIFE,
1870S–1920S

In 1916, the director of a free prenatal clinic in Seattle named Armenouhie Tashjian Lamson published a chronicle of her unborn baby's nine-month struggle to develop from an egg to a zygote to an embryo to a fetus to a baby boy.[1] Although *My Birth: The Autobiography of an Unborn Infant* went out of print in 1936 and has largely been forgotten, it was popular and well-received in its time.[2] The book's narrator was Lamson's unborn baby who, in addition to detailing his process of development, explained repeatedly that the good food and safe environment helping him grow would also help the American nation grow healthy, strong, and just. Lamson was an Armenian immigrant who in 1902 had come to the United States to attend Johns Hopkins University Medical School, one of the few programs open to women.[3] After completing her coursework, Lamson moved with her husband to Seattle, where she founded and directed her clinic, wrote extensively in local newspapers and magazines about her work with expectant mothers, and served as the chair of the Washington chapter of the National Woman's Party.[4] In *My Birth*, Lamson used the story of fetal development to comment on an era in which industrialization and immigration had fundamentally reshaped the political economy, social structures, and cultural and intellectual life of the United States.

Between the 1870s and 1920s, the places people lived and the jobs they worked, the clothes they wore and the foods they ate, the values they held and the facts they believed, the ways they spent their time and the ways they spent their money, the concerns they had and the hopes they held, all metamorphosed in ways that historians have characterized as the birth of modern industrial society.[5] This transformation required the careful negotiation of new social relationships as well as the inauguration of new identities, such as "white-collar" workers, "teens," the "New Woman," and the "New Negro."[6] Another emergent identity, albeit a less-heralded one, was the fetus. Although Lamson's explanation of the mechanism of fertilization, the transmission of heredity, and the process of embryonic and fetal development would most likely have been new to her readers, those same readers would have been accustomed to the idea that an unborn child could be used as a symbol in discussions about the history and future of America.

In 1902, noted Scottish embryologist Dr. John William Ballantyne came to teach for a year at Johns Hopkins Medical School, where he well might have taught Armenouhie Lamson. While at Johns Hopkins, he noted what he characterized as an "increase in the value set upon foetal life" and suggested that "economic, practical, and political" factors were more responsible than medical advances for this "increased attention to matters of antenatal interest."[7] Lamson's book was one example of the growing public interest he describes.[8] When the first-person narrator expresses his desire to be born in an America in which "all barriers of sex, religion, race and color should be forever obliterated and the gates of equal opportunity opened to all," he—and presumably Lamson—is articulating a vision for society in a changing world and is participating in a trend in which doctors, political activists, social theorists, and the lay public frequently invoked the unborn in their efforts to define, explain, and solve social problems.[9] In the late nineteenth and early twentieth centuries, physicians like Ballantyne interpreted the biological life of the fetus and authors like Lamson created a biographical life for the fetus in ways that highlighted how "economic, practical, and political" forces intersected with medical advances to intensify and shape public interest in what Ballantyne called the "prenatal epoch," and the "embryological view of life."[10]

To Progressive Era reformers embarking upon the "search for order" and struggling to reconcile "drift" with "mastery," the fetus offered the dual possibilities of order and mastery.[11] Arguing that the complexities of modernity demanded that "conscious intention" replace "unconscious striving," and that "purpose" replace "tradition," journalist Walter Lippmann challenged Americans to "be awake in during our own lifetime . . . by watching ourselves and the world outside . . . [to draw] the hidden into the light of consciousness, record it, compare phases of it, [and] note its history."[12] From this perspective, the fetal body was a perfect metaphor for the body politic. Controlling the fetus through reproductive policies like criminalizing abortion and advocating eugenics offered Americans a way to control the future, whereas interpreting the fetus through laws, medical texts, or literature became a way for Americans to interpret their changing world. But before it could be conceptualized as a social subject with political significance, the fetus needed to be materialized as a scientific specimen with physical substance.

That materialization was made possible, in part, because of developments in embryology in the late nineteenth century.[13] Historian and animal behaviorist Matthew Cobb explains that the "link between copulation and pregnancy was firmly established by observing domesticated animals when humanity invented agriculture around nine thousand years ago . . . slowly, over thousands of years, but with growing certainty, mating and generation—at least in domesticated animals and humans—became linked in humanity's collective knowledge."[14] But although it was understood that a woman could become pregnant only if she had sexual intercourse with a man, and that a woman's menstrual flow ceased when she was pregnant, less understood was the relationship between those facts.

Western explanations of this process can be traced back to the fifth century BC, when Hippocrates posited that human generation resulted through the interaction between two kinds of semen—a man's ejaculate and a woman's menstrual blood. In the fourth century BC, Aristotle elaborated upon that idea, theorizing that the "dynamic and creative male semen" transformed the "passive, plastic" menstrual blood into what he called an "embryon."[15] After observing a chick's embryonic development for three weeks, Aristotle concluded that what began as a "fleshlike substance resolved itself into its distinct parts" over a period of time—forty days for a embryon to become a formed male fetus, and ninety days to become a formed female fetus.[16] Prohibitions against human dissection prevented Aristotle from observing the same process in humans, but he felt sure that they underwent this same process of embryonic development, which he called epigenesis.

Aristotle's theory of reproduction remained essentially intact for nearly two thousand years, at which point the technological advances, epistemological shifts, and political imperatives of seventeenth-century Europe called it into question.[17] In the 1640s, anatomist William Harvey rejected Aristotle's theory that male semen transformed female blood into an embryo, suggesting instead that female ovaries produced eggs that were propelled into the womb by the magnetic force of male semen.[18] But although Harvey rejected Aristotelian theories of embryonic origin, he embraced Aristotelian theories of embryonic development, concluding that embryos began "as a homogenous mass, from which the organs derive one after another by the process of formation, or epigenesis."[19] As anatomy underwent a methodological shift from the gross dissection of dead bodies to the microscopic analysis of live organisms, and an epistemological shift from Aristotelian-Galenic explanations of the workings of the human body through elemental forces and humors to Cartesian explanations of those workings through mechanical laws and principles, Harvey's claim inaugurated a debate between epigenicists and "preformationists" that would last into the late nineteenth century.[20]

The preformationists were a new generation of anatomists and embryologists who dismissed as unscientific and old-fashioned Harvey's Aristotelian theories of epigenesis. Using new microscopic technologies that made visible that which had only been imagined, anatomist Marcello Malpighi claimed in 1673 to have "perceived the entire fetus" inside a chicken egg, and in 1694 Niklass

Hartsoecker claimed that he could see "an already formed embryo" within spermatazoids.[21] All preformationists—both the "ovists" who saw embryo in the egg and the "spermists" who saw the embryo in sperm—agreed that embryos existed before conception as complete, miniaturized versions of themselves needing only to be stimulated into growth.[22] Quickly, if temporarily, preformationism replaced epigenesis as the leading scientific theory explaining human reproduction.[23]

Although the microscope provided visual evidence to support theories of preformation, it does not explain the readiness of intellectual and political elites to endorse this new idea, a readiness that stands in stark contrast to their responses to other changes in scientific thought, particularly astronomy. Whereas the world viewed through a telescope posed serious challenges to religious and political authority based on a geocentric world, the world viewed through the microscope provided evidence that seemed to justify traditional political systems and social hierarchies. As historian Clara Pinto-Correia explains it, "Preformation made it seem inevitable that servants would always originate from servants, just as kings would always originate from kings. By putting lineages inside each other, preformation could also function as a 'politically correct' antidemocratic doctrine, implicitly legitimizing the dynastic system."[24] But although they were scientifically modern, visually persuasive, and politically useful, theories of preformation were also completely wrong.

Nonetheless, the debates between epigenicists and preformationists continued until the mid-nineteenth century, when German embryologist Karl Ernst von Baer's identification of the mammalian egg in 1827, combined with the development of cell theory in the 1830s, allowed scientists to understand that the spermatozoa and egg were two cells that combined to create a new embryonic cell.[25] In 1875, German zoologists Oscar Hertwig and August Weissman clarified that process further, explaining how the genetic material from an egg and sperm combined to form a zygote, which then underwent the complex process of cell division through which organ systems form and develop.[26] The final piece in this puzzle—a piece that would be further refined by James Watson and Francis Crick's 1953 discovery of DNA and subsequent advances in molecular biology—was provided by Weissman's explanation that individual inheritance was transmitted through chromosomes carrying genetic information through the egg and sperm cells.[27] It turned out that what the preformationists had "seen" was wrong, whereas what Aristotle and other epigenesists had "imagined" was closer to the truth.

Understanding conceptually the process of reproduction and development, embryologists became motivated to observe and document the developmental stages of the embryo. In 1883, after obtaining his medical degree from the

University of Michigan, Dr. Franklin Paine Mall embarked upon his lifelong project of collecting human embryos and fetuses when he went to Leipzig to study with the leading embryologist Dr. Wilhelm His.[28] His had been involved with a controversy within the scientific community with Ernst Haeckel, an anatomist, embryologist, and ardent evolutionist whose biogenetic law and recapitulation theory was expressed in the famous, if inaccurate, phrase "ontogeny recapitulates phylogeny." Haeckel had illustrated that theory, using wax embryo models to show that all vertebrates begin the same way, to show that "noblemen were—for the first two months—hardly distinguishable from dogs."[29] His felt that Haeckel was exaggerating the commonalities in order to make a political argument for evolution, and attacked his embryological illustrations as being "in part highly unfaithful, in part, nothing short of invented."[30] In contrast to Haeckel's evolutionary model of embryology, His wanted to demonstrate the complexities of development within individual species. The conflict between His and Haeckel represents another example of how competing understandings of embryological development and the visual presentations of those understandings become politicized. Whereas that politicization emerged in the late nineteenth century in debates over evolution, it emerged in the seventeenth century in debates between preformationists and epigenesists, and in the late twentieth century in debates about abortion, frozen embryos, embryonic stem cells, and still, in debates about evolution.

Perhaps because of his disagreement with Haeckel, His became increasingly committed to using actual embryo specimens rather than wax models to illustrate his conclusions. Mall's first task under His was to persuade gynecologists who "wasted or ruined valuable specimens through insufficient analysis" to donate these "precious objects" to scientific research. To reward those who agreed "to collect material and in the interest of research to sacrifice it on the altar of science," His and Mall promised to name each embryo after its donor, which was understood to mean the contributing doctor rather than the woman who had been pregnant.[31] The painstaking and laborious process by which His and Mall materialized embryos—obtaining them, sectioning them, staining them, classifying them, fixing them in paraffin for slides—illustrates the complex steps through which the modern embryo was not discovered, but was constituted and produced through Progressive-Era technologies and assumptions.[32]

After returning to the United States, Mall taught at Clark University and the University of Chicago until 1893, when he was appointed to chair the anatomy department at Johns Hopkins School of Medicine. There he dedicated his career to a "massive scientific embryo collecting project," believing that embryology could "establish certain points of great value to medicine and to the race."[33]

Anthropologist Lynn Morgan details the phenomenon in which "tens of thou-sands of dead human embryos, fetuses, and infants were collected by hospitals and universities for research purposes. The remains and tiny bodies were col-lected by the scores, retrieved from miscarriage, induced abortion, surgery, and autopsy. They were shipped across state lines and national borders, dissected, dismembered, eviscerated, and sliced into sections for scientific research."[34] Physicians around the country responded to Mall's requests for help "procuring more material... to further the study of human embryology." By the time he was appointed to head the Carnegie Institute's Department of Embryology in 1913, Mall was in possession of "about a thousand young embryos and young foe-tuses" and was well on his way to chronicling a "complete account of the human body."[35]

Embryologists had to walk a fine line in their collection efforts. On the one hand, they needed to convince gynecologists and obstetricians that human embryos were scientifically valuable objects requiring embryologists' unique expertise. On the other hand, they did not want to encourage laypeople to view human embryos as socially significant subjects with moral value. Embryologists' desire to solidify their professional legitimacy by maintaining exclusive access to human embryos resulted, according to Morgan's case study of Baltimore, in legislative compromises in which "embryologists agreed to produce scientifically based knowledge about human development for the benefit of improving social policy and clinical practice" in exchange for juris-dictional autonomy.[36]

This jurisdictional autonomy was not, however, uncontested. For example, complaints like the one from the Baltimore commissioner of health that "city residents buried miscarried fetuses in their backyards or threw them down their privies" heightened public health officials' concern about hygiene and sanita-tion and resulted in regulations that required death certificates and burial per-mits for fetuses.[37] When Mall asked Maryland's attorney general whether "all embryos and fetuses, no matter how early, would require a permit," he was informed that the regulation "should be given as broad an interpretation as pos-sible and should be held to include any foetus that had at least assumed any definite shape."[38] While navigating these new regulations, embryologists continued their collection efforts, and by 1944, the Carnegie Institute had more than nine thousand human embryos.[39]

As embryologists worked to construct the embryo as a specimen, a second group of physicians who were fighting to criminalize abortion worked to con-struct the fetus as a subject. And as the embryo moved from the scientific labo-ratories to the public stage, it became clear that not only was the embryo body produced through the intersection of technique and ideology, but so too were the meanings and values ascribed to that body. The first statutes governing abortion practices in the United States were enacted in the 1820s and 1830s, when, claiming concern for women's safety, state legislatures began prohibiting the advertising and sale of abortifacient drugs.[40] In the 1840s, as surgical abortions began to replace drug-induced abortions, physicians gave free lectures and circulated popular tracts delineating the physical dangers posed to women by both medical and surgical abortions.[41] In 1857, ten years after its inception, the American Medical Association embarked upon a more organized movement to prohibit abortion, appointing Dr. Horatio Robinson Storer to lead the AMA's Committee on Criminal Abortion. Under Storer's leadership, the "antiabortion crusade" accomplished the twin goals of elevating physicians' prestige while simultaneously circumscribing women's options.[42]

Everything in Storer's training and early career indicated that he would follow his father's professional path and become a professor of obstetrics and gynecology at Harvard Medical School. When a series of conflicts with leading Harvard physicians ended that dream, Storer accepted an appointment at the New England Hospital for Women and Children. According to biographer Frederick Dyer, Storer's lifelong effort to criminalize abortion was motivated by personal tragedy, including the death of his first two wives and a young daughter; according to historian Janet Farrell Brodie, Storer's motivation was his desire to "gain recognition and to make his own mark."[43] Wherever the truth lies, it is clear that Storer was a man whose inconsistencies—he worked closely with several women physicians while opposing training women as physicians; he dedicated his life to women's health while limiting their reproductive choices—shaped his multipronged attacks on abortion.

In *Why Not? A Book Intended for Every Woman*, for which he received the 1867 AMA award for the best antiabortion book intended for the lay public, an award established as part of the AMA's antiabortion movement, Storer emphasized the dangers that abortions posed to women.[44] Storer made little distinction between abortion and contraception, arguing that the "systemic prevention of conception"—either through abortion or contraception—was the principal cause of women's medical problems, including lame backs, disabled limbs, cramps and paralysis, general hypochondria and despondency, uterine problems, and nervous disease.[45] Perhaps because he worried that medical problems resulting from abortion might be insufficient motivation for legislators and physicians to join his crusade, perhaps because he realized that his arguments were based on weak evidence, or perhaps because he was merely using those problems to mask less altruistic reasons for his activism, Storer introduced a second line of argument in his campaign against abortion, focusing attention on the fetus rather than the woman.

Public acceptance of abortion was, Storer believed, premised on the assumption that quickening represented the onset of fetal life, and his campaign focused on convincing physicians and laypeople that fetal life began with conception. "Quickening is as unlikely a period for the commencement of foetal life as those others set by Hippocrates and his successors, varying from the third day after conception to that of the Stoics, namely birth, and as false as them all," Storer wrote. "Common sense...would lead us to the conclusion that the foetus is from the very outset a living and distinct being."[46] It is, Storer explained, impossible for one body to contain two lives, or for two bodies to represent only one life. Therefore, "[t]he mother and the child within her...must be entirely identical from the conception of the latter to its birth, or entirely distinct." Storer located a crucial moment of distinctness that, in his formulation, made "indisputable" the fact that "independent life dates from no other epoch than conception." Because, he said, "the ovum does not originate in the uterus; that for a time, however slight, during its passage through the Fallopian tube, its connection with the mother is wholly broken...it is not rational to suppose that its total independence, thus once established, becomes again merged into total identity."[47] Insisting that conception was the starting point for independent life required Storer to understand the fallopian tube, in contradistinction to the uterus, as being disconnected from the woman's body, a convoluted piece of reasoning that suggested, perhaps, that his argument was less scientific than political.

Dr. Hugh Lenox Hodge, Chair of Obstetrics at the University of Pennsylvania Medical School and another physician actively involved in the campaign to criminalize abortion, made a similar argument:

> From the moment of conception [the ovum] is separated...from the ovary, where it was generated, and travels, some three or four inches through a narrow tube or canal, to the uterus, as much disconnected from the mother as a chick in ova is separated from the parent hen. Its subsequent attachments to the mother, by means of the placenta and uterus, are so indirect...that we are justified in ascertaining that the mother has little more influence upon the child in utero than the parent bird has upon its offspring in the egg.[48]

For Storer, and for Hodge, the implications of the "indisputable" fact that independent life began at conception were obvious. "If there be life," Storer wrote, "then also the existence, however undeveloped, of an intellectual, moral, and spiritual nature, the inalienable attribute of humanity, is implied.... Then we are compelled to believe unjustifiable abortion always a crime."[49] Hodge had made a similar argument thirty years previously, when he had published a lecture titled "An Introductory Lecture to a Course on Obstetrics," attacking abortion "on the grounds that embryos could think and perceive right and wrong."[50]

An argument that had little traction in 1839 met an entirely different response in 1872, when Hodge republished that same lecture, with a new title, "Foeticide, or Criminal Abortion." This lecture began by praising the medical profession's new conventional wisdom about fetal life. "If," he wrote, "the profession in former times, from the imperfect state of their physiological knowledge, had, in any degree, undervalued the importance of foetal life, they have fully redeemed their error and they now call upon the legislatures of our land...to stay the progress of this destructive evil of criminal abortion."[51] Growing references in medical literature to "intrauterine murder," "medical respect of foetal life," "infant murder," and "ante-natal infanticide," and similar language in the mainstream press, support Hodge's claim that the idea that fetal life began at conception had gained significant currency.[52] During the summer of 1871, a year before the publication of Hodge's pamphlet, the New York Times ran a series of lurid articles about abortion. One reader responded to those articles in a letter to the editor, mourning the fact that "thousands of human beings are thus murdered before they have seen the light of the world," and praising the paper's "high valuation of foetal life."[53]

Whereas medical journals may have been predisposed to the cutting edge, and newspapers may have been predisposed to the sensational, the fact that medical textbooks identified conception rather than quickening as the starting point for fetal life indicates that this was indeed the new consensus. In his widely used *Manual of Obstetrics,* Dr. William A. Newman Dorland dismissed the argument that "the child is not viable until the seventh month of gestation, hence there is no destruction of life." Dorland easily links medical professionalism with moral authority, praising "the truly professional man's morals...because he sees in the germ the probable embryo, in the embryo the rudimentary foetus, and in that, the seven months viable child and the prospective living, moving, breathing man or woman, as the case may be."[54] What distinguishes professional men from nonprofessionals and from women is, according to Dorland, both their greater expertise and their higher moral sensibilities.

Hodge similarly emphasized the "indifference" of pregnant women, who "seem not to realize that the being within them is indeed—that it is, in verity, a human being—body and spirit; that it is of importance, that its value is inestimable, having reference to this world and the next. Hence, they in every way neglect interest. They eat and drink; they walk and ride...utterly regardless of unseen and unloved embryo."[55] To compensate for "mothers [who] have no wish to preserve the intra-uterine being," Hodge argued that those "who have devoted themselves to the pursuit of a science so exalted, so noble, so useful as that of medicine," have an obligation to act "as the guardians of the rights of... the invisible product of conception."[56]

For Hodge, that obligation resulted from the mutually reinforcing power of medical expertise and religious values. "[H]uman existence," he writes, "corporeally and spiritually, commences, not with the birth of the foetus and the first inspiration, but at conception. Nutrition, growth, the development of organs, the successive display of organic, animal, intellectual, moral, and spiritual functions, are but the successive manifestations of that mysterious principle of life, the gift of the Creator."[57] In connecting the corporeal with the spiritual, in emphasizing not just the sanctity of an individual's rights but the sanctity of God's creation, claims about the inviolability of fetal life frequently linked biological knowledge with theological authority.

An editorial in the *Boston Medical and Surgical Journal,* for example, argued that "no sophistry can do away with the fact that, whether the lamp of life is extinguished in the womb or at any period after birth, with an avowed and wilful [*sic*] intention to taking the life of the foetus or infant, it is murder, and the perpetrator of it cannot expect to escape the vengeance of offended heaven."[58] Despite efforts by antiabortion physicians to link theological and biological definitions of life, historian Carl Degler has suggested that in the early stages of the antiabortion movement, "[n]o churches of any denomination were especially interested in the matter."[59] Perhaps this lack of interest reflected a concern that movement was contradicting the earliest Christian teachings about fetal life.

Embracing the Aristotelian concept of "delayed ensoulment," St. Augustine believed that a human soul cannot live in an unformed body, and that an abortion performed early in pregnancy was not murder because no soul was destroyed. Christian theologians also believed that women had the power to determine the moment of "ensoulment" through the experience of quickening. In his "Treatise on the Soul," the third-century theologian Tertullian appealed to the "mother's experience of the being within her," arguing that "[i]n this matter, there is no more fitting teacher, judge, witness, than one of this sex. Reply, you mothers, you bearers of children, let the sterile and the masculine be silent, the truth of your nature is sought."[60] When the twelfth-century monk Gratian compiled the authoritative canon law in the *Decreten,* he concluded that "abortion was homicide only when the fetus was formed."[61] This idea was confirmed as Catholic dogma in 1312, when the Council of Vienne adopted St. Thomas Aquinas's endorsement of Aristotle's theory of ensoulment, or "delayed hominization." Not until 1869, when Pope Pius IX dropped the distinction between "fetus animatus" and "fetus inanimatus" and made abortions performed at any stage in pregnancy excommunicable, did religious leaders in the United States publicly endorse the antiabortion movement.[62] In *Criminal Abortion*, Storer quotes Bishop John Joseph Williams of Boston, who described his pleasure that "the American Medical Association has turned its attention to the prevention of criminal abortion, a sin so directly opposed to the first laws of nature, and to the designs of God, our Creator, that it cannot fail to draw–down a scourge upon the land where it is generally practiced."[63]

Religious leaders wanting to reject distinctions between prenatal and post-natal life as meaningless needed to reconcile the facts of science with the teachings of religion. Reverend James E. Kelly explains that "with the exception of respiration, all the functions are performed in early foetal life." Therefore, he writes,

> The conclusion at which we must arrive, a conclusion corroborated by the teachings of religion, is that from the instant at which impregnation occurs and the ovum first receives life, the foetus is human, and at all periods differs in degree and not in kind from the infant and the adult. Therefore, we must regard it as a "human being," with an inalienable right to life, and that its destruction is homicide.[64]

Locating the fetus at the intersection of medical knowledge and religious teachings and ascribing to it "inalienable rights," Kelly uses what could be called a discourse of bio-theology to justify a new political identity for the fetus. In her 1884 MD thesis about infanticide, Mary Mitchell similarly imbricates fetus with nation, arguing that "every life is of political value and ought to be made a source of wealth to the country."[65]

Notwithstanding Mitchell's rhetorical claim, the historical reality that every life was not considered to have equal political value was manifestly evident in the strain of antiabortion rhetoric that linked the well-being of the fetus to the well-being of the nation through the trope of "race suicide." The criminalization of abortion took place at a time when, as cultural theorist Nathan Stormer puts it, "the growing white bourgeoisie in the United States was experiencing significant anxiety about its overall health, fitness, and vitality."[66] In the late nineteenth century, as non-Protestant immigration rose and the rate of white, native-born births declined, physicians exploited the growing nativist sentiment by connecting the problem of abortion to the problem of race. European-American fertility rates declined from 7.04 children in 1800 to 3.56 children in 1900, a decline historians attribute at least in part to a dramatic increase in induced abortion.[67]

Antiabortion physicians exploited anxieties about the precarious state of the racial and gendered order of Victorian America to argue that white, Protestant, native-born, middle-class women had a responsibility to maintain that order, a responsibility they could uphold by performing their obligations as citizens by having babies.[68] Hodge, for example, bemoaned the fact that the "low estimate of the importance of foetal life is by no means restricted to the ignorant, or to the lower classes of society. Educated, refined, and fashionable women—yea, in many instances, women whose moral character is, in other respects, without reproach...are perfectly indifferent respecting the foetus in utero."[69]

Horatio Storer was even more direct. Determining "that the average number of births to each Protestant family is less than it was half a century ago," Storer championed the idea that the upsurge of induced abortion threatened the nation's future and put "Americans" at risk.[70] "Look westward," he exhorted. "The great territories of the far West, just opening to civilization...offer homes for countless millions yet unborn. Shall they be filled by our own children or by those of aliens?... This is a question our women must answer. Upon their loins depends the future destiny of our nation."[71] This rhetorical strategy connected women's reproductive obligations to the nation's manifest destiny, and constructed the fetus as an "emblem of the cultural responsibilities of women and the future of the nation and race."[72] Echoing Storer and anticipating Theodore Roosevelt's concern that race suicide was the "greatest problem of civilization," one doctor wrote in 1874 that "the annual destruction of foetuses [was so] truly appalling" among native-born American women that "the Puritanic blood of '76 will be but sparingly represented in the approaching centenary."[73] Reverend Brevard Sinclair similarly worried that Catholic immigrants would soon "possess New England," because of their opposition to abortion and Protestant women's declining birthrate.[74] Following Stormer's reading of antiabortion politics as an ideological project to "optimize cultural life, not only multiple biological lives," by the end of nineteenth century, the fetus represented not only individual personhood, but also the cultural survival of the nation.[75]

Despite these purportedly high stakes, and the fact that the AMA had succeeded in criminalizing abortion by the beginning of the twentieth century, abortion continued to be widely practiced and rarely prosecuted, suggesting that the AMA's ability to change laws had exceeded its ability to change minds or behavior. Acknowledging this discrepancy, J. M. Sheehan, the attorney for the medico-legal committee of the Chicago Medical Society, suggested that "the law as it stands is further advanced than apparently the public demand for its enforcement would require."[76] Dr. Rudolph Holmes, also of the Chicago Medical Society, had "come to the conclusion that the public does not want, the profession does not want, the women in particular do not want, any aggressive campaign against the crime of abortion."[77] The Reverend Sinclair had put it more bluntly in an 1891 sermon. When it comes to abortion, he said, "society is indifferent, the Church asleep, and the public conscience is dead."[78]

Frustrated by this indifference and by women's refusal to accept their responsibility and their physicians' authority, antiabortion physicians intensified their efforts to persuade the public that fetal life began at fertilization and to convince women to carry their pregnancies to term. People needed to be taught that "the fertilized egg contains all the hopes and possibilities of a mature foetus," said Dr. Charles B. Reed, a member of the Chicago Medical Society's abortion committee.[79] It was hard, Dr. Palmer Findlay wrote, "to convince the lay person that life begins at the moment of impregnation."[80] Dr. Holmes attributed this difficulty to wishful thinking, suggesting that "many now make themselves believe that there is not life until the movements are felt."[81] But even when they were able to change common beliefs about the beginning of human life, physicians failed to change how people acted upon these new beliefs. Dr. E. E. Hume bemoaned the fact that only rarely did telling a woman "this is a life" dissuade her from obtaining an abortion.[82] Dr. Frederick Taussig proposed that physicians begin showing patients and audiences "an enlarged picture of an embryo of six weeks," suggesting that "pictures like that of the six weeks' embryo will keep many women from having an abortion done."[83] Dr. Joseph Nix regretted that although "few...still believe that life does not exist in the human embryo from the moment of conception...countless thousands value this life so little and their own morals so much less that they sacrifice this fetus animated by an immortal soul to lust, to gold, to convenience."[84] But the physicians' efforts to make indisputable the fact that fetal life began at conception continued to face resistance both from women who still sought abortions and physicians who still performed them, and also in an entirely different arena of debate, the courtroom.

As physicians were focusing on the need to recognize and protect fetal life in the context of abortion politics, lawyers and judges were reaching different conclusions about fetal personhood in the context of tort law. The first attempt to make a legal claim on behalf of a fetus was in 1884, when a woman from Northampton, Massachusetts, slipped on a public road, went into premature labor, and subsequently sued the town for negligently causing the wrongful death of her unborn son. In the case of *Dietrich v. Inhabitants of Northampton*, Massachusetts Supreme Court Justice Oliver Wendell Holmes rejected this woman's claim, explaining in his majority opinion that because the fetus was "a part of the mother," it was not "a person for the loss of whose life an action may be maintained."[85] At the same time that physicians were organizing around their new definition of the fetus as a separate living being and embryologists were collecting and studying human embryos, the decision emphasized the indivisibility rather than the individuality of the fetus and mother. Holding that "a child...is so intimately united with its mother as to be a 'part' of her and as a consequence is not to be regarded as a separate, distinct, and individual entity," Holmes set a powerful precedent for subsequent decisions.[86]

In 1900, for example, a pregnant woman, after being badly injured in an elevator accident at St. Luke's Hospital, gave birth to a "wasted, withered, and atrophied" child who was "sadly crippled for life."[87] She sued the hospital for damages on behalf of her child, and in the case of *Allaire v. St. Luke's Hospital,* the Illinois Supreme Court rejected her claim, finding that "an action for injuries could not be maintained by a plaintiff who at the time of the injury was a pre-natal infant with no separate legal existence."[88] Citing the *Dietrich* precedent, the decision held that "when the act of negligence occurred, the plaintiff was not in esse, was not a person, or a passenger, or a human being.... At that time, the plaintiff had no actual existence.... That a child before birth is in fact, a part of the mother, and is severed from her only at birth cannot we think be successfully disputed."[89] Unlike the *Dietrich* decision, however, the opinion was not unanimous. In his dissenting opinion, Justice Boggs held that "it is but to deny a palpable fact to argue that there is but one life and that the life of the mother. Medical science and experience have demonstrated that at a period of gestation, in advance of the period of parturition, the foetus is capable of independent and separate life, and that, though within the body of the mother, it is not merely a part of her body." But although Boggs's dissent would be recalled and relied upon in later decisions recognizing separate fetal life, Holmes's decision that the fetus was "not to be regarded as a separate, distinct, and individual entity" would stand for the next half-century.[90]

Some physicians used the same logic of the *Dietrich* and *Allaire* decisions to challenge the dominant strain of antiabortion rhetoric. Dr. Maximillian Herzog, for example, described calling "an embryo four weeks old a human being" as "an exaggerated view."[91] In *Fewer and Better Babies,* Dr. William J. Robinson, an activist in the early birth control movement, argued that "there is no right to be born," and that "it was better to permit the removal of a few animate cells" than to have "more and more unwanted children born in an already overpopulated world."[92] Robinson's support for abortion as a eugenic response to overpopulation can be read as a mirror image of Storer's opposition to abortion as a crusade against "race suicide." Whereas Storer had emphasized the declining birthrate of "desirable" babies, Robinson emphasized the rising birthrate of less desirable babies. Both worried less about overpopulation in the terms of the economist Thomas Malthus, and more about the changing racial composition of the population in the terms of social Darwinist Herbert Spencer.

These arguments resonated deeply with a public deeply worried about immigration and urbanization. The proliferation of books analyzing pauperism, feeblemindedness, alcoholism, prostitution, rebelliousness, and criminality testify to the trend in which public fears about social change were articulated in demographic and reproductive terms. The titles of some of these books—*A Plea for the Unborn, The Right to Life of the Unborn Child, The Color Line: A Brief in Behalf of the Unborn, Race Culture or Race Suicide? A Plea for the Unborn, The Melting Pot: A Plea for the Unborn Children in America, The Right of the Child to Be Well Born, The Rights of the Unborn Race,* and *The Rights of Unborn Children*—highlight the metaphoric jurisdiction of the unborn as a synecdoche for a white, Protestant nation besieged.[93] Efforts to solve these social problems through controlling reproduction were seen as closely connected to the fight for the future of the white, Protestant nation. Whereas some physicians committed to criminalizing abortion had framed those problems through the language of "race suicide," Progressive Era reformers advocating a wider range of policies and reflecting a broader range of motives identified the "right to be well born" as the key to saving a nation.

In the 1890s, the fluid and contested concept of heredity intersected with the fluid and contested set of ideas constituting the protean movement called "Progressivism."[94] The new sciences of genetics and heredity invigorated old debates about the degree to which individual character was a product of inheritance and was, therefore, predetermined and immutable, and the degree to which it was a product of environment and was, therefore, fluid and subject to influence. The historical argument about the relative merits of preformation and epigenesis had been reformulated into a modern argument about the relative influence of nature and nurture, and, more specifically, an argument among the competing theories of prenatal culture, eugenics, and euthenics. Eugenics was by far the dominant theory of the three, but the other two were expressed in a variety of places in the early twentieth century. Prenatal culturists argued that heredity could be influenced by a pregnant woman's thoughts and behavior; therefore those thoughts and behavior must be controlled. Eugenicists argued that heredity was immutable; therefore reproduction must be controlled. Euthenicists argued that heredity could be improved by fixing external environmental conditions; therefore those must be controlled. The understandings of heredity embedded in theories of prenatal culture, eugenics, and euthenics contained within them descriptions of and responses to changes in racial demography and gender roles, as well as unarticulated assumptions about the power of science, religion, or politics to explain and solve social problems. Representing different responses to radical social change while sharing the belief that reproduction was the linchpin in the nation's future, prenatal culturists, eugenicists, and euthenicists debated those problems through the trope of the "right to be well born."

One site for those debates was the 1893 World's Columbian Exposition in Chicago.[95] Friedrich Ziegler, the German artist-scientist famous for his hand-crafted wax models of embryos, brought to the fair his glass display of wax models of starfish, sea urchin, beetle larvae, trout, chick, frog, and human embryos, as well as models of developing hearts, brains, skulls, eyes, ears, and teeth.[96] Offering an evolutionary and developmental illustration of the fair's theme of "progress," Ziegler's exhibit won the fair's highest prize. Although this exhibit was the only one featuring human fetuses and embryos, it was not the only exhibit focused on the significance of prenatal life.

At the World's Parliament of Religions, Theosophist Annie Besant lectured on the power of prenatal culture.[97] As the leader of the Society of Theosophy, a group committed to seek "eternal truth" through spiritual ecstasy or direct intuition, Besant talked about the power of "prenatal culture" to protect "the greatest right of which we can conceive—the right of a child to be well-born."[98] Mothers, she insisted, "must commence the training of their children before they are born" because "at the moment of birth there is no doubt that a child's whole moral disposition is contained within."[99] Like Besant, most prenatal culturists imposed stringent demands and responsibilities upon pregnant women.

For example, poet and Theosophist Ella Wheeler Wilcox, commissioned by the Columbian Exposition to write an essay imagining what the world would look like in 1993, predicted that "women will be financially independent of man, and this will materially lessen crime. No longer obliged to rifle her husband's pockets for money, she will not give birth to kleptomaniacs or thieves."[100] Like Besant and Wilcox, most prenatal culturists came from offshoots of nineteenth-century spiritualist movements, particularly Theosophism, Christian Science, Practical Metaphysics, and "New Thought."[101] One of the major principles embraced explicitly or implicitly by all these philosophies was that internal powers could influence external conditions. Katherine Tingley, leader of the American Theosophical Society, described her belief in "the possibility of conscious participation in evolution; the power of thought to affect one's self and surroundings."[102] New Thought leader Sarah J. Farmer defined her movement this way: "It is simply putting ourselves in new relation to the world about us by changing our thought concerning it ... we are not creatures of circumstances; we are creators."[103]

Prenatal culturists believed that the fetus was a blank slate upon which the mother's feelings, thoughts, and actions inscribed the future of the child, and thus the nation. They believed that the mental, physical, and spiritual health and well-being of a baby were transmitted through the mother's feelings and beliefs, and that most personal traits and many social problems could be traced back to something that the mother did or failed to do, thought or failed to think, throughout her pregnancy. As Dr. R. Swinburne Clymer put it, "The will, feeling, desire, and active effort on the part of the pregnant woman may completely reverse heredity and natural tendencies."[104] A convert to Christian Science, Clymer went on to explain: "The secret of a mother's ability to transmit to her children any desired quality, goodness, greatness, talent, potentiality and possibility, even though the desired quality is not possessed by the pregnant woman, is the greatest of all the phenomena in the universe and is based on her desire and love for that which she is engaged in creating."[105] Advocates of the power of prenatal culture attributed social problems, and implicitly, the power to solve those problems, almost exclusively to "maternal influences." Charles Bayer explained that since "the chief influence over one's entire life is due to the mental and physical condition of the mother during the year preceding its birth, more depends upon the pre-natal environment than on pre-conception or post-birth conditions."[106] He gave the following example:

> The money-making mania seems to be increasing, and desire to accumulate gold, stocks, bonds, and all the various forms of wealth, pervades the very air of the large centers of commerce.... [W]hat is the cause of this speculative mania? Our theory is that the prospective mother, who overhears the exciting stories of the day's success in making money on the Board of Trade, which engrosses the mind of husband, father, or brother, and the plans which are formed for a further accumulation of wealth in her hearing, necessarily influences the mentality of the unborn child, just as if the mother should every night listen to a good musician, she would produce a musical brain.[107]

More examples were provided: a woman who was frightened during pregnancy would likely give birth to an anxious and easily frightened child; a woman who drank alcohol or engaged in sexual intercourse during pregnancy would likely give birth to an alcoholic or promiscuous child. Accompanying Bayer's argument that problems such as crime, poverty, alcoholism, and materialism were caused by a pregnant woman's thoughts and actions was his belief that the solutions to those problems lay within women's control: "It is a certainty that by a proper education and diffusion of the knowledge of maternal impression and its effects, the prospective mothers will be able to reduce the number of paupers and criminals; also the production of physically imperfect human beings could be largely averted."[108]

Just as there were countless activities that women needed to avoid during pregnancy, there were also duties women needed to perform from the moment of conception. Believing that "the power of prenatal influence which a mother possesses is inspiring," Ella Wheeler Wilcox argued that "every expectant mother should direct her mind into wholesome and optimistic channels; she should read inspiring books and think loving and large thoughts.... [T]he moulding of a noble human being is surely worth eight or nine months of concentrated though and unflagging zeal of purpose."[109] Arthur Smith insisted that prenatal education was the most effective way to form a child's character:

> The nine months of a child's prenatal life are the most momentous of its career, especially as far as its character is concerned, and this period can be used by its mother not only in doing away with or reducing to a minimum, any probable bad traits which she may think it has inherited, but also in implanting into it other tendencies and also increasing those already there, which she may consider calculated to be for its future good.[110]

Smith warned pregnant women to be "careful of the books they read," "the thoughts they think," and "the company they keep."[111] Even subconscious thoughts could endanger the unborn child. E. I. Champness warned that "the influences... might possibly be either through the conscious mind of the mother of the future child—that is, by creating a vivid idea on which her mind dwells... or through her subconscious mind—that is, by vibratory influence acting on the embryo through the mother's nervous system, and without her having any consciousness of the fact."[112]

A small minority of prenatal culturists retained the more radical politics of Free Thought spiritualism and believed that women's role in ensuring the well-being of the unborn gave them unlimited freedoms. Moses Harman, editor of the once-spiritualist-now-anarchist paper *Kansas Liberal,* and advocate for free love and birth control, was also a prenatal culturist:

> Nine-tenths of the education of every human being is received by him before the hour of birth; that is the training he gets through suggestions made upon the maternal mind during the period of embryonic growth tremendously outweighs all the work of teachers, and of the environment generally, after he enters upon the stage of post-natal existence, or all of the work of genetic inheritance, before he is conceived.[113]

But Harman rejected more conservative renderings of prenatal culture that insisted women retreat from public activities, refrain from unpleasant thoughts, and avoid "immoral" behavior. Rather, he insisted that the "power of prenatal impression in giving form and character to the unborn" is proof of "the overshadowing need that women should be free and self-owning, so that she may choose her conditions."[114] But efforts to translate ancient beliefs in maternal impressions and nineteenth-century practices of spiritualism into a twentieth-century vernacular, whether conservative or radical, reinforced the idea that the responsibility for the unborn was exclusively the mother's.

After hearing Besant's lecture about prenatal culture, visitors might have headed to the main fairgrounds by taking a steamship down Lake Michigan, alighting near the fisheries building, and walking a few steps east to the impressive Midway Plaisance. After seeing a model of the Eiffel Tower and St. Peter's Basilica, taking a balloon ride, riding a Ferris wheel, or watching "Little Egypt" do her famous belly dance, those walking the midway could see exhibits replicating villages from around the world. These exhibits featured real people performing daily activities and cultural practices that purportedly reflected their lives in places including Algeria, Dahomey, Java, Moscow, China, Cairo, and Lapland. Reflecting the fair's theme of "human progress," these exhibits embodying a complex of assumptions and arguments about the racial and national evolution of civilization had originally been conceived as part of the Department of Anthropology before being moved to the midway.[115] Whether intended to introduce the public to different cultures and races from around the globe, or to make the case that Anglo-American civilization represented the highest step on the evolutionary ladder—or both—these exhibits, designed by a protégé of P. T. Barnum and located adjacent to Hagenbeck's Zoo, highlight how turn-of-the-century evolutionary discourses developed in tandem with and as justifications for imperialism and inequality. Critics of the midway, like the journalist who bemoaned the fact that "amusement of cheap and even vulgar sorts, is being substituted for education," would have preferred the Anthropological Building, where exhibits made similar, if less sensationalist, arguments about the relationship between heredity, culture, and civilization.[116]

These arguments were illustrated visually in Ziegler's display case of embryos. Other nearby exhibits included one on criminal anthropology that illustrated the use of "'selective genetic prevention' to identify potential criminals," and one on experimental psychology that focused on the measurement and meaning of individual differences, capacity, gender, and race. University of Wisconsin psychologist Joseph Jastrow, with assistance from G. Stanley Hall and Franz Boas, organized the psychological laboratory to introduce this new science and distinguish it from the mystical practices of mind reading, phrenology, and séances. The focal point of the exhibit was a testing room replicating Francis Galton's Anthropometric Laboratory. Galton, a second cousin of Charles Darwin, believed that "essences" and "innate physical and mental abilities" could be measured, and that a statistical analysis of these measurements explained the hierarchical evolution of nations, cultures, and races. Strongly influenced by Galton, Jastrow also believed that "men differ widely" in their possession of "original, inborn characteristics" not subject to outside influence, and wanted to collect for research purposes a large sample of the averages and statistical deviations of the U.S. population.[117]

Visitors willing to contribute to this research, and anxious to have their own abilities tested and measured, paid 10 cents to undergo a series of tests measuring their "innate physical and mental abilities," after which each was encouraged to "find his place upon the chart or curve for each form of test and from a series of such comparisons obtain a significant estimate of his innate proficiencies and deficiencies."[118] As the perfect example of the Progressive Era commitment to make the "work of experts open to the critical gaze of citizens," the exhibit both reflected the explicit assumption that presumed genetic inheritance could be measured through standardized testing and contributed to the increasingly popular belief that heredity could and should be regulated through eugenics, the belief that controlling the reproduction of individuals or populations could improve the human race.[119]

The practice of eugenics in the United States had yet to become popularized or codified into law, but the ideas behind those practices can be traced back to some time before the Columbian Exposition. Worried about what he described as the "involuntary and random propagation" of the human race, John Humphrey Noyes founded a "perfectionist" community at Oneida, New York, in 1848. Oneida was based on the practices of "complex marriage," free love, group families, and shared property, as well as a program called *stirpiculture*— Latin for "race culture"—that was intended to perfect the human race through controlling reproduction. In his youth, influenced by religious leader Charles Finney and radical social reformer Frances Wright, Noyes had striven for perfection on earth through the spirit. As an adult, influenced by Charles Darwin and Francis Galton, Noyes strove for perfection on earth through science. In the words of Galton, "what Nature does blinding, slowly, and ruthlessly" through natural selection "man may do providently, quickly, and kindly" through eugenics.[120] Admiring Galton's demonstration "by elaborate statistics that genius and all other good qualities are hereditary in human families," Noyes described with pride the "very encouraging success" the Oneida Community had in attempting to "reduce the theory of Scientific Propagation to practice."[121] Between 1869 and 1880, fifty-eight children—"stirps"—were born at the Oneida community, their parents having been carefully selected by Noyes and a committee of elders on the strength of their physical and intellectual attributes.[122]

Oneida, though, was too small and marginal a movement to have had much influence on the spread of eugenic thinking, and scholars typically mark the beginning of American eugenics at the turn-of-the-century shift away from the belief that human nature was malleable and responsive to environmental influences to the belief that it was fixed and predetermined by genetic inheritance.[123] This shift, made possible by genetic research in the late nineteenth century that was slowly displacing Jean Baptiste de Lamarck's theory of "acquired character-istics" with August Weismann's theory of the "continuity of germplasm," was embraced with particular passion by Harvard-trained biologist Charles Benedict Davenport.[124] Combining Galton's *eugenics*, a term Galton coined in 1883, based on the Greek for "good in birth" and defined in 1904 as "the science which deals with all influences that improve the inborn qualities of a race," with Mendel's *genetics*, the theory that specific traits were transmitted by specific genes, Davenport professionalized and popularized the practice of eugenics in the United States.[125] Davenport headed the Eugenics Record Office, founded in 1910 in Cold Spring Harbor, New York, and funded by the Carnegie Institute of Washington—the same Carnegie Institute that housed Dr. Franklin Mall's Department of Embryology—where Davenport chaired the Committee to Study and Report on the Best Practical Means of Cutting off the Defective Germplasm in the American Population.[126] The committee was charged with examining various churches' attitudes towards sterilizing "persons known to possess defective germ plasms," and with "eugenical limitations of marriages by the ministry."[127] "Positive eugenics," the kind practiced at Oneida through stirpi-culture and the kind articulated by Horatio Storer in his attacks on "voluntary motherhood" and "race suicide," was intended to ensure that people with desir-able mental and physical traits had more children. "Negative eugenics," the kind encouraged by Davenport, was intended to ensure that people with undesirable traits should have fewer.[128] Combining the Progressive Era's value on science with its concern about the problems of rapid urbanization and massive immi-gration, advocates of eugenics endorsed coercing sterilization of "unfit" popula-tions, as well as restricting immigration and segregating the mentally ill.[129]

Uncomfortable with the racist elements of the eugenicists' belief in the scientific truth of immutable heredity, as well as with the mystical elements of the prenatal culturists' belief in the spiritual power of maternal impressions, were the euthenicists, who believed that mental, temperamental, and moral traits were determined by environmental factors, rather than genetics.[130]

At the World's Fair, euthenic arguments were made most explicitly by Ellen Swallow Richards, a chemist from the Massachusetts Institute of Technology who ran the fair's restaurant, which provided more than ten thousand people a 30-cent lunch as well as free pamphlets about the principles of cheap and nutri-tious cooking.[131] Believing that that "environmental poisons or personal habits acquired over the course of a lifetime could be transmitted, for good or ill, to the next generation," and hoping to minimize the transmission of poisons and max-imize the transmission of good habits, Richards developed the science of *euthenics*, which she defined as the "science dedicated to improving the human race by changing heredity through improving environmental conditions."[132]

Explicitly advocating euthenics over eugenics, Richards concluded that "euthenics precedes eugenics, developing better men now, and thus inevitably creating a better race of men in the future."[133]

Although he did not call himself a euthenicist, Frederick Jackson Turner's argument that Americans' individual and collective identity was shaped by the frontier depended on many of the same assumptions about the relationship between environment and character that Richards expressed in an entirely different context. In the speech he gave at the fair, "The Significance of the Frontier in American History," he argued that that Americans' social, intellectual, and political traits were not divinely ordained or genetically predetermined, but were environmentally produced.[134] In Turner's words, "this perennial rebirth, this fluidity of American life, this expansion westward with its new opportunities, its continuous touch with the simplicity of primitive society, furnish the forces dominating American character."[135] If eugenicists believed that heredity shapes the environment, Turner, like euthenicists, believed that the environment shapes heredity. Literary critic Christine Holbo has analyzed the ways that a group of architects, economists, urban planners, home economists, and sanitary engineers in the Progressive Era who shared Turner's belief in the formative influence of the frontier and his concern about its closing decided "to model new urban and suburban life on the aesthetic of the frontier, interiorizing the process of rebirth and evolution to create society with features supposedly productive of individualism, Americanism, and democracy."[136] Although euthenicists did not equal eugenicists in numbers or power, advocates of euthenics included important liberal leaders such as Clarence Darrow, the lawyer and leading member of the American Civil Liberties Union, and Julia Lathrop, the Hull House Reformer who in 1912 was appointed by President William Howard Taft to became the first head of the newly created Children's Bureau, giving the movement a legitimacy and influence that exceeded its numbers.

If the urban and suburban home, as managed and regulated according to the euthenic principles of Ellen Richards, offered one possible new frontier, the pregnant body offered another ideal site for Turner's "rebirth" of "individualism, Americanism, and democracy." In 1916, in *My Birth*, Armenouhie Lamson constructs the uterine environment as a frontier of sorts, one where the nation's newest pioneer, the fetus, becomes an individual and an American.[137]

In imagining a biographical history to accompany the biological process of development, Lamson presented a carefully edited version of her own identity; negotiated debates about the degree to which character, temperament, and intelligence were fixed or malleable; rejected the racist arguments of eugenicists and the mystical arguments of prenatal culturists; and argued that the values of democracy and individuality would be best achieved through equal rights for women and healthy and safe living conditions for everyone. Writing in the voice of the fetus, Lamson chose to obscure her own personal identity beneath what she posits as the universalizing experience of motherhood. In her introduction, Lamson made no mention of her immigrant status, medical training, professional experience, or political commitments. Identifying herself only as a "mother and author," she describes the personal experience that motivated her to write the book:

> It was in my fourth month of approaching motherhood when I felt the little guest move freely within the hidden chamber which was in me and part of me.... These mysterious jerky motions, which are spoken of as "Quickening," were the first communications I had received from that new life.... With quickening my suspected baby became a reality.[138]

Rather than present herself as a trained professional who had studied embryology and obstetrics at Johns Hopkins and ran a clinic for pregnant women, Lamson identified with her readers rather than with the experts. "Like most young mothers of my time," she writes, "I was quite ignorant of the conditions under which this baby of mine was existing.... I could not understand the medical books which my doctor kindly gave me...because of the many scientific terms utterly foreign to me."[139]

The following two questions intrigued her: "[w]as it true that the thoughts and actions of an expectant mother affect the progress, perhaps retard that great creative work?" and "[w]as the fetus a mere parasite, living on its mother, or was it already an independent being, endowed with all the attributes of life?"[140] As if in answer to her questions, Lamson heard "the insistent calling of my little infant...whispering into my soul all that was taking place in him and about him."[141] The reader holds in her hands, Lamson writes, not the medical profession's interpretation of fetal development, but an "exact transcription" of that whispering, an explanation of human development from the source itself. After this introductory preface, readers are introduced to the voice "from the land of the unborn."[142] That unnamed narrator begins by expanding the time frame of a story generally bounded by conception and birth, and by making a distinction between biological life and human personhood. "When my mother was born I happened to be living in her left ovary," readers are told.[143] But fertilization— an event he characterizes as "the greatest miracle of life, beyond the reach of scientific understanding, understood by no one but God"—made him a "potential citizen of earth."[144] The moment of fertilization, the moment when "the heroic act of the spermatozoon" saves the "wandering ovum from destruction and death," was the turning point in his journey from life to personhood: "There is no day in my life more worthy to be remembered or perchance celebrated that the day when the two primary germ cells—the spermatozoon and the ovum—met, and united gave birth to a new being. Rightfully, that day should be considered my birthday."[145] Elaborating upon this claim that his "future self" was established at the moment of fertilization, the narrator explains that "[i]n the act of fertilization of the ovum…the character of my species, sex, and appearance were decided upon, and the corner stone of my mental, moral, and spiritual life was laid."[146]

Carefully striking a balance between characteristics that are mutable and immutable, Lamson explains that the development of mental and moral characteristics "can also be influenced by experience, environment, and education.… My life will be the result of the interaction of my inherited equipment with a long series of influences with my environment."[147] And later she is even more attuned to the inextricability of genetic inheritance and environmental influence, explaining that particular inherited mental and moral traits may not develop in an unhealthy environment. Lamson explains *environment* as "the soil that gives food and impetus to dormant qualities which when sufficiently exposed to the sun rays of education and experience may bloom according to their native splendor," and concludes that "[n]ature and nurture, environment, education, experience, and schooling hold the destiny of the individual as well as that of a race."[148]

The next step in his personal history, cell division, offers Lamson an opportunity to have her unborn narrator explain prenatal development with metaphors that would resonate with readers in an industrializing nation. One of the metaphors was the specialization of labor that defined factory work. Although the cell workers "seemed alike—each possessing a nucleus and a body filled with required building material and charged with an indefatigable urge to build," Lamson notes that they were actually "equipped to do a definite work and no other. Some were destined to make bone, others muscular bundles, some nerve fibers, others connective tissues." Labor relations was another metaphor. The narrator describes that in his case, "development was directed by a most Harmoniously working unit. Not a cell went on strike, not a single working force refused to do its utmost in the accomplishment of that great task—the construction of my body."[149] Lamson's story of the reproduction and development of the individual human body can be read metaphorically as her prescription for the "Harmony" necessary for the reproduction and development of the body politic.

An active suffragist, Lamson also uses the story of human reproduction to make her case for women's equality. After admitting that he was relieved when he realized he was going to be male "because the world still believes and depends on the myth of physical and mental supremacy of manhood, and because it still gives man greater opportunities for service and achievement," the narrator critiques that myth: "If you are a man and truly believe in the inferiority of women, blame man-made forces that control her training, education, and bringing up."[150]

Although advocating women's equality, the narrator carefully defends women as nurturing and maternal, describing his experience of being "welcomed and comfortably housed within the uterus [where] all was done that could be done for my welfare and protection."[151] Weighing in on the important question of the nature of the maternal-fetal relationship, he invokes his authority that derives from personal experience to trump the authority of scientific expertise: "There took place no fight between me and my mother's tissues, as is often stated by scientists.... My new dwelling place responded willingly to all my needs."[152] He concludes his autobiography with a discussion of his birth, reiterating his position toward women's inequality:

> The most remarkable feature of this act, which merely consists in the changing of my temporary dwelling place, is the fact that from the moment I am born the attitude of all people toward me will completely change. To-day, while yet a fetus, I am thought of as a mere parasite, living in my mother, giving her nothing in return. But as soon as I am born, I shall be considered an independent personality, and because of my sex, automatically all the rights of citizenship will be invested in me. I shall not have to beg or fight for them in later years.[153]

In Lamson's hands, fetal personhood was a vehicle for challenging society's refusal to grant women's equality:

> Among the great lessons we are learning during World War I is that men and women—fathers and mothers, sons and daughters, are equally responsible for the well-being of a nation and the progress of civilization.... Tranquility, happiness, and prosperity sought by all is not won on the battlefields but at home in the hearts of every father and mother who believes, practices, and preaches the right of all to be, to strive, and to achieve. Therefore the time is at hand when all barriers of sex, religion, race, and color should be forever obliterated and the gates of equal opportunity opened to all.[154]

Fetal personhood also became a vehicle for her to argue that society should provide safe and healthy conditions for everyone. Unlike the eugenicists, who believed that heredity was permanent but equally derived from the mother and father, and unlike the prenatal culturists who believed that heredity was mutable but only through the influence of the mother, Lamson insisted that parents are equally responsible for the well-being of their children, and that heredity is most affected by external environmental factors, like nutrition. She made the first point in her introduction, when she told "every girl and every boy that in future motherhood and fatherhood…every act of each day in their life may add a straight or crooked, a true or false line to the moral pattern of that new life, which will come into being through them and in them."[155] She made the second point in her conclusion, when she praised the Children's Bureau's annual manual on prenatal care written by doctors for expectant mothers, which "increasingly rejected any discussion of mother's emotional and psychological state, and instead emphasized the importance of diet, rest, exercise, and regular visits to the doctor."[156]

At the same time that she was writing *My Birth*, she was also campaigning for legislation funding prenatal health centers like the one she started. When Congress passed the Sheppard-Towner Maternity and Infancy Protection Act in 1921, it would be the first federally funded health-care program to be implemented in the United States.[157] The Sheppard-Towner Act was acclaimed by women's groups across the country, and women's magazines began devoting significant attention to the importance of prenatal care. *The Woman Citizen*, originally dedicated to the cause of suffrage, had found a new issue and began publishing a new column on "Mother and Child."[158] Dr. Gulielma F. Alsop's first column was on "The Right to Be Well Born":

> The achievement of this right will depend upon both its father and its mother. The mating of the parents determines the hereditary characteristics of the child. So much is fixed at birth by the choice of the parents; but an equally great degree depends upon the condition of the choice of the parents.…If the first half of the condition of being well-born depends upon a successful and suitable mating of healthy parents, the second half depends as much upon the condition of the mother during pregnancy.[159]

According to Alsop, in addition to food and medical care, active participation in all aspects of life was the crucial variable in ensuring a healthy pregnancy and healthy baby: "The Anglo-Saxon custom of housing a pregnant woman is most cruel and pernicious. She ought to go about freely, both to work and to amusements. A healthy woman need not discontinue her work, unless for physical discomfort until term. The longer she works, provided her work does not exhaust her, the better."[160] The transition from insisting that pregnant women remain cloistered in her private sphere to arguing that women's participation in the public sphere was contingent on their reproductive contributions to the state, to celebrating pregnant women at work and play, offers a stark rendering of the transition from the Victorian world of separate spheres to the modern emergence of the New Woman.

But in arguing that reproduction should be understood as a job in service of the state, arguments for euthenic policies often merged with arguments for eugenic policies, placing the physical fetus and the metaphorical unborn at the intersection of three Progressive Era themes—scientific racism, the regulatory state, and professionalization. The Second International Congress of Eugenics, held in New York City in 1919, capitalized on growing fears about heightened immigration and labor radicalism in the postwar era. President of the American Museum of Natural History Henry Fairfield Osborn opened the meeting by warning delegates that "the melting pot" had failed, dangerously weakening the "germplasm of the nation.... The selection, preservation, and multiplication of the best heredity is a patriotic duty of the first importance.... We are engaged in a serious struggle to maintain our historic republican institutions."[161]

The exhibits at the conference made explicit Osborn's concerns. A booth devoted to "the races of man" explained that "[h]umanity is composed of many races, differing widely in physical, mental, and moral qualities.... A democracy, in common with the science of eugenics, recognizes the aristocracy of personal ability, physical, mental, and moral. A democratic nation, in order to live, must foster good blood and hereditary talent, just as assiduously as an undemocratic country fosters special privileges."[162] An exhibit organized by A. H. Schultz, an embryologist at the Carnegie Institution, and Alex Hrdlicka, curator of physical anthropology at the American Museum of Natural History, featured fourteen plaster casts of "caucasian" and "negro" fetuses intended to "illustrate the chief points of difference in fetuses of the two races." A text panel explained that "the brain part is proportionally smaller in the negro fetuses than in the white."[163]

In contrast to the social Darwinists who advocated laissez-faire state policies in order to allow society to be governed by the laws of natural selection, eugenicists advocated state intervention in regulating immigration and reproduction. By 1924, that intervention resulted in twenty-eight states prohibiting interracial marriage, the passing of an immigration bill intended to prohibit immigration of "dysgenic" groups from Southern and Eastern Europe, and more than three thousand people undergoing involuntary sterilization. In the case of *Buck v. Bell* (1927), Chief Justice Oliver Wendell Holmes, author of the 1884 *Dietrich* decision, upheld a Virginia statute instituting compulsory sterilization of the mentally retarded for "the protection and health of the state." Finding that Carrie Buck "is the probable potential parent of socially inadequate offspring, likewise afflicted," Holmes wrote that "she may be sexually sterilized without detriment to her general health and that her welfare and that of society will be promoted by her sterilization." He went on to justify his decision with the language of negative eugenics:

We have seen more than once that the public welfare may call upon the best citizens for their lives. It would be strange if it could not call upon those who already sap the strength of the State for these lesser sacrifices, often not felt to be such by those concerned, in order to prevent our being swamped with incompetence. It is better for all the world, if instead of waiting to execute degenerate offspring for crime, or to let them starve for their imbecility, society can prevent those who are manifestly unfit from continuing their kind.... Three generations of imbeciles are enough.[164]

For Holmes, men fulfill their citizenship obligations by serving in a war and women fulfill theirs by reproducing, or not reproducing.

People advocating a wide range of policies repeatedly invoked the right to be well born. A small group of physicians in the late nineteenth and early twentieth centuries built their campaign to outlaw abortion around the newly articulated "right to be born." For eugenicists, a related commitment to "the right to be well born," would lead to calls for laws regulating marriage and reproduction among the "unfit." For prenatal culturists, that same commitment to "the right to be well born" would lead to calls for pregnant women to be watchful of their every thought and emotion. For euthenicists, a commitment to "the right to be well born" would lead to the Sheppard-Towner Act. Each of these categories of fetal discourses—abortion, eugenics, prenatal culture, euthenics—encompassed a wide range of interpretations of social problems, but deployed similar rhetorical strategies. Those strategies began by claiming to protect the "right to be well born" and quickly moved on to debate the meaning of fetal life and define the relationship between the mother and fetus. Fetal life was now commonly understood to begin not with quickening but at conception, or even before conception. By the 1920s, the fetus as a blank slate upon which the mother makes her mark, both through heredity and behavior, had given way to the idea of the fetus as an independent being who does not develop and exist merely as a function of the mother. The idea that the maternal-fetal relationship was primarily a moral one in which the mother transmitted values and character to her unborn child was rearticulated as primarily a physiological and biological one in which the mother was primarily a source of nutrition and shelter for the fetus. Just as the economic, practical, and political imperatives of early twentieth-century America shaped fetal meanings in the Progressive Era, those same imperatives would reshape fetal meanings for the next generation.

CHAPTER 2

INTERPRETING FETAL BODIES, 1930S–1970S

Visitors to the 1933 Century of Progress World's Fair in Chicago were presented with two opportunities to view exhibits of human embryos and fetuses. Although Friedrich Ziegler had exhibited wax models of human embryos at the 1893 Columbian Exposition, these 1933 exhibits displayed the real thing.[1] The self-proclaimed "masters of the midway" Lew Dufour and Joe Rogers created a midway sideshow called "Life," featuring a "graduated set of human embryos and fetuses" preserved in bottles of formaldehyde to "illustrate the development of an unborn baby from the first month to the eighth."[2] Drawing fairgoers into the show of "babies in bottles" was Dufour's "pickled star," a two-headed fetus in a jar, hanging outside the entrance in a basket held by a wooden stork. In a *New Yorker* profile of the duo, A. J. Liebling explained that Dufour came up with the idea for his show at a state fair in Ohio, where he had seen large groups of people gathered in front of a medical pitchman walking around with a bottle of formaldehyde containing a pig embryo. "I felt the strength of the thing right away," Dufour said. "There was money in the facts of life. A scientist may know a lot about embryology and biology, but it don't mean anything at the ticket window because it's not presented right."[3] At 10 cents a customer, Dufour and Rogers took in more than $110,000.[4]

At the same fair, some twenty million visitors attended the Hall of Science to view human embryos and fetuses presented in "The History of Man: Embryology."[5] In an exhibit sponsored and designed by Loyola University's School of Medicine, forty embryos and fetuses ranging from a few days to almost nine months of gestational age were displayed in glass containers preserved in a mixture of glycerin, formaldehyde, and oil of wintergreen. (figure 2.1). Adjacent to the containers were text panels describing the week-by-week development of fetal physiology and X-ray images of *in utero* embryos and fetuses at the same developmental stage. Hall of Science curator Eban James Carey explained the exhibit's purpose this way:

> The public was entitled to share in the discoveries continually being made in scientific laboratories of the world. Newer methods were introduced to

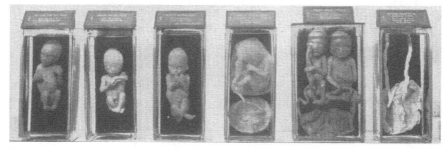

Figure. 2.1 "The History of Man: Embryology" exhibit, 1933 Chicago World's Fair

medical students in the teaching of the development and structure of the human body a few years ago. It was believed that the subjects dealing with the development and structure of the human body were not only the most fascinating of all studies but they also illustrated many points of practical value to humanity.[6]

Both exhibits had obtained their specimens from the same source—Chicago hospitals—but through dramatically different means. Liebling describes how Dufour and Rogers bought theirs on the black market:

> While it is true, as Lew sometimes roguishly observes, that you cannot buy unborn babies in Macy's or Gimbel's, there are *sub-rosa* clearing houses for them in most large cities. The embryo business even has its own tycoon, to borrow a word from graver publications, a man in Chicago who used to be chief laboratory technician at a medical school. The specimens are smuggled out of hospitals by technicians or impecunious internes [*sic*]. Hospitals have a rule that such specimens should be destroyed, but it is seldom rigidly enforced; no crime is involved in selling one.... Once you have bought the specimens, it is a cheap show to run. The actors need no rehearsal and draw no salary.[7]

The Loyola exhibit obtained their specimens from a more traditional source. Carey had asked Dr. Helen L. Button, a graduate of Loyola Medical School and obstetrics resident at Cook County Hospital, to donate some specimens from her collection.

Button was one of many physicians who collected and preserved the miscarried and aborted fetuses of her patients. Cook County Hospital had been disposing of them in a potter's field until Button decided to collect and preserve specimens in various stages of development.[8] Like Armenouhie Lamson, Button was a medical pioneer, becoming one of the very few women surgeons in the 1930s, and practicing and teaching medicine in Chicago for more than fifty years. Also like Lamson, Button was a strong advocate of women's health. When she described her work in the 1930s, she focused on the poverty-induced malnutrition and poor health of the women whose fetuses she preserved, and also on the limits of what she could do for her patients. "It was pathetic to watch helplessly as women died from infection after childbirth, simply because we had no treatment for them," she said. Remembering her experience as head of the Cook County Hospital gynecological clinic, she described the countless women who had "performed all types of abortion on themselves, many with dire results."[9] For Button, understanding and explaining the process of prenatal development was inextricably linked to her commitment to women's health.

These two World's Fair shows were shaped by quite different impulses. Motivated by profit, the sideshow presented the embryos and fetuses as cultural oddities and medical curiosities, inviting fairgoers to "come see the two-headed baby!"[10] Motivated by science, the Loyola exhibit presented them as scientific specimens, inviting fairgoers to come to "a celebration of man's progress in understanding the human body."[11] Carey was desperate to differentiate his show from Dufour and Rogers,' and he insisted that the popularity of the Hall of Science exhibit was not "mere morbid curiosity on the part of the public." But *Hygeia* magazine, published by the American Medical Association, explicitly connected the two, suggesting that "the crass freak shows occurring outside the confines of the lofty Hall of Science shared with it an ability to bring to the general observer some of the fascination of the unusual that is provided by a study of medical science."[12] This shared "fascination of the unusual" was revealed in the ways that the embryos and fetuses were presented as curiosities or specimens, rather than as people or babies. There is no indication that the public was in any way disturbed by the exhibits, or that anyone found it odd that a Catholic medical school would be involved in displaying fetal bodies obtained through abortions.

Fetal bodies were interpreted quite differently in 1977 than they had been in 1933. At the 1977 Lake County Fair in Illinois, Ward Hall was arrested for exhibiting a "pickled fetus" at a show he modeled on Dufour and Rogers.' The police

raided the freak baby show and charged me with illegal transportation of human remains. The idea is that you can't just go out and pick up a dead body and take it around unless you're a mortician....It was a little local thing, [but] all of a sudden it hit the wire services, so it went all across the country....Preliminary hearing, wire services. And then the county coroner, his name was Mickey, did one more shot. They lined up 12, 14 little coffins. And he had a priest, a minister and a rabbi and Mickey standing there with the coffins at the cemetery having the burial for the carnival babies. This hit the wire services and came out during the New Orleans [carnival trade] convention and the New Orleans paper carried a picture [of the burial] about 4 columns by 8 inches.[13]

That same year, Chicago's Museum of Science and Industry completed its renovation of the "Miracle of Growth" exhibit. The museum retitled it "Prenatal Development" and posted the following disclaimer at its entrance: "The forty specimens in this exhibit show the stages of human development before birth. They offer a unique look at the journey we all made from a fertilized egg to a complete human being. To the best of our knowledge, their survival was prevented by natural causes or accidents."[14]

Over the more than forty-year period between the Chicago World's Fair and the arrest of Ward Hall, fetal bodies had been transformed from curiosities and specimens inspiring wonder and awe into "babies" and "human bodies" deserving sympathy and burial.[15] Although the politics of abortion played a significant role in this transformation, the process of transforming a biological entity into a social one, of imbuing a scientific specimen with individuality, personhood, and rights, began long before the 1973 *Roe* decision. The ways that physicians researched the fetus, the ways that the public learned about the fetus, and the ways that the law regulated the fetus from the 1930s through the early 1970s reveal how inchoate anxieties about the future of humanity, the meaning of individuality, and the well-being of society influenced fetal discourses. Shaped by the lessons of World War II, the political culture of the Cold War, and the tenets of postwar liberalism, these anxieties transformed the fetal body from a scientific specimen into a symbolic subject vulnerable to the dangers threatening American families and emblematic of the values and ideals at the heart of American democracy.

Before the fetal body could be transformed from a specimen to a symbol, it had to be transformed from the metaphysical and metaphorical idea it had been in the Progressive Era into the physical and visible presence it became in the 1930s. That transformation was made possible, in part, because of the developments in classical embryology.[16] By 1940, the Carnegie Institute had more than nine thousand human embryos, each of which, according to director Dr. George Washington Corner, "was an honored and cherished gift upon the altar of truth."[17] The specimens had been collected through donations from a wide network of physicians around the country, like Helen Button, who sent the institute well-preserved aborted fetuses, both normally and abnormally developed ones. Some of these specimens were displayed at fairs and in museums, but most of them were used in college classrooms teaching zoology and human biology, in medical schools teaching developmental anatomy, and most frequently, in scientific laboratories researching reproduction, genetics, and endocrinology.[18]

Two of the most renowned embryo collectors were Dr. John Rock, an obstetrician, and Dr. Arthur Hertig, an embryologist and pathologist. In 1938, Rock and Hertig began collecting human embryos as part of their research on in vitro fertilization. A devout Catholic and father of five whose religious beliefs deeply informed his research, Rock was committed to helping families have the children they wanted to have. Running a fertility clinic at the Brookline Free Hospital for Women in the 1920s, he had been moved by the stories of women who were unable to conceive because of blocked fallopian tubes. Building on Gregory Pincus's experimental research on rabbit fertilization, Rock began researching the possibility of bypassing blocked fallopian tubes through in vitro fertilization. In a 1937 editorial in the *New England Journal of Medicine* describing the potential of his research, Rock concluded, "[W]hat a boon for the barren woman with closed tubes!"[19] He hired Pincus's lab technician, Miriam Menkin, and together they embarked upon this ambitious project.

Rock and Menkin asked patients scheduled to have hysterectomies at the Brookline Free Hospital for Women to engage in unprotected sexual activity in the days and weeks preceding the operation. After the surgery, Menkin would locate and extract unfertilized eggs within the ovaries that Rock had surgically removed and would try to fertilize them. Over six years, Menkin attempted to fertilize 138 ova, with no success. While Menkin was working with the unfertilized eggs, Hertig searched the uterus for fertilized eggs and embryos. From the 211 women who agreed to participate in the study, Hertig recovered 34 embryos.[20] After using these embryos for their own research, Hertig and Rock donated them to the Carnegie Institute of Embryology. Dr. George Washington Corner celebrated their donation of a two-cell human embryo as a "veritable jewel of science," and championed Hertig and Rock's successful efforts to "watch for and preserve early human embryos obtained from the operating room" as worthy of a Nobel Prize.[21]

Although Corner characterizes Hertig and Rock's specimens as being obtained from the operating room rather than from women's bodies, it is nonetheless true that each embryo and fetus—whether displayed at a fair, used in a classroom, or studied in a lab—once lived in a woman's body. We know very little about these women. We don't know why they needed the surgery. We don't know their age, race, class, or marital status. We don't know if they had any children. We don't know if they were scared or relieved about the procedure. We don't know if they were glad to participate in a scientific study or if they felt unable to say no to their physician. We do know, from Rock's notes, that most of the women gave their consent and that he continued to provide care for those who did not consent to participate in the study. And although we don't know if these women thought of the fertilized eggs and embryos that Hertig would study as their babies, or of the procedures Rock would perform as abortions, the fact that one woman wrote to Rock after her surgery, asking, "[B]y the way, did you get an embryo?" suggests that at least some of the women understood that the purpose of having unprotected sex was to become pregnant before the procedure.[22]

As embryologists were gaining a detailed understanding of embryological development, they were also becoming increasingly interested in the applications of their research. Corner explains how, once Hertig and Rock had obtained embryos from every day of the first three weeks of development, the "classical embryology of the human species was about to become, practically a finished subject" and was being replaced by a growing interest in experimental embryology.[23] And for other physicians in the field of reproduction, the emphasis shifted from understanding fertilization and fetal development to facilitating it. As a result of this work, fertility was becoming less mysterious and more responsive to human control.

In 1938, reproductive endocrinologists had developed a pregnancy test that could determine the existence of fetal life in the first month following fertilization, and by the 1950s, they had developed a sixty-minute "Q-test" that made it possible for a woman to learn if she was pregnant while in the doctor's office.[24] Doctors championed this new test, saying "aside from its speed, simplicity, and convenience, the Q-test permits pregnancy determination at an early date, thereby enabling prenatal care to begin weeks earlier than was heretofore believed possible."[25] In 1944, *Newsweek* published a story about Rock's work, focusing on his success in becoming the first to artificially fertilize the human ovum in a test tube.[26] In 1953, *Science News Letter* heralded another important achievement in the study of human reproduction—artificial insemination. Under the headline "Frozen Sperm Pregnancies!" the article discussed the phenomenon of three women who "are pregnant by artificial insemination with frozen spermatozoa in what is believed to be the first successful clinical application to human beings of the method used widely in animal breedings."[27] All of this research succeeded where Horatio Storer had failed in convincing the lay public that fetal life preexisted fetal movement.

Americans were also becoming increasingly familiar with what the fetus looked like. When the Century of Progress World's Fair closed in 1934, Dufour and Rogers took their bottled fetuses on the road to other state fairs until they went out of business in 1946. Loyola donated theirs to the Museum of Science and Industry in Chicago, where they have been displayed since 1947.[28] When the Century of Progress World's Fair's organizer Rufus Dawes became the president of Chicago's Museum of Science and Industry in 1934, he announced that one of his first goals would be to reconstruct the fair's "History of Man" exhibit as one titled "The Miracle of Growth." While Loyola's exhibit had celebrated "man's progress" in understanding the human body, and whereas Corner celebrated the embryo as a "jewel of science" while seeming to forget the women who made his work possible, the MSI exhibit, which opened in 1947, makes central the biological, cultural, and political relationship between mothers and fetuses. The different futures of these two exhibits suggest that the fetus had become less an example of a carnival curiosity or a paean to scientific curiosity than an icon of motherhood and democracy, and the relationship between the two.

Welcoming visitors to the MSI exhibit was a transparent pregnant female mannequin, which the museum staff nicknamed *Beulah*, meaning "mother" in ancient Hebrew. By tracing the "miracle of growth" from conception through adolescence, the exhibit emphasized the continuity between prenatal and post-natal life, as well as the responsibility of mothers to ensure the healthy physical and psychological development of their children, before and after birth. This theme was part of the larger postwar culture of pronatalism, expressed most quantitatively in the baby boom, and more qualitatively in the tightening link between "family values" and national security.[29] The American home and family became the bulwark protecting the nation from outside threats like Communism and nuclear war and inside threats like dissent, homosexuality, and feminism.[30] The MSI exhibit can be seen as an example how the postwar pronatal culture contributed to the heightened interest in prenatal culture.

The 1947 exhibit featured wax models of fetuses and embryos rather than the real ones used in at the 1933 fair. The museum saved the real specimens, and it is not clear why they were not used in the exhibit. Perhaps it was because the wax models could be presented *in utero*, making explicit the biological relationship between the mother and the fetus that might be less obvious with the real spec-imens displayed in bottles. In reviewing the exhibit for *Parents* magazine, Kit Hildebrand described how two imagined viewers—one an eleven-year-old boy named Johnny, the other a fourteen-year-old girl named Mary—might approach the exhibit differently, with Johnny imagining himself as the fetus, and Mary imagining herself as the mother. For Johnny, the exhibit allows him to "take a long step toward maturity. He learns the secret of birth. . . . He knows that he, as a baby, like every other baby, made a dramatic entrance into this world. He walks out of the exhibit, his curiosity well satisfied, his mind at ease, his emo-tions proud." Mary has a different experience. "She learns the significance of her menstrual period, and how she can some day bear a child," Hildebrand writes. "She walks out content with her start toward womanhood."[31] These imagined responses highlight the gendered message of this exhibit, which makes the implicit argument that all girls and women are future mothers and all fetuses are future boys and men.

The "Miracle of Growth" exhibit presented the maternal-fetal relationship as both biological and political, making clear that relationship's connection to American democratic values. The exhibit catalogue explained that since the exhibit's installation, "thousands of visitors, including high school boys and girls who are parents of the future, have gained a new insight into the significance of marriage, of family, and of children. And so, the exhibit serves the democratic way of life."[32] The book goes on in even more heightened language:

> In a democracy, as conceived by the Declaration of Independence and interpreted by Abraham Lincoln, there are three inalienable rights: life, liberty, and the pursuit of happiness. These rights apply to children, as well as to men and women. Each child is endowed by Nature with certain potentialities of growth. A democratic culture seeks to recognize these potentialities and to foster them in a manner which will safeguard the dignity of the individual.[33]

Because the exhibit blurred the distinction between prenatal and postnatal life, the reader could likely assume that those same rights applied to the fetus. The catalogue made clear that this exhibit was about far more than a biological process, but was also about a cultural and social process that connects an individual's physiological development, as facilitated by his mother, to the nation's political development.

The exhibit's self-conscious significance obscured, or perhaps was explained by, the museum's concern about possible negative public reactions. The concern, though, was not about the politics of the unborn, but about the age appropriateness of an exhibit about the "facts of life." Museum historian Herman Kogan explained that the museum considered "opening the exhibit on separate days for women and men, and for barring children under seven."[34] These fears went unmet, and the public reaction to the exhibit was enthusiastic. In the first year, ten thousand school children and more than two million other visitors attended the exhibit. The *Parents* magazine article "How to the Tell the Story of Birth" heaped praise on the exhibit, describing it as "simple, beautiful, and impressive" and a wonderful experience for families.[35]

The *Parents* article, which was accompanied by several photographs of the exhibit, was only one example of how, beginning in the 1940s and 1950s, the vast majority of Americans who had not seen the embryos and fetuses at the Century of Progress exhibitions, in college classrooms, at state fair sideshows, or at Museum of Science and Industry exhibits were able to see embryos and fetuses. In 1946, *Newsweek* published a study finding that a fetus of twelve weeks gestational age and weighing 1.5 ounces could breathe and swallow, and included a photograph of a three-month-old fetus.[36] In 1949, *Time* published a photograph of a human embryo at forty days of development, writing that, "[I]t is at this stage, during the sixth week of life, that the embryo first shows all the human characteristics."[37] In 1950, the museum's exhibit catalogue was published as a book, which was available in bookstores, classrooms, and libraries across the country. That same year, *Life* published a series of photographs of the human embryo between three and thirteen weeks of growth, tracing its development from "a single cell to a fully formed baby."[38] Three years later, *Life* published a photograph of an embryo's face, taken by Swedish photographer Lennart Nilsson, after six weeks of development, with the following caption: "Its length is only about half an inch and it weighs about 1/25 of an ounce, yet it has already begun to take on a human appearance."[39]

As the fetus became detectable and visible at progressively earlier stages, it was understood to be vulnerable to very specific dangers transmitted through the mother. Researchers determined, for example, that women who had had German measles, or rubella, during their pregnancy, were significantly more likely to give birth to children with birth defects, particularly congenital cataracts, bad teeth, heart disease, deafness, or mental retardation.[40] Studies on pregnant women caught in the radiation area of the atomic blast at Hiroshima suggested that the X-rays that doctors had long recommended for their pregnant patients posed serious dangers to the fetus.[41] And the U.S. Public Health Service issued a pamphlet titled "Protecting the Unborn Baby," which focused on the dangers of transmitting syphilis *in utero*. Although the pamphlet was about prenatal health care, its cover featured a smiling baby, another example of the fusion between the unborn and born.[42]

The emphasis on the human appearance and increasing vulnerability of the fetus was accompanied by an emphasis on the human experience of the fetus. The Samuel S. Fels Research Institute for the Study of Prenatal and Postnatal Environment was founded in 1935 as an important interdisciplinary center where experts in embryology, child development, and psychology worked together to explore the fetal experience of life *in utero*.[43] The institute's mission was to "prevent, lesson, or resolve contemporary social problems," and to "initiate and to assist any activities or projects of a scientific, educational or charitable nature which tend to improve human daily life and to bring the average person greater health, happiness, and a fuller understanding of the meaning and purposes of life."[44] The fact that the Fels Institute saw prenatal development as fitting within the parameters of that mission during the Great Depression, when the problems of hunger and housing might seem more relevant, only emphasizes the growing belief that understanding fetal development was central to ensuring the well-being of individuals and the nation.

In the late 1940s, the Fels researchers began asking what the embryo or fetus did, rather than just exploring what happened to it, during the nine months of gestation. This interest in fetal behavior—including social, emotional, psychological, and physiological behavior—grew out of the then popular Gestalt school of psychology, defined as "the study of perception and behavior from the standpoint of an organism's response to configurational wholes," and was premised on the belief that perception and behavior "are present before birth."[45] Although its study sample of seventy-three families was small, the Fels Institute received a great deal of press coverage. In the first of a 1952 series of articles on prenatal life, *Coronet* magazine heralded "the new questions being asked at the Fels Institute: What happens to a baby before he is born? Is he sometimes uncomfortable? Does he feel motions? Can he hear? Can he think? Is he capable of learning?" as going far beyond the work that had come out of the Carnegie Institute:

> Up to now, medicine has not had time to answer questions such as these. It has had its hands full just figuring out how an unborn baby grows during these first nine months of its existence. At that, the doctors did so well that they were able to piece together an exact week-by-week picture of that miraculous period of life before birth. Medicine now knows just how a baby looks and acts at any stage of prenatal development. They can tell you, for instance, that the tiny heart of a four-week-old embryo, just one-tenth inch in length, is already beginning to beat; that an eight-week-old fetus, one inch long, already shows signs of developing facial features, arms and legs, a brain, and will even respond to tickling; that by the time it is twenty weeks old, it has several accomplishments, among them the ability to pout, clench its fist, and move enough to make its mother aware of its presence.[46]

Developmental details hailed as extraordinary discoveries only a few years earlier had been relegated to matter-of-fact descriptions of peripheral importance to the work of the Fels Institute.

In addition to having a biological and physiological life, the fetus was also presented as having a biographical and psychological life. In 1948, psychologist and child development expert Dr. Arnold Gesell founded the Gesell Institute of Child Development. Gesell described his work this way: "We are asking new questions. What happens to a baby before he is born? Can he think? Can he feel? Can he learn? Can he remember? Can he dream?"[47] The possibility of prenatal consciousness and unconsciousness intrigued psychologists working in the emerging field of prenatal psychology.

Although it had antecedents in the early-twentieth-century theories of prenatal culturists, the field of "prenatal psychology" got a modern stamp of approval in 1948, at the American Psychological Association's annual meeting where one prenatal psychologist gave a talk explaining to his audience how he was helping patients recover their "experiences in the prenatal state, as recorded and reproduced in dreams."[48] At the same meeting, Drs. J. G. N. Gushing and Mary McKinniss Gushing offered an analysis explaining why babies hate their mothers. "The hatred," they explained, "begins even before the child is born; it hates confinement in the womb, but it hates being born even more." They showed the audience images of the fetuses they had studied, explaining the "avoidance reactions" they detected as early as fourteen weeks after conception. They characterized one facial expression as "having all the elements of a sneer," and described "one fetus with the stance of a John L. Sullivan who warded off stimulations with what appeared to be aggressively defensive movements." The prenatal experience is, they said, so traumatic that "the store of hostility in the child is so great that it cannot be entirely compensated."[49] The following year, in his influential *The Search for the Beloved,* Dr. Nandor Fodor argued that "experiences in the prenatal state are recorded and reproduced in dreams....These experiences influence postnatal psychical development. They form the base of several neurotic symptoms of the adult."[50] The study of the "fetal psyche" and "prenatal mind" had particular implications for mothers.

While dismissing "maternal impressions" as old wives' tales to be discarded in light of new medical knowledge, doctors identified a new danger transmitted by the mother to her unborn child—neurosis. Dr. Sontag of the Fels Institute diagnosed "prenatal neurosis" in eight of the fetuses he observed, describing how the infant "has not had to wait until childhood for a bad home situation or other cause to make him neurotic."[51] A concerned mother wrote in to *Today's Health* magazine with the following query: "My doctor told me there is no connection between the nerves of an expectant mother and the nerves of the child. How can the mother's emotions affect the child?" The answer tried to make clear the distinction between maternal impressions and prenatal psychology: "Dr. Sontag isn't talking about the mother's mental images, he's talking about her emotions."[52]

At the annual meeting of the American Medical Association in 1953, Dr. William S. Kroger of the University of Illinois Medical School led a session on prenatal neurosis. He argued that "a new baby may be destined to be a neurotic child if his mother was the victim of disturbed feelings during the months before birth," and that "the expectant mother, if sufficiently upset, may lose her baby through spontaneous abortion." He went on to explain that "the psyche has also been implicated in the early and late toxemias of pregnancy. Such entities may, in part, be due to the stress of modern living."[53] His arguments, and similar ones, were heralded in articles with titles like "Baby May be Neurotic if Mother Is Disturbed," "Expectant Mothers' Emotions May Have Bearing on Child," and "Fears and Babies."[54] This trend paralleled the popularization of psychoanalytic explanations of infertility, leading some physicians to attribute a woman's inability to get pregnant to her "unconscious desires to avoid parenthood."[55] A woman's neurosis could, evidently, both damage the fetus and prevent a pregnancy—both being examples of a woman failing to fulfill her natural role, with implications for the nation as a whole.

These concerns about the impact of a mother's feelings on the development of a fetus echoed a growing trend of blaming overprotective and suffocating mothers for raising weak and neurotic men.[56] Articles like "Protecting against Mother Love," "Are American Moms a Menace?" "What's Wrong with American Mothers?" "Doting Mother," "Overprotective Mother," and "You Can Love a Child Too Much" all suggested that many of society's problems could be attributed to the problem writer and social critic Philip Wylie had characterized as "momism"—a term describing the undeserved worship given to mothers—in his *Generation of Vipers*.[57] In *Their Mothers' Sons,* war psychiatrist Edward Strecker argued that two million men had been rejected by draft boards or discharged from the war for psychiatric reasons because their mothers, unable to "untie the emotional apron string," had raised immature and neurotic sons. Adopting Wylie's neologism, Strecker concluded that "momism was the product of a system veering toward matriarchy."[58] Strecker had elevated momism from mere social commentary to medical condition, a condition afflicting some during their prenatal months. At the same time that some psychiatrists were attributing the problem of a population "unable to face life, live with others, think for themselves, and stand on their own two feet" to mothers transmitting neuroses to their born and unborn children, some embryologists were interpreting the prenatal experience as providing the foundation for individuality.[59] Coming at these problems from different perspectives, psychologists and embryologists shared the belief that an individual's psychological well-being was ensured or deterred *in utero,* and that mothers were responsible for creating a psychologically toxic or healthy fetal environment.

In addition to explaining psychological and social problems, life *in utero* also became a subject for exploring political and philosophical questions. Students of embryological and prenatal life were increasingly interpreting their work in the context of pressing questions about the relationship between individuals and society, emphasizing the ways in which fetal development was simultaneously a unique experience for every individual as well as a universal experience shared by all human beings. In the context of heightened interest in the origins of difference and the fragility of life that pervaded the collective consciousness during and after World War II, the fetus became a symbol in the struggle to define and defend individuality.[60] In 1944, Dr. George Washington Corner published *Ourselves Unborn: An Embryologist's Essay on Man,* a collection of lectures he had given at

Yale University.[61] Describing the nine months of "prefatory life" as a "pilgrim's progress," and noting the "miraculous" relationship among "the universal biological process, the particular environmental influence, and the singular genetic inheritance, that combine to create the individual human being that is you," Corner explained that the story he is telling is "your history… and mine, and that of my own child and of yours."[62] In Corner's words, "Life is a paradoxical career in which the individual must both accept and contend with his environment, at once struggle for independence and adapt himself to cooperative action."[63] This story, for Corner, "will tell us much about the nature of our perplexing race and something perhaps of human fate and foreordination."[64]

Others identified this same struggle at the heart of the meaning of personhood. In the "Miracle of Growth" exhibit catalogue, author Arnold Sundgaard makes the similar point that the status of personhood is attained through the attributes one person has in common with all people, as well as through the attributes unique to that one particular individual:

> Yet in all the world—all over the entire face of the globe—there are no two people exactly alike. Out of the generations we have each of us derived our own particular heredity. And by the very nature of living in a particularized environment, we are made completely and irrevocably individual. All of us are linked, out of necessity and choosing, one to the other. Our fulfillment as human beings rests deep within ourselves and even deeper within each other.[65]

In *The Person in the Womb*, zoologist Dr. Norman J. Berrill wrote that "no two humans are exactly alike. No one is like oneself. Recognition of this gives a unique value to the person and also demands recognition of the uniqueness of others. Such is the basis for tolerance."[66]

For Corner, Sundgaard, and Berrill, the uniqueness of humanity was in the balance between the persistence of individuals' general forms and their potential for random variation, and the challenge of contemporary society was to simultaneously recognize one's independence and interdependence. These authors used stories about fetal development to argue that individuality was both the most personal as well as the most universal aspect of every person, to dissolve the contradiction between believing that every individual is completely unique and all human beings are deeply connected.

Berrill's emphasis on "tolerance" points to a related theme in books about fetal development, which is the idea of racial liberalism. In her 1938 bestseller *The Biography of the Unborn: The First Nine Months*, Margaret Shea Gilbert concluded that "the manifold changes occurring during this period form the personal history of each member of the race. It is the one phase of life we all have in common; it is essentially the same for everyone, of whatever race, creed or condition."[67] Sidonie Matsner Gruenberg's 1952 children's book, *The Wonderful Story of How You Were Born* begins with the following statement:

> Everybody you know started to be and started to grow from just such an egg. Your mother did and your father did, and your sisters and brothers, and your cousins and your teachers and your friends. No matter how big anyone is now or how small, he began in exactly the same way. No matter whether a person has white skin or brown skin or yellow skin, whether he lives in America or India or Africa or China, he began as a tiny little egg.[68]

In emphasizing that the universal human experience of embryological development transcends racial differences, Gilbert and Gruenberg's books are two examples of how the story of fetal development could offer an explanation of a common humanity that was starkly different from the early-twentieth-century belief in biologically determined racial differences.

The proliferation of mass media coverage of prenatal life from the perspectives of biology, sociology, psychology, and politics—and the overlapping of those domains—were part of a larger pattern in which science was becoming an increasingly powerful part of American culture. The growing consensus valuing the authority of scientific knowledge was accompanied by a concern that scientists take seriously their moral, social, and political obligations. Professional scientific journals published articles arguing that scientists needed to recognize their social responsibility and increasing public role.[69] Exploring the emerging cult of the expert following the war, particularly the increasingly influential role of science and scientific experts, historians have suggested that an unarticulated anxiety about the consequences of scientific progress and expertise underpinned the rhetorical and ideological invocation of that authority.[70]

Much of this anxiety revolved around the atomic bomb, which was heralded as an extraordinary scientific achievement and identified as a moral problem. *Ladies Home Journal* insisted that "the shaping of atomic policy is not just a scientific question, but a political, moral, and even religious question... [that] has to be answered by you and me."[71] In an article in *American Home* titled "Parents: Architects of Peace," Louisa Randall Church suggested that addressing that problem was the responsibility of parents:

> Out of the smoke and smoldering ruins arose a great cry for leadership equipped to guide the stricken people of the world along the hazardous course toward peace... Upon the shoulders of parents everywhere, rests the tremendous responsibility of sending forth into the next generation men and women imbued with a high resolve to work for everlasting peace.[72]

Rhetorical and analytical links between the nuclear bomb and the nuclear family, a term coined in 1947, were easily drawn, as the atomic sciences and the science of embryology became at least loosely linked in the public imagination.

After viewing the "Miracle of Growth" exhibit, psychologist and pediatrician Arnold Gesell immediately connected the two realms, commenting that "there are many things to understand. At one extreme, is the atom; at another extreme is the child."[73] Physician and philosopher Albert Schweitzer also linked atomic and fetal culture, with an additional nod toward the rhetoric of the American Revolution, lamenting that in a case of "annihilation without representation," nuclear war would destroy the "rights of the unborn."[74] The rights of the unborn were first recognized not, as Schweitzer would have hoped, through a commitment to world peace, but in the much more limited realm of prenatal tort law. Altered assumptions about the maternal-fetal relationship and heightened concerns about the meaning of individuality intersected with developments in legal culture to produce what one judge characterized as "perhaps the most rapid reversal of a common law tradition."[75]

Prenatal torts—or the right of a child to recover for damages imposed through a wrongful act and incurred prenatally—were first recognized in 1946 in the case of *Bonbrest v. Kotz*. In 1939, Bette Gay Bonbrest was delivered with forceps, and as a result incurred serious injuries during birth. Her mother had died during delivery, and seven years later, Bette Gay's father, on behalf of his daughter, successfully sued the delivering obstetrician for negligence. The case established for the first time the right of a child to recover for harm incurred when it was a viable fetus *in utero*. The court held that "a child *en ventre sa mere* is regarded as a human being from the moment of conception."[76] In overturning a sixty-year precedent that had explicitly disallowed recovery for negligently inflicted prenatal injuries, the *Bonbrest* decision represented a significant legal shift in the recognition of fetal personhood.

The first attempt to make a legal claim on behalf of a fetus had been in 1884, in the case of *Dietrich v. Northampton* discussed in the previous chapter, in which a woman sued the town for negligently causing the wrongful death of her unborn son, when she slipped on a public road and went into premature labor.[77] At the same time that physicians were organizing around their new definition of the fetus as a separate living being and embryologists were beginning to model and collect human embryos, Massachusetts Supreme Court Chief Justice Oliver Wendell Holmes found that "a child *en ventre sa mere*... is so intimately united with its mother as to be a 'part' of her and as a consequence is not to be regarded as a separate, distinct, and individual entity."[78] That the *Dietrich* decision was not in keeping with the contemporaneous medical interest in the separate life of the fetus suggests that late-nineteenth-century legal theory did not depend upon medical and scientific arguments.[79]

Between 1884 and 1946, parents had continued to make legal attempts to recover damages incurred by their children before they were born. In the late 1930s, courts continued to base their decisions on the precedent of *Dietrich,* but some began expressing their uneasiness with the 1884 decision. In 1938, Mrs. Theresa Joller Smith was given a series of X-ray treatments designed to destroy what her physician thought was a tumor but turned out to be a pregnancy. When she subsequently gave birth to a child born "crippled and feeble-minded," she sued Dr. Albert E. Luckhardt.[80] In the case of *Smith v. Luckhardt,* the court denied the right of the child to claim for prenatally inflicted damages. But when the presiding Judge Harry M. Fisher was interviewed by *Time* magazine for an article titled "Fetal Rights," he expressed his hope that the case would be appealed to a higher court. He said that he thought the court had reached the "right legal decision, but personally, I think that Justice Holmes was wrong."[81]

In a similar case four years later, Pauline Stemmer's doctor diagnosed her with a uterine tumor. She underwent three separate X-ray treatments as part of her treatment. Six weeks after her third X-ray treatment, she and her doctor were surprised when she went into labor and delivered an infant, born five weeks prematurely. Doctors described the infant as "a microcephalic idiot, prematurely born. It hasn't the power to walk, talk, hear, or see."[82] Stemmer sued her doctor. Although the jury determined that the X-rays were the cause of the infant's condition and found that the doctor had acted negligently, the court determined that that the doctor could not be held liable for "negligently causing harm to an unborn child."[83] The court expressed its discomfort with their decision:

> Written in 1884, it [the *Dietrich* decision] concludes by saying no cause of action was accrued because at the time of the happening, the child was part of the mother. With that premise stated as a fact it was easy enough to come to the conclusion arrived at: but the premise is not true as a matter of elementary physiology. While it is a fact that there is a close dependence by the unborn child on the organism of the mother, it is not disputed today that the mother and the child are two separate and distinct entities. It is not the fact that an unborn child is part of the mother, but rather in the unborn state it lived with the mother, we might say, and from conception on developed its own distinct, separate personality.[84]

In 1946, that purportedly indisputable fact—which was being discussed and presented in museum exhibits, prescriptive literature, popular magazines, and medical literature—found its legal expression in a decision that would set the foundation for fetal rights in the postwar era.

The logic and precedent of the *Dietrich* decision were overturned in 1946, when the District Court of the District of Columbia explicitly rejected both in their decision in the *Bonbrest* case:

The argument that the child is "part" of its mother seems to me to be a contradiction in terms. True, it is in the womb, but it is capable now of extra-uterine life—and while it is dependent for its continued development on sustenance derived from its peculiar relationship to its mother, it is not a "part" of the mother. It has, if viable, its own bodily form and members, manifests all of the anatomical characteristics of individuality, possesses its own circularity, vascular and excretory systems, and is capable *now* of being ushered into the world.[85]

When the *Bonbrest* decision rejected the pattern set by *Dietrich*, it did so by arguing that scientific advances had enabled the recognition of individual fetal personhood. Justice McGuire, author of the *Bonbrest* decision, characterized Holmes's decision as a "legal fiction long out-moded," and criticized those who gave it such precedential authority for having a view that was "static and inert," "arid and sterile," and "myopic and specious." He went on to say the following:

The absence of precedent should afford no refuge to those who by their wrongful act have invaded the rights of an individual....And what right is more inherent, and more sacrosanct, than that of the individual in his possession and enjoyment of his life, his limbs, and his body. The law is sufficiently elastic to meet changing conditions....The law is presumed to keep pace with the sciences.[86]

Although the case had nothing to do with abortion, McGuire did go out of his way to express his opposition to "therapeutic abortion...the unborn child is an individual human being, not an unjust aggressor."[87]

Contemporary law journals pointed to the significance of the *Bonbrest* case, emphasizing, with a greater or lesser degree of approval, the rejection of precedent in favor of science. The *Chicago-Kent Law Review* reported this decision as one without precedent, based "upon the concept that judges were free to mold the common law to meet changing conditions or to keep pace with progress in other sciences." The article concluded with some displeasure that "the infection of that bold disregard for fundamental doctrines...seems to be spreading through the federal judiciary."[88] In contrast, the *Nebraska Law Review* praised the decision, finding that "a system of law that disregards scientific advancements cannot presume to be practical."[89] The *Cornell Law Quarterly* similarly acknowledged that with "the advancement of modern science and with the safeguards of requiring adequate proof of the injury, there appears to be no sound reason for not permitting the infant to attempt to prove his cause of action."[90] The debate over the *Bonbrest* decision was part of a larger legal debate about whether and how to balance developments in science, social science, and social values with the standing precedent of previous decisions.[91] That legal debate, which would be at the heart of the *Brown v. Board of Education* decision in 1954, emerged nearly ten years earlier in a case about prenatal torts.[92]

As legal scholars analyzed the *Bonbrest* ruling, other courts cited that 1946 decision as justification for recognizing fetal personhood in the context of tort law. An idea that had taken almost sixty years to be accepted quickly became a matter of common sense, as indicated by the Minnesota Supreme Court's finding in the 1949 case of *Verkennes v. Corniea*. Asked to decide if the estate of an unborn infant that had died prior to birth as a result of another's action could sue under the state's wrongful death statute, the Minnesota court held that "it seems too plain for argument that where independent existence is possible and life is destroyed through a wrongful act, a cause of action rises."[93] By 1960, eighteen states had awarded damages for prenatal injury or death. An examination of the arguments, evidence, and language of tort cases recognizing fetal personhood between 1946 and 1960 suggests that even as scientific advances were cited as crucial evidence in constructing a new framework for determining fetal personhood, that framework was simultaneously shaped by Cold War anxieties about individuality, motherhood, and democracy.

In 1949, in a decision whose language reflects these anxieties, a prenatal tort case was concluded after eight years in the courts. On April 4, 1941, Ruth Williams had fallen off of a bus. Williams was seven months pregnant, and she immediately went into labor, delivering a baby girl, Mina Margaret Williams, several hours later. Born two months prematurely, Baby Williams suffered from heart trouble, anemia, spasms, and epilepsy—problems her physicians attributed to the trauma of her mother's fall that incurred while Baby Williams was *in utero*.[94] In May 1947, six-year-old Mina Margaret Williams sued the bus company for negligence and carelessness in causing her injuries. Citing the *Dietrich* decision as support, the court rejected her claim. Under appeal, however, the Supreme Court of Ohio upheld Williams's claim for prenatal damages. Concluding that Mina Williams incurred her injuries when she was "an existing viable child," the court found that "an infant who is an existing viable child...is a 'person.' Injuries wrongfully inflicted upon an unborn viable child capable of existing independently of the mother are injuries done him in his person."[95] In the *Dietrich* case, the standard of legally recognizable fetal life had been established only at birth, when the baby became physically separate from the mother. In the *Williams* case, the standard of legally recognizable fetal life had become the fact of viability. In this scenario, the fetus was considered an independent life and person when it was determined to have the capacity to live separately from the mother.

The *Williams* decision received even more notice and praise from legal scholars than had the *Bonbrest* decision. The *Ohio State Law Journal* wrote that "the Supreme Court of Ohio has commendably broken away from precedents based on dicta and outmoded medical ideas."[96] The *University of Illinois Law Forum* also praised the *Williams* decision: "The Supreme Court of Ohio seized an opportunity to grasp an enlightened tort doctrine recently rekindled, coordinating and integrating the law with the scientific facts of life."[97] Although they carefully acknowledged and traced precedent in their decision, and made particular reference to the 1884 *Dietrich* decision, the *Williams* court ultimately rejected historical tradition in favor of scientific progress:

> It is to be hoped that the law will keep pace with science and certainly there has been some progress in medical science since 1884. To hold that the plaintiff in the instant case did not suffer an injury in her person would require this court to announce that as a matter of law the infant is a part of the mother until birth and has no existence in law until that time. In our view such a ruling would deprive the infant of the right conferred by the Constitution upon all persons, by the application of a time-worn fiction not founded on fact and within common knowledge untrue and unjustified.[98]

The decision concluded with the claim that "the law should keep abreast with the marvelous advancement of science and the readily changing conditions of the world."[99]

The Ohio Supreme Court articulated a new vision of the role of law in society and a new vision of the role of science in law. But what exactly was the advancement that so impressed them? Certainly the process of embryological and fetal development was understood with increasing complexity in the 1930s and 1940s, due largely to the research at places like the Carnegie Institute and the Fels Research Institute. But although this work added important details and supplied a larger set of data, it did not substantively challenge the broad outlines of what had been known about human reproduction and fetal development decades earlier.[100] In fact, discussions about fetal development in medical textbooks in the 1940s were remarkably similar to those same discussions in the earlier part of the century. For example, the section on "Signs of Fetal Life" in the 1903 edition of *Williams Obstetrics* matches verbatim that same section in the 1945 edition.[101] The 1949 decision in the *Williams* case cited this 1945 textbook as evidence of medical breakthroughs in the knowledge of human embryology, but jurists in the early twentieth century had access to identically phrased information and reached opposite conclusions.

Understanding why the *Dietrich* line of reasoning was rejected after more than sixty years, then, requires examining the increasingly influential role played by scientific evidence in the courtroom.[102] The authority of science in the legal system, and the related willingness of the courts to reject tradition and precedent and to embrace progress and change illustrated in the *Williams* decision, were part of a larger mid-century trend in medical jurisprudence. The *Bonbrest* and *Williams* decisions rested on the changed value placed by the courts on scientific evidence, rather than on the changed content of that scientific evidence.[103] An additional, and perhaps even more important, factor shaping these rulings was the cultural and historical lens through which the courts viewed these cases.

The transformation from separability to viability was linked to and rooted in the ways the court interpreted the available medical evidence within the changed ideological framework and historical context of the late 1940s. The Ohio court made that very point as it not only invoked science but also referenced "changing conditions of the world" to justify its decision: "The law is progressive and expansive, adapting itself to the law of new relations and interests which are constantly springing up in the progress of society. Precedents on which counsel set such great store, despite their glaring illogic and pitiable results are valuable only so long as they do not obstruct justice and destroy progress."[104] What exactly were these new relations and interests? What justice and progress was at stake in their decision? The Ohio court described them:

> Everybody today talks about the welfare of the nation, the safeguarding of human rights and the various freedoms but all these things are useless and of no avail to a certain class if the future persons for whom these things are to be preserved are not protected and safeguarded while *en ventre sa mere*, and their rights preserved when they are of all times most helpless.[105]

In 1949, the linchpin in the mission to protect the welfare of the nation, human rights, and freedom was democracy. Historians Mary Dudziak and Thomas Borstelmann have explored the links between this language of freedom and rights—language shaped in the crucible of World War II and the Cold War—and the emergence and limitations of the civil rights movement, arguing that the United States became increasingly concerned with the possibility that their international struggle for democracy was compromised by their domestic refusal to grant full citizenship to African Americans.[106] That same language was used to suggest that not recognizing independent fetal life would similarly compromise the country's commitment to democracy. This rhetoric echoes arguments made by child development experts Dr. Benjamin Spock and Dr. Leo Kanner, who explained to their readers that the ideal relationship between parent and child, or mother and child, is democratic, not despotic.[107] Kanner describes the relationship between child development and democracy:

> There is a fallacy abroad that democracy does not begin until the voting age is reached. This would be all right if democracy were merely a political concept. But real democracy is far more than that. It is a way of living. And life begins not at forty, not at twenty-one, but at the beginning. Therefore, true democracy begins not in the polling booth, but at home, in the nursery, in the living room, at the dinner table, in the earliest relations between parents and their children.[108]

The consequence of a "tyrannical parent is a tyrannical child," or an "infantile dictatorship," he warned.[109] For readers who had attended the "Miracle of Growth" exhibit, read the exhibit catalogue, or read articles about prenatal psychology, it would not have been a stretch to assume that those "earliest relations" began *in utero*. The Kanner and Spock model embraced the individuality and independence of the child in the same way that Gilbert, Corner, Berrill, Gruenberg, and others embraced it in the fetus.

Whereas it took a half-century or more to shift the starting point of fetal personhood from birth to viability, the shift from viability to conception occurred within a decade. In 1956, in the case of *Hornbuckle v. Plantation Pipe Line*, the Georgia Supreme Court endorsed conception as the determining factor in allowing claims for prenatal personal injury.[110] *Hornbuckle* was immediately recognized as the first case to reject the "legalistic" distinctions made between conception, viability, and birth. *Fordham Law Review* endorsed the "more logical" view taken by the *Hornbuckle* court, writing that it "sensibly recognized that a legal separability begins with biological separability, that is at conception."[111] The *Cornell Law Quarterly* praised this approach as "more modern as well as more just."[112]

Why did the law suddenly embrace conception rather than viability as the more biologically sound standard for personhood? The *Hornbuckle* court identified the importance of the 1953 decoding of DNA, the protein molecules of which genes are comprised. That discovery would reinvigorate the genetic thinking of the early twentieth century. Understanding that the "secret of life" resided in DNA meant that one's identity was determined primarily at the moment of fertilization between egg and sperm, and secondarily at the moment of meiosis, the moment of genetic division and recombination between egg and sperm.[113] Viability could now be understood as a developmental stage, rather than a foundational one.

A related change was the heightened interest in the legal implications of atomic energy. In 1951, a group of legal scholars at the University of Michigan began a project studying those implications and published their findings in 1959, in *Atoms and the Law.* In a chapter examining how to determine negligence in tort liability cases, the authors devoted more than twenty pages to the issue of radiation in causing postconception and genetic prenatal injuries. Although attentive to the epidemiological and legal issues involved, the authors were insistent that the question of whether to allow damages to unborn children, a question that they believed "the greatly accelerated use of radiation will bring into very sharp focus," was ultimately one of social policy rather than law or science.[114] Recognizing the issue as a political rather than a scientific one helps explain the rapid acceptance of the idea that personhood begins at conception.

The shift in the legal standard for individuality to conception was roundly praised by legal scholars. The courts presented the logic and impetus of their decisions as relatively uncomplicated. The logic was science, the impetus justice, and the relationship between the two was supportive and unproblematic. The courts repeatedly cited advances in medical science, a commitment to progress and modernity, and the interests of social values and common sense as the reasons for their decisions. There is, in these decisions, a striking absence of specific examples of new medical knowledge in favor of vague allusions to scientific progress. This suggests both that the new information was common knowledge that did not require explication, and that the mere invocation of science was seen as particularly persuasive. Both of these statements are, to some extent, accurate. Certainly the intricacies of embryonic and fetal development were becoming increasingly publicized, through museum exhibits, books, and magazine articles. And what is equally true is that the recognition of fetal personhood relied on the authority of science but did not necessarily use the facts of science.

What was true in legal decisions was oddly enough also true in medical literature, as a comparison of two medical textbooks suggests. Compare the illustrations of the cardiovascular system of a fetus *in utero* in the 1945 and 1956 editions of *Williams Obstetrics.*[115] The 1945 illustration is a graphic of the cardiovascular system on a blank background (figure 2.2). The 1956 illustration uses that same graphic, but superimposed it on a large baby (figure 2.3). Granting that certain medical advances had been made in those ten years, the large baby portrayed in the 1956 illustration bears little resemblance to the then available *in utero* photographs of fetal development. The contrast between these illustrations is particularly surprising given that the textual description of fetal development is identical in both editions. Clearly, this visual personification of the fetus was more than a response to new scientific knowledge.

If the fetus was a symbol that could somehow represent particular American commitments to the value of individuality and the protection of personal rights,

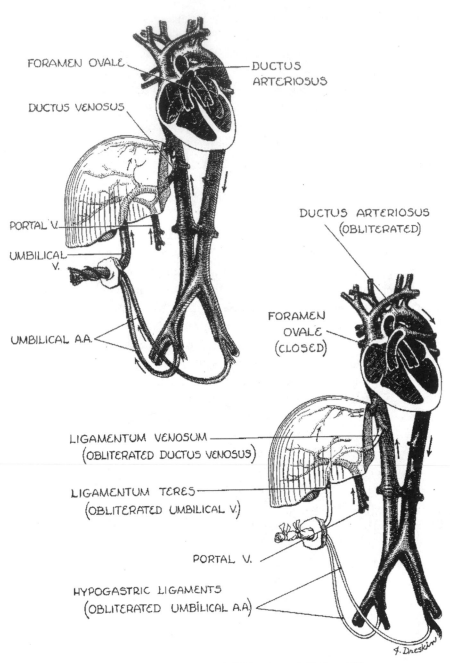

FORAMEN OVALE

DUCTUS ARTERIOSUS

DUCTUS VENOSUS

DUCTUS ARTERIOSUS (OBLITERATED)

PORTAL V.

UMBILICAL V.

UMBILICAL A.A.

FORAMEN OVALE (CLOSED)

LIGAMENTUM VENOSUM (OBLITERATED DUCTUS VENOSUS)

LIGAMENTUM TERES (OBLITERATED UMBILICAL V.)

PORTAL V.

HYPOGASTRIC LIGAMENTS (OBLITERATED UMBILICAL A.A.)

F. Dreskin

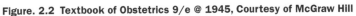

Figure. 2.2 Textbook of Obstetrics 9/e @ 1945, Courtesy of McGraw Hill

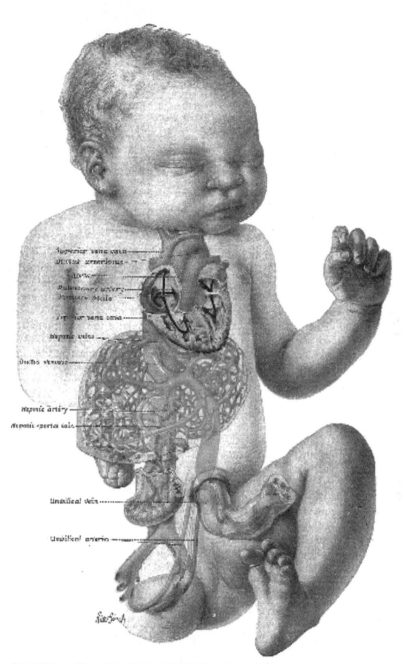

Figure. 2.3 Williams Obstetrics 11/e @ 1956, Courtesy of McGraw Hill

and could, in the terminology of the cold war, "contain" a set of cultural anxieties, it also contained within it the potential to inaugurate a new set of social conflicts. The legal profession was largely supportive of the spate of legal decisions ascribing individuality to the fetus, and few legal scholars suggested any downside to this trend. One exception, though, was an article in the *Indiana Law Journal* that supported the *Bonbrest* decision but also raised the specter of a maternal-fetal conflict. "It might be argued," the article suggested, "that a mother's contributory negligence should be imputed to the child." Making no judgment as to whether that would be a good or bad argument, the article explained the problem in the legal context of parent-child immunity: "The real issue is whether an unborn child should be treated as a very young child under the doctrine of imputed negligence. It appears, then, that the success of the defense of imputed negligence will depend upon the willingness of the particular jurisdiction to impute a parent's negligence to a born child."[116]

When, in 1900, the *Allaire* decision had raised this same possibility of parental culpability, writing that "if the action can be maintained, it necessarily follows that an infant may maintain an action against its own mother while pregnant with it," it was offered as an example of the worst-case scenario.[117] And in 1957, for the first time, a parent—in this case, a father—was found culpable for pre-natal neglect. That year, a California Appellate Court found Donald L. Clarke guilty of failing to "furnish necessary food, clothing, shelter, or remedial care for minor child, including child conceived but not yet born."[118] The statute at issue was meant to "place upon father of minor child, born or unborn, legitimate or illegitimate, responsibility of providing basic needs for preservation of life of child."[119] Finding Clarke guilty of a misdemeanor offense, Justice Richards wrote the following:

> One old enough to father a child may be presumed to know that the way by which the human embryo and fetus is nurtured during gestation is through the intermediary of the mother and that to sustain the life of an unborn child, the mother herself must be sustained with food, clothing, and shelter.... As to the method or means of furnishing the unborn child's necessaries, the statute does not require that they be furnished "to" the child, but "for" the child.[120]

Whereas the *Clarke* decision expanded a father's obligations to the unborn, subsequent debates in the late 1960s and early 1970s about defining the term *dependent child* in determining Aid to Families with Dependent Children (AFDC) benefits would contract the state's responsibilities to the unborn.

Since 1941, the Social Security Board, which was responsible for administering AFDC, had held that "unborn children were technically eligible for assistance," allowing but not requiring states to provide benefits on behalf of the unborn. Premised on interpreting the term "dependent child" in section 406(A) of the Social Security Act as including an unborn child, the policy was formalized in the Department of Heath, Education, and Welfare's 1946 *Handbook of Public Assistance.*[121] In the late 1960s, litigation brought by women claiming that they were being unjustly denied benefits for their unborn children resulted in ten district court decisions finding that Congress had intended to include the unborn in the definition of "dependent child." Five circuit court decisions upheld those findings, thus requiring the states to provide benefits to pregnant women on behalf of their unborn children.[122] One of the states now required to provide AFDC benefits for the unborn was Mississippi. Responding to the decision, Mississippi attorney general A. F. Summer said, "[T]he time for payments has been moved backward from birth to conception. I hope they decide to stop there. If we have to begin with the gleam in the eye, who will do the counting and the certifying?"[123]

While state and federal courts were interpreting the statute, Congress was considering rewriting it. In 1971 and 1972, Congress was debating proposed amendments to the Social Security Act, including the issue of whether or not the unborn should be eligible for AFDC benefits.[124] In those debates, both the Senate Finance Committee and the House Ways and Means Committee concluded that "an unborn child would not be included in the definition of a child.... Only children who have actually been born would be eligible for Aid to Families with Dependent Children."[125] Congress seemed motivated, at least in part, by the economic implications of the issue. The House report noted the "geometrically increasing costs and caseloads in the 1960s" and characterized the AFDC program as "completely out of control."[126] The Senate report noted that the unborn constituted 2 percent of the recipient caseload in California.[127] The bill was not passed into law, but the difference between the proposed amendment and the lower court rulings reveal a real conflict of opinion. In 1975, in *Burns v. Alcala,* the Supreme Court settled the issue and overturned the five circuit court decisions. The court found that "the term 'dependent child' as so defined, does not include unborn children, and hence States receiving federal financial aid under the AFDC program are not required to offer welfare benefits to pregnant women for their unborn children."[128]

The debates about AFDC benefits did not focus on determining the moral status of the unborn but focused on interpreting the intent of the original statute. Given the timing of them, it is notable that the congressional debates, district court decisions, and the Supreme Court decision made no reference to abortion. All sides of the issue most likely wanted to avoid making that connection. Those who supported legalized abortion might also have supported providing benefits to pregnant women for their unborn children, whereas those opposed to legalized abortion might also have felt that not defining the unborn as a child in this context might be a way to limit the expansion of welfare benefits. What this suggests is that determining the status of the fetus in the actual policy depended on political goals and values rather than on questions about fetal life.

Determining the status of the unborn in the middle of the twentieth century—whether in medical research, museum exhibits, tort law, or debates about Social Security benefits—revealed some disagreements. But whereas those disagreements had, for the most part, been relatively contained, abortion politics was about to change that. Subsequent to the 1973 *Roe v. Wade* decision legalizing abortion, disagreements over the status of the unborn would erupt and transform American political culture in ways previously unimagined.

For most of the twentieth century, abortion was simultaneously proscribed and practiced.[129] In 1953, Alfred Kinsey reported that nine out of ten premarital pregnancies ended in abortion and that 22 percent of married women had had an abortion while married.[130] In 1955, the continuing demand for abortion motivated Planned Parenthood's medical director Dr. Mary S. Calderone to organize a conference featuring women testifying about the hardships of dangerous and unwanted pregnancies, and physicians advocating for liberalized abortion restrictions.[131] Whereas the American Medical Association (AMA) had led the nineteenth-century movement to criminalize abortion, it was now in the vanguard in an incipient movement to legalize it. In 1960, physicians at the AMA annual convention argued that laws against abortion were unenforceable, thus undesirable, and in 1962 the American Law Institute (ALI) endorsed the liberalization of abortion laws.[132] Yet abortion remained largely out of the public sphere until two events in the early 1960s—Sherri Finkbine's abortion in 1962 and the rubella epidemic in 1963–1964—focused national attention on the issue and triggered grassroots movements to fight for legalizing abortion.

As the host of public television's *Romper Room*, Sherri Finkbine was a minor television celebrity in Phoenix, Arizona, when she became pregnant with her fifth child. Suffering from insomnia and morning sickness, Finkbine took a sleeping pill her husband Robert had obtained while vacationing in Europe. When she asked her obstetrician if it was safe for her to take sleeping pills, he assured her that most sleeping pills were not dangerous and asked her what kind she had taken. Learning it was thalidomide, he advised her to apply to the hospital's abortion board for permission to have a therapeutic abortion.[133] Developed in Germany in the 1950s to treat chronic insomnia, thalidomide quickly became popular with pregnant women throughout Europe as a way to ameliorate morning sickness. By the time it was realized that thalidomide taken during pregnancy caused severe birth defects to the fetus—most famously *phoc-omelia,* a deformity in which babies are born with tiny flipper-like stumps instead of arms and hands—more than 16,000 "thalidomide babies" had been born. Sherri Finkbine was one of the very few women in the United States who had obtained the drug, which had not been approved by the Food and Drug Administration.[134]

Finkbine's doctor scheduled her surgery and wrote a letter recommending the procedure to the hospital's abortion board. In the late 1940s, hospitals had established "abortion boards" to adjudicate women's requests for "therapeutic abortions." Initially, the list of medical indications justifying a therapeutic abortion was long and ambiguous, and the board rarely challenged a physician's recommendation that a woman undergo an abortion. But scholars have shown that the medical indications justifying an abortion and the rate of therapeutic abortions declined dramatically throughout the 1950s.[135] Despite this trend, Finkbine's doctor assumed that the clear dangers posed by thalidomide would be sufficient cause for the board to approve his recommendation. Concerned about other pregnant women who might be taking the drug, Finkbine called a journalist friend, who promised to publicize the danger without revealing Finkbine's identity. But somehow her name was leaked, whereupon the hospital immediately rejected her application for an abortion, claiming that her case did not fall within the necessary Arizona statute permitting abortion only "when necessary to preserve the mother's life." Her doctor's request for a court order requiring the hospital to allow the abortion was denied, and Finkbine went to Sweden for the procedure, which revealed that the fetus was so deformed that it would not have survived. Finkbine's case triggered national debate, and a Gallup poll taken shortly after this case revealed that 52 percent of Americans supported Sherri Finkbine's abortion, whereas only 32 percent opposed it.[136]

Several months later, a second story focused national attention on the issue of abortion. In early 1963, an epidemic of rubella (German measles) swept the country, afflicting eighty-two thousand pregnant women in their first trimester of pregnancy. As a result of the epidemic, the American College of Obstetricians and Gynecologists estimated that as many as thirty thousand babies were born dead or died in infancy, and another twenty thousand suffered from major abnormalities. The publicity generated by the Finkbine case and the rubella epi-demic intensified physicians' efforts to liberalize abortion laws and generated political pressure on states to change their statutes.[137] In April 1967, Colorado passed the nation's first abortion reform law, which permitted hospital commit-tees to authorize abortions not only to save the woman's life but also in cases in which continued pregnancy would "gravely impair" the mother's physical or mental health or in pregnancy caused by rape or incest. Colorado's example was followed that same year by North Carolina, California, and Oregon, and then by Georgia and Maryland.[138] Not satisfied with reforms that kept the power to grant or refuse an abortion in the hands of doctors and hospital boards, grassroots activists began advocating for the repeal of all abortion restrictions. In 1969, the National Association for Repeal of Abortion Laws (NARAL) was founded at the First National Conference on Abortion Laws, and the radical feminist group Redstockings held the first speak-out on abortion.[139] In 1970, the New York state legislature legalized abortion, an act endorsed by Republican governor John D. Rockefeller.[140] In 1971, a national poll showed that more than half of Americans favored legalizing abortion, the American Bar Association issued a statement supporting the legalization of abortion up to the twentieth week of pregnancy, and the Supreme Court heard the first round of oral arguments in *Roe v. Wade*.

On January 22, 1973, the Supreme Court ended the nearly century-long prohibition against abortion in the United States.[141] In his majority opinion, Justice Harry Blackmun made clear the Court's desire to remove the abortion question from the abstract realms of philosophy, theology, and morality and place it in the concrete realm of law: "We need not resolve the difficult question of when life begins. When those trained in the respective disciplines of medicine, philosophy, and theology are unable to arrive at any consensus, the judiciary, at this point in the development of man's knowledge, is not in a position to speculate as to the answer."[142] Locating abortion within the doctor-patient relationship, the Court argued that it was protected by the woman's constitutional right to privacy, a right that the state could, subsequent to the viability of the fetus, override in order to protect its interest in "potential human life."[143] But in skirting a set of questions about the origins of human life, the court had implicitly raised a second set of questions about the meaning and determination of viability. The court had, perhaps, hoped to simplify and depoliticize the issue of abortion by stripping it of its metaphysical meanings, but as the history of fetal discourses should have made clear, and as the post-Roe years quickly showed, it would prove difficult to separate theological questions about life from biological questions about physiology from political questions about personhood.

CHAPTER 3
DEFINING FETAL PERSONHOOD, 1973–1976

On April 11, 1974, following an eight-month investigation by the district attorney's office, a grand jury in Suffolk County, Massachusetts, indicted four doctors affiliated with Boston City Hospital, charging them under the 1814 Massachusetts statute against the "violation of sepulture."[1] This "grave-robbing" statute—similar to the one that officials would use in Illinois in 1977 to arrest Ward Hall for exhibiting his "pickled fetus"—had originally been intended to stop the growing black market for cadavers, bought, sold, and stolen by physicians wanting to dissect them.[2] For participating in a study on the effects of certain antibiotics on the fetus, a study that began with transferring aborted fetuses from the pathology department to their research laboratories, these four physician-researchers were indicted on charges of "willfully removing and carrying away from a building known as BCH Gyn. Bld., a certain human body of a decedent with the intent to dispense of said body for the purpose of dissection not being lawfully authorized by the proper authorities."[3] Later that day, the same grand jury indicted for manslaughter a fifth BCH physician, Kenneth Edelin, for his actions in performing a second-trimester abortion on a seventeen-year-old daughter of West Indian immigrants.[4] Charges against the researchers were dismissed in 1978, but Kenneth Edelin was not so lucky.[5]

In another time and place, these cases might have attracted little public notice, but in the wake of the recent Supreme Court decision in *Roe v. Wade*, they escalated into local and national dramas featuring debates over fetal life, fetal personhood, and fetal rights. The incidents reflected a backlash against second-wave feminism focused on abortion and the Equal Rights Amendment; highlighted tensions of race, class, and ethnicity; and exploited growing concerns about the unchecked authority of physicians and scientists. Examining these two cases, this chapter explores how pro-life activists mobilized a grassroots movement to produce a newly vulnerable fetal subject requiring protection and how these dramas highlight the political and cultural conflicts that erupted nationally subsequent to the *Roe* decision. The unusually prominent role of the Catholic Church and the medical profession, as well as the particularly explicit racial and class tensions manifested in the school busing crisis then going on in the city, combined in ways that make Boston far from typical of the rest of the nation. But in highlighting the increasingly tight links between the politics of abortion and the politics of race and exposing the fracturing of New Deal liberalism and the coalescence of New Right conservatism, these events in Boston both illuminate the articulation and deployment of fetal meanings in one particular time and place, and anticipate debates later in the century.

The Boston City Hospital researchers had begun their antibiotic study in 1971, before the *Roe* decision. Medical researchers had been exploring the therapeutic possibilities of using tissue from aborted fetuses since the early twentieth century, including possible applications for diabetes treatment in the 1920s and 1930s.[6] Although those efforts did not succeed on their own terms— doctors would not successfully transplant fetal tissue cells into humans until 1985—they did trigger further research into the possible uses of human embryonic and fetal tissue.[7] The 1954 development of a polio vaccine through growing a polio virus in tissue cultured from fetal kidney cells sparked further excitement about the possibilities of this research.[8] In 1961, the University of Washington established the Laboratory for the Study of Human Embryos and Fetuses, institutionalizing the procurement and distribution of human fetal tissue for research purposes.[9] Following the rubella epidemic of 1963–1964, researchers across the country obtained from the Washington laboratory tissue from an infected aborted fetus to develop a Rubella vaccine.[10] Other researchers used fetal tissue to develop tests for Rh incompatibility and to develop amniocentesis screenings for other genetic anomalies.[11]

Working within the context of this long-standing and as-yet uncontroversial tradition of fetal research, Agnita Philipson, a Swedish physician and visiting researcher at Boston City Hospital's Thorndike Memorial Laboratory, and Dr. Leon Sabath, a professor at Harvard Medical School and researcher at Thorndike, devised a study to determine the differential effects on the fetus of erythromycin and clyndamycin taken by pregnant women allergic to penicillin. Needing to use intact aborted fetuses in order to compare the levels of these two different antibiotics in specific organs, they decided to make their study group women who were already planning to have an abortion. Sabath explained that "the safest course would be to get pregnant women who were going to have abortions anyway.... There was no reason to think that either antibiotic would be harmful to the fetus—each is widely used—but it seemed wrong to take any chance."[12] This study was one of many like it that followed the thalidomide scare and the discovery that the Sabin polio vaccine made from monkey fetal tissue was significantly less successful than the Salk vaccine made from human fetal tissue, two events that highlighted the value of studying the impact of drugs on the fetus and the benefits of using human fetal tissue in the research protocol.[13]

After receiving funding from the National Institutes of Health and approval from the BCH review board, Philipson and Sabath invited Dr. David Charles, director of BCH Department of Obstetrics and Gynecology, and Dr. Leonard Berman, a visiting pathologist at BCH, to join their study.[14] Charles would identify women who were planning abortions and would obtain their consent to participate in the study, and Berman would examine the tissue of the aborted fetuses for traces of the antibiotic. On June 7, 1973, the doctors published their findings in the *New England Journal of Medicine* in an article titled "Transplacental Passage of Erythromycin and Clyndamycin." The study concluded that both antibiotics would be reasonable alternatives to penicillin in treating intrauterine infections, expressing a slight preference for clyndamycin.[15] At any other time, only those physicians interested in the issue would have been likely to read this article.[16] But in June of 1973, mere months after the *Roe* decision, the *NEJM* article precipitated a thirty-year political struggle over fetal research that intersected with the abortion battle and continues today in contemporary debates about embryonic stem cell research.[17]

Between January 22, 1973, when the *Roe* decision rendered all existing Massachusetts laws regulating abortion unconstitutional, and August 1974, when the state passed its first state statute regulating abortion in compliance with *Roe*, abortion in Massachusetts was completely legal, restricted only by the availability and willingness of individual doctors and hospitals. During that eighteen-month period, Boston City Hospital, the only public hospital in the city, was inundated with patients requesting elective abortions. Located in the heart of the South End, adjacent to Roxbury, Charlestown, and South Boston, BCH served a population of mostly low-income West Indian immigrants and African-Americans, and its staff consisted largely of Irish-Catholic nurses.[18] Before the *Roe* decision, the hospital performed two to four therapeutic, medically recommended, abortions a week. After the decision, the hospital was performing between eighteen and thirty elective abortions a week.[19]

The hospital's "conscience clause" allowed any doctor to refuse to perform abortions, and in 1973, only two doctors at BCH, one of whom was Kenneth Edelin, performed abortions.[20] The conscience clause did not, however, apply to nurses, some of whom were becoming increasingly uncomfortable with the number of abortions done at their hospital. Elective abortions were producing a larger supply of healthy aborted fetuses ideal for research purposes, and, disturbed by what happened to these aborted fetuses, a group of nurses began writing letters to Boston city councilman Albert "Dapper" O'Neil about their concerns months before the *NEJM* article was published.[21] After reading about the antibiotic study (it isn't clear how he came across it), Thomas Connelly, director of the Massachusetts Citizens for Life, a pro-life organization founded in 1970 that had close to forty thousand members in the spring of 1973, immediately wrote to Massachusetts State Representatives Raymond Flynn and William Delahunt. Connelly sent the *NEJM* article, along with a letter in which he described doctors "performing abortions just to get their hands on the fetuses" and researchers "jabbing needles into unborn fetuses," "experimenting on fetuses that had been kept alive deliberately after abortion," and "cutting off fetuses' heads and keeping blood circulating through their bodies.'"[22]

Delahunt, Flynn, and O'Neil responded to the letters in ways characteristic of their relationship to their constituencies, their personal beliefs, and their political ambitions. A Democrat and a Catholic, Delahunt had been elected in 1973 to the statehouse from Quincy, a city with a small Catholic population and a history of moderate politics. Elected to the U.S. House of Representatives in 1996 by the 10th Congressional District of Massachusetts, Delahunt is currently a strong supporter of reproductive rights and stem cell research.[23] But in 1973, his public, and perhaps his private, position toward abortion and fetal research was less defined. After seeking advice from his friend and Boston College law professor James Smith, who told him that "a fetus scheduled for abortion should not be the subject of experiments because there is no one to look after its interests," Delahunt decided to write a bill that would allow most fetal research, while banning all research on any fetuses that were the subjects of planned abortions.[24]

Dr. Jack Ewalt, associate dean for clinical affairs at Harvard Medical School, had concerns about the implications of Delahunt's bill, particularly about whether amniocentesis and genetic screening tests would be excluded under this restriction. More generally, he questioned the consequences of allowing the complex issues of medical research to be regulated in the political arena by "people who don't remember their high school biology."[25] Ewalt asked Dr. Arthur Hertig, emeritus professor of anatomy and embryology at Harvard Medical School and the Carnegie Institute for Embryological Studies, to testify at the hearings, where opponents of fetal research repeatedly shouted him down during his presentation.[26] Delahunt, however, was impressed by Hertig's testimony. He subsequently invited Ewalt, Dr. Thomas Weller, who had helped develop the polio vaccine, Dr. David Nathan, professor of pediatrics at Harvard and chief of hematology and oncology at Children's Hospital, and Dr. Kenneth Ryan, chair of obstetrics and gynecology at Harvard and chief of obstetrics and gynecology at Brigham and Women's Hospital, to meet privately with his committee to discuss possible compromises.[27]

Nathan was particularly concerned about restrictions that might impinge on his own research into the hemoglobin disorder beta-thalassemia.[28] His studies relied on using fetal blood, which he could obtain only by using the newly developed amnioscope, a tiny cannula with a lens at its tip, inserted into the pregnant woman's uterus to visualize the fetus.[29] The technology was so new that it was impossible to know whether it posed any risk to the fetus, and Nathan worked to convince Delahunt that even though he was "personally not in favor of abortion," it made more sense to test it on fetuses already slated for abortions because, as he said, "if I could diagnose sickle cell anemia, and thalassemia, and other disorders *in utero*, I'd be preventing more abortions than they ever could. We have women who have an abortion because they don't want to risk having an afflicted child. With antenatal diagnosis, I could tell them, three times out of four, to go ahead and have the baby."[30] Nathan persuaded Delahunt and his committee. Although the final bill allowed research only on those fetuses not intended to be aborted, it explicitly exempted all "diagnostic or remedial procedures the purpose of which is to determine the life or health of the fetus involved or to preserve the life or health of the mother involved."[31] The bill was signed into law on June 26, 1974, and although scientists were not completely happy with the idea of having any regulations on their research, they were also relieved that the original, more restrictive bill had not gone through.[32]

In contrast to Delahunt's willingness to work behind closed doors to reach a compromise between the researchers and the pro-life movement, Flynn's response polarized the two sides even more dramatically. Flynn, a Democrat representing the Irish-Catholic enclave of South Boston, had, like most of his constituents, vehemently opposed *Roe*.[33] On July 30, 1973, Flynn forwarded the letters he had received from Massachusetts Citizens for Life to O'Neil, who was the chair of the Health and Hospital Committee and an Irish-Catholic Democrat from South Boston. Flynn included his own letter decrying the "inhumane procedures" practiced at BCH. He explained that he shared "your [O'Neil's] views and the views of all right-thinking people that abortions should not be permitted under any circumstances," and asked O'Neil to hold hearings on the matter.[34] Flynn knew that handing the fetal research issue to O'Neil was tantamount to waving a red flag in front of a bull and, predictably, O'Neil was happy to put on a show. "Abortion letters were just pouring in, and I decided to call an open hearing to look into what was going on down there," he said. "I set the hearing for September 19, 1973."[35]

The beginning of the 1973 school year was unusually tense in Boston. Just as O'Neil was beginning his hearings, Judge W. Arthur Garrity was concluding the case of *Morgan v. Hennigan*, a class action suit brought by the NAACP on behalf of fifty-three black children and their parents claiming that the racially segregated Boston schools violated the 1965 Racial Imbalance Act.[36] Irish-Catholics in South Boston and Charlestown feared, rightly as it would turn out, that Garrity's decision would disproportionately impact their communities, while exempting the wealthier white communities surrounding them. Many were also troubled by the recent *Roe* decision. Like Flynn, O'Neil was both a vocal supporter of Massachusetts Citizens for Life and of the antibusing movement, led by Louise Day Hicks, a one-time Democratic congresswoman and longtime member of the Boston city council, who, along with hundreds of mothers from Charlestown and South Boston, had recently organized an antibusing group called Restore Our Alienated Rights (ROAR).[37] Having long represented the antibusing interests on the city council, O'Neil was eager to give his constituents a venue to express their anger about abortion, and he orchestrated hearings on fetal research to provide one.

Focused on Delahunt's committee, few doctors attended O'Neil's hearings, which they perceived as a show trial with little power to effect policy. Dr. Leon White, commissioner of health and hospitals and member of the BCH board of trustees, did not attend the O'Neil hearings, but sent a letter to Council President Patrick F. McDonough explaining that the research had complied with all necessary guidelines, had been approved by the hospital's Committee on Human Experimentation, and was funded by the Milton Fund, Harvard University, and the U.S. Public Health Service. "I can assure you," he concluded, "that no abortions have, or ever will be performed at Boston City Hospital for experimental purposes, nor does the Hospital permit any attempt to keep aborted fetuses alive."[38] His letter was read aloud at the hearing, as was one from Dr. Charles, which read as follows:

> The charges concerning thousands of deaths per year of unborn babies at Boston City Hospital are untrue…the authors [of the *NEJM* article] had nothing to do with causing the pregnancies, influencing the women in their decision to terminate the pregnancies, nor influencing the Supreme Court of the United States in their decision that women have the right to have abortions.[39]

These letters, along with the doctors' absence from the hearings, illustrate the Boston medical community's conviction that their authority and credibility as doctors would be sufficiently impressive to end debate. The doctors significantly misread a changing political culture, in which professional expertise was being displaced by personal testimony, and in which class tensions in Boston were expressed as antielitism.[40]

At the vanguard of that cultural shift, the pro-life movement was learning that appealing to that antielitism could mobilize their supporters, and that grassroots power wielded through public protest and moral authority could trump Harvard credentials. The hearings were dominated by pro-life activists from MCL, Massachusetts Youth for Life, the Value of Life Committee, and the Catholic Church. Connelly testified first, illustrating the MCL strategy of evoking graphic images that elided the difference between fetal tissue and actual babies. Attacking the BCH researchers for destroying "innocent human beings number[ing] in the thousands," Connelly described in detail the process by which "the unborn babies are subsequently killed, then the various organs, brain, liver, bones, etc. are removed, and ground up to detect the presence of the administered drug."[41]

Representing the Boston Archdiocese, Monsignor Paul Harrington accused the researchers of treating the "babies like experimental animals."[42] It was highly unusual to have such an elevated religious official attend a city council hearing, and Harrington's presence indicates something about the tenuous position of Boston Archbishop Humberto Cardinal Medeiros. Portuguese-American Medeiros had been named archbishop in 1970, replacing the popular and powerful Richard Cardinal Cushing. The first non-Irish archbishop in Boston in 122 years, Medeiros was perceived as an outsider who was soft on busing. He had a fraught relationship with his Irish constituency, and perhaps saw these hearings as a way to establish his credentials with this community.[43] Possibly hoping to reach out to the more conservative members of the archdiocese whom he might have alienated with his moderate stance on racial issues, he had recently given an address titled "A Call for a Consistent Ethic of Life and Law," in which he expressed his support for the *Humanae Vitae* ("of human life"), Pope Paul VI's 1968 Encyclical Letter reaffirming Vatican II's position that abortion was "an unspeakable moral crime" and prohibitions on artificial contraception.[44]

Reflecting the growing influence of conservative women in grassroots social movements and the recognition that pro-life women might be more persuasive than pro-life men was the testimony of Sister Sheila, an administrator of a Catholic social service agency, and Dr. Mildred Jefferson, vice-president of the MCL and a director of the National Right to Life Committee.[45] Sister Sheila's testimony focused on emphasizing the personhood of the fetus, and she circulated a series of color photographs of fetal development. In contrast, Jefferson positioned herself as an advocate of women who, she argued, had been taken advantage of by powerful doctors who had not asked them what they wanted done with their "dead children" and had not consented to the research done on their aborted fetuses.[46] A series of BCH nurses gave compelling and graphic testimony about what they had seen and about how the male doctors and researchers ignored their concerns. The hearings concluded with testimony from the BCH obstetrics nurse who had written the original letter to O'Neil. She testified that she had been directed to dispose of "still breathing" live fetuses. Instead, she delivered them to the nurseries: "When I have taken live aborted babies to the nurseries during this time, I have gotten a lot of harassment...you know, things like 'Why are you bringing us these specimens?' 'You were supposed to get rid of them.'"[47]

Dapper O'Neil adjourned the hearings with these words: "I am going to go to the district attorney. I want him to assign a couple of men to me, and I am going through that hospital with a fine-toothed comb to find out the truth."[48] O'Neil sent the minutes of the hearings to the district attorney's office, hoping that some of the acts described at the hearings might be prosecutable crimes. District Attorney Garrett Byrne and Assistant District Attorney Newman Flanagan had already been following the hearings and had received many phone calls from MCL members about the hearing.[49] When a reporter asked Flanagan how his office had gotten involved in this case, Flanagan pointed a finger at him and said, "[S]uppose you dropped dead right now and I carted you off to someplace and dissected your body. That's an illegal act and a felony. . . . We had no alternative but to look into the matter and either confirm it or make a statement that said it was nonsense."[50]

The political ambitions of Byrne and Flanagan figured heavily in the DA office's eagerness to pursue the issue. An aging incumbent with an increasingly tenuous hold on his position, Byrne had nearly been beaten in his most recent election by antibusing leader Louise Day Hicks, who had won large majorities in South Boston and Charleston as a candidate for district attorney. Byrne also suspected, rightly, that forty-four-year-old Flanagan was planning to challenge him in the next election.[51] In contrast to Byrne, who was relatively circumspect about his personal beliefs about abortion, Flanagan was a devout Catholic and an outspoken opponent of abortion, and Byrne realized that this issue could be used against him in the next election.[52] Byrne and Flanagan were equally eager to respond to the interests of their Irish-Catholic constituents, and prosecuting the researchers seemed a logical next step.[53]

The arrests shocked the medical community of Boston. "I just can't believe that I've been arrested, fingerprinted, and mug shot for trying to find a way to prevent congenital syphilis," Nathan said.[54] Others characterized the suspensions as a capitulation to the politically motivated actions of the DA's office. "They [the doctors] are being made scapegoats by Massachusetts' politically potent anti-abortion forces," one unidentified doctor said.[55] The *New York Times* described how the "outraged medical community" believed that the indictments were "brought in response to heavy pressure from antiabortion forces, which are politically potent in heavily Roman Catholic Massachusetts."[56]

The publicity surrounding the case and the indictments themselves had quite tangible costs for the doctors themselves as well as for women seeking abortions at Boston City Hospital. In December 1973, responding to the public outcry following the O'Neil hearings, BCH had halted construction on their planned outpatient abortion clinic and banned all research involving fetal tissue. Following the indictments, the doctors were temporarily suspended "without prejudice" from BCH, whereupon Dr. Philipson returned to Sweden and Dr. Charles resigned and took a new position in Canada.[57] On March 10, 1974, the hospital went even further, temporarily suspending all nontherapeutic abortions.[58] Almost immediately, local chapters of the League of Women Voters, the Civil Liberties Union of Massachusetts, the National Organization for Women, Americans for Democratic Action, Pregnancy Counseling Service, Zero Population Growth, the Boston Women's Health Book Collective, and the Massachusetts Organization for the Repeal of Abortion Laws organized protests, calling the hospital's policy a violation of women's civil rights.[59] "We believe that women who rely on BCH for their gynecological care should be able to obtain safe, legal abortions on the same basis that they qualify for other medical services," said Lynn Salisbury of the League of Women Voters.[60] *Time* magazine noted the disparate impact of the decision: "This case has also worked a particular hardship on the poor.... Overworked BCH has been one of the few places in the city where those who could not afford to pay could end unwanted pregnancies. As a result of the indictments, the hospital has forbidden abortions except in medical and psychiatric emergencies."[61] Responding to these concerns, Commissioner White issued a statement recognizing that "BCH has a special responsibility to provide abortions to the community that City Hospital serves" and BCH Board of Trustees chairman Herbert Gleason assured the public that the board planned to "resume abortion services at the hospital as soon as possible."[62] Although the official ban was lifted in July, elective abortions at BCH were, for the most part, approved only in cases in which the life or health of the mother was at stake. In November 1974, *Science* magazine reported that "while the hospital used to do up to 30 elective abortions a week, since the trouble began there have been none."[63] Cheering their success, MCL reported that women seeking "abortion on demand" were being referred to private clinics, an option that they recognized was not feasible for the typical patient seeking an abortion at BCH.[64]

The Boston case prefigured what was developing into a national debate about fetal research, and just as the particularities of local politics shaped the BCH case, the complexities of national politics would shape the national debate. "Doctors everywhere are proceeding with caution," the *New York Times* commented. "The Boston indictments, legal action threatened elsewhere, and the anticipated Federal guidelines for human experimentation are said to have curtailed much fetal research already."[65] Fetal research had not been completely hidden from the public before the publicity surrounding the BCH indictments. It had been at the periphery of public attention since 1968, when following the first successful transplantation of fetal cells into patients with DiGeorge syndrome, Senator Walter Mondale (D-MN) initiated what he called a "national dialogue" on the ethics of medical research, particularly fetal research, organ transplantation, and genetic engineering.[66] On February 8, 1968, Mondale announced that his Subcommittee on Government Research would hold hearings to explore the possibility of establishing a President's Commission on Health Science and Society to oversee and advise the government on these new technologies.[67] Mondale's hearings quickly became polarized between those who feared that unregulated advances in biomedicine and technology would lead to the horrors of science fiction or Nazi Germany, and those who feared that public interference in biomedicine and technology would prevent future miracles like the discovery of penicillin and invention of the polio vaccine and enable more tragedies like the most recent thalidomide disaster. An exchange between Senator Abe Ribicoff (R-CT) and Dr. Arthur Kornberg, winner of the 1959 Nobel Prize for his work on the biochemistry of DNA illustrates that tension. Asked by Ribicoff whether he saw any possibility that in the wrong hands, his work could lead "to the creation of a master race," Kornberg replied that he "would like to be part of a 'master race' relieved of some of the scourges that have plagued people for centuries."[68]

These hearings represent an early example of a growing public discomfort with the unregulated power of scientists and physicians. A spate of troubling stories about unethical medical research using human subjects transformed that discomfort into active resistance. In the late 1960s and early 1970s, the public learned about the Tuskegee syphilis studies, in which African-Americans suffering from syphilis were studied but not treated; a study in which half of the study group of Mexican-American women in San Antonio were given placebos instead of contraceptives; a study in which doctors dispensed Depo-Provera and DES as contraceptives to their patients on welfare without informing them of potential side effects or obtaining informed consent; and a study in which children institutionalized at the Willowbrook State School for the Retarded were injected with live hepatitis viruses.[69] Each of these stories fed the general concerns about medical research using human subjects, and the more specific concerns about the ways in which these studies exploited particularly powerless populations. A Harris Poll revealed that between 1962 and 1972, public confidence in the medical establishment had dropped from 73 to 42 percent.[70] The emergent disability rights movement was also articulating their concern about the questionable ethical decisions made possible by new medical technologies, arguing that the increasing ability to diagnose disabilities prenatally would increase pressure to abort "imperfect" fetuses.[71] These fears were expressed in debates over whether and how the power of doctors and scientists to explore the frontiers of scientific knowledge should be regulated, and how to protect the rights of individuals participating in scientific research, debates at the heart of the discipline of bioethics.[72]

In the aftermath of World War II and in the light of new knowledge about scientific and medical experiments performed by Nazi physicians on concentration camp prisoners, the Nuremberg Code of 1949 established a set of ten basic principles for research conducted on human subjects, principles further refined in the World Medical Association's 1954 Declaration of Helsinki.[73] The United States endorsed both documents, but without mechanisms of enforcement, these principles remained abstract ideals more than concrete practices.[74] In the 1960s, theologians, philosophers, and scientists organized a series of conferences to discuss issues raised by doing research with human subjects, conferences that would lead to the establishment of bioethics institutes and think tanks, most notably the Hastings Center, established in 1969, and the Kennedy Institute, established in 1971.[75]

As stories of research improprieties and scandals mounted, the growing body of bioethics professionals—a new elite that emerged despite and because of the general trend against expertise—demanded a larger role in analyzing and regulating the ethical implications of scientific advances at the same time that the lay public demanded the right to participate more actively in decisions previously left to the professionals and experts. Hoping to avoid being dragged into a public, and inevitably political, debate, the NIH began in 1970 to develop internal guidelines regulating fetal research.[76] The NIH debate about these proposed guidelines remained out of the public eye until April 10, 1973, when the *Washington Post* reported that the NIH was planning to adopt a policy that "encouraged the use of newly delivered live fetuses for medical research before they died."[77] If delivered intact, the article reported with inflammatory language, "these tiny infants...may often live for an hour or so with beating heart after abortion...artificial aid—fresh blood and fresh oxygen—might keep them alive for three or four hours."[78] After reading about the proposed policy in the *Washington Post,* students from a local Catholic high school planned a protest march on the grounds of the NIH campus. NIH deputy director for science Robert Berliner called for an open meeting with the students, hoping to defuse their anger. In front of nearly two hundred students, Berliner insisted that "there are no circumstances at present or in the foreseeable future which would justify NIH support of research on live aborted human fetuses."[79] On April 14, 1973, days after the *Washington Post* first reported on the NIH debate in an article that had not clarified that it was a debate still in process rather than a final proposal about to be adopted, the NIH issued a statement that they "will not fund research on live aborted fetuses anywhere in the world."[80] In November 1973, the

Department of Health, Education, and Welfare incorporated the NIH recommendations into their regulations titled "Protection of Human Subjects: Policies and Procedures."[81]

Despite the NIH's best efforts to keep the decisions about fetal research in the hands of researchers, the lay public, pro-life activists, and bioethicists had forced the issue out of the private domain of hospital committees and research laboratories into the public arena. In Boston, those debates led to criminal charges; in Washington, they led to congressional hearings. In May 1973, in the wake of NIH controversy, just as the BCH case was about to erupt, and while the NIH and HEW continued their private deliberations, Congress held a series of debates about medical research, which quickly became a proxy for arguments about abortion. The House proposed a bill that included a provision "prohibiting federal funding of any research in the United States or abroad that would violate any ethical standards adopted by the NIH," but that language was not strong enough for Representative Angelo Roncallo (R-NY), who attached to the bill an amendment "prohibiting any research on a fetus with a beating heart."[82] Following a heated floor debate, the House passed the amended bill by a vote of 354–9 and sent it to the Senate, where the debate was also appropriated by pro-life forces. Senator James Buckley (Conservative Party-NY) rejected the idea that pregnant women had the right to consent to procedures done on an aborted fetus, and proposed permanently banning federal funding for any research using selectively aborted fetuses:

> Where the mother has already consented to the killing of her unborn offspring, it seems to me that she has abrogated any right that she might otherwise consent to any medical procedure on her child. These children should not become guinea pigs. Let them, I say, die in peace, unmolested by prying hands, electrodes, and chemicals of those who would play God in the laboratory.[83]

Hoping to get a bill passed before it turned into a referendum on *Roe,* Senator Ted Kennedy (D-MA) proposed amending the bill to include a moratorium on all fetal research until a commission established guidelines regulating fetal research.

On July 12, 1974, in one of his last acts as president, Richard Nixon signed into law the National Research Act, establishing the National Commission for the Protection of Human Subjects of Biomedical and Behavioral Research and imposing a temporary moratorium on all fetal research.[84] The three physicians, three lawyers, three ethicists, two biomedical researchers, and one public representative who comprised the commission were directed to "investigate and study research involving the living fetus, and to recommend whether and under what circumstances such research should be conducted or supported by the Department of Health, Education, and Welfare."[85] Their report titled *Fetal Research* outlined five ethical principles to which all fetal research must adhere: first, that research on animal models and nonpregnant humans must precede any research on the fetus; second, that the potential knowledge must be important and obtainable no other way; third, that the risks and benefits to mother and fetus must be explicitly acknowledged and explained; fourth, that the mother must give her informed consent; and fifth, that the research subjects must be selected so that "risks and benefits will not fall inequitably among economic, racial, ethnic, and social classes."[86] The report also held that research interests should never "determine recommendations by a physician regarding the advisability, timing, or method of abortion"; that "decisions made by a personal physician concerning the health care of a pregnant woman or fetus" should not be compromised for research purposes; that no "inducements, monetary or otherwise" should be "offered to procure an abortion for research purposes"; and that "no individual shall be required to perform or assist in the performance" of any part of fetal research if it was "contrary to his religious beliefs." Finally, the commission recommended an immediate end to the moratorium on fetal research established by Senator Kennedy's amendment.[87] Approved on July 29, 1975, these recommendations became the first federal regulations governing fetal research.[88]

While Dapper O'Neil was holding hearings on the goings-on at Boston City Hospital and the U.S. Congress was debating fetal research, the Suffolk County district attorney's office continued its investigations into Boston City Hospital, responding to the letter they received from O'Neil and to several anonymous phone calls claiming that there were "two big babies in bottles down at the Boston City Morgue."[89] When state medical examiner Dr. George T. Curtis investigated, he found two fetuses preserved in formaldehyde, both of which he estimated to be more than twenty weeks of gestational age. Massachusetts law required a birth and death certificate for any fetus born alive after twenty weeks, and when he determined that neither fetus had either certificate, Curtis declared them evidence of a possible crime. Believing that the *Roe* decision had left undecided the question of a doctor's responsibilities toward a still-living fetus following an abortion, Byrne and Flanagan seized upon the possibility that the fetus had been born alive and asked Curtis to conduct an autopsy on the larger of the two fetuses. Flanagan explains that they were particularly interested in "the biggest one.…I wondered if possibly that baby had been alive at the time it was taken from the mother and, if so, if there was some way that Dr. Curtis could tell that. If it were alive, then we had a whole different ball game."[90] The autopsy identified a "partial expansion of some of the alveoli [air cells of the lung]," evidence to Curtis that the fetus had "sucked amniotic fluid," "taken in room air through the uterine incision," or breathed "after delivery clear of the uterus."[91] Flanagan reacted immediately. "Now instead of just an abortion case," he said, "we were dealing with a case of murder or at least manslaughter, and there was only one honest thing to do—prosecute the person who had committed the crime.[92]

That person was Dr. Kenneth Edelin, who, in 1973, at the age of thirty-five, had been named the hospital's first African-American chief resident. For Edelin, the issues of women's reproductive health and racial justice were inextricably linked. The youngest of four children, Edelin had grown up in segregated Washington, D.C., went to high school at the progressive and integrated Stockbridge School in Great Barrington, Massachusetts, and graduated from Columbia University in 1961. He taught math and science at the Stockbridge School for two years before moving to Tennessee to attend Meharry Medical College, the only private black medical school in the country. After completing a one-year internship at the U.S. Air Force Hospital at Wright Patterson Air Force Base in Ohio and serving three years at a U.S. Air Force base in England, Edelin moved to Boston with his wife Ramona and two young children to begin his residency at BCH. In his memoir, *Broken Justice*, Edelin traced his commitment to women's health to watching his mother die of breast cancer when he was twelve and she was forty-six, describing how that experience made him "all the more determined to be a doctor—a woman's doctor—to save lives and perhaps spare some other woman's son the anguish I had to go through."[93] He also related the story of his girlfriend getting pregnant in 1962, and the difficulties they had in finding a physician who would perform the illegal abortion, their struggles to find $600 to pay for it, and his fears about the danger and criminality of what they were doing. He described how his experiences at Meharry and the clinics of Nashville further convinced him that he wanted to work at a public urban hospital. He also recounted having to explain to an African-American patient at BCH that when she had undergone a caesarean section in North Carolina, she had been sterilized without her consent. All of these experiences contributed to Edelin's commitment to urban medicine, women's health, and racial equality. As he explained to *Boston Phoenix* reporter Connie Paige, "I've gone through the whole argument of when life begins....I've seen too many women sick and sterile from hysterectomies and women who eventually die from abortions....The problem is, the women who die are poor women, and mainly black women."[94]

Although they had charged Edelin with "assaulting and beating a certain person, to wit, a male child...and by such assault and beating did kill said person," the DA's office was not arguing—and few would have believed—that

Edelin literally assaulted a baby, beating it to death.[95] There was, in fact, a general sense of confusion about what they were actually accusing Edelin of doing. This lack of clarity contributed to an unusual aspect of the subsequent trial, which was the fact that much of the testimony revolved around determining whether or not there was an actual victim and an actual crime, rather than on proving that the defendant was guilty. And just as there was little consensus about the nature of the crime, there was little agreement about the basic narrative of events that led up to the trial.

Sometime in April or May 1973, the seventeen-year-old daughter of West Indian immigrants, identified in court only as Alice Roe, became pregnant. Afraid of her strict father's reaction, she had concealed the pregnancy until September, when she was confronted by her mother, who accompanied her to BCH for an abortion.[96] Dr. Hugh Holtrap, the chief of the ob-gyn clinic at BCH, performed the initial physical exam on Alice Roe. Noting on her chart that, despite the fact that she gave a last menstrual date indicating that she was seventeen weeks pregnant, he estimated her to be closer to twenty-one weeks pregnant, Holtrap recommended a saline procedure that was the most common method for second-trimester abortions.[97] He called Edelin into the room, and Edelin examined the patient and agreed to perform the abortion. Alice Roe agreed to participate in a study Holtrap was conducting on aminoglutethamide, a protein intended to increase the hormone production of the placenta. She was told to come to the hospital a day before her scheduled abortion to undergo an intravenous infusion of the protein and a subsequent urine analysis.

Alice Roe was admitted to the hospital on September 30, 1973. The next morning, third-year Boston University medical student Alan Silberman took her medical history and performed another exam. Silberman had started his obstetrics rotation at BCH only three days earlier, and he noted "looks 24 weeks pregnant?" in the margins of the chart, as a reminder to ask someone more experienced to recalculate his estimate of the gestational age of the fetus.[98] Dr. Enrique Gimenez-Jimeno, a second-year resident who refused to perform abortions under the conscience clause, confirmed Silberman's estimate of twenty-four weeks.[99] Later that day, Dr. Holtrap came to begin Roe's aminoglutethamide infusion. Noting the discrepancy between her estimated last menstrual period, his estimate of gestational age, and Silberman's and Gimenez-Jimeno's estimate of gestational age, Holtrap conducted a fourth exam. Concluding that his estimate of twenty-one weeks was correct, he noted that again on her chart, and completed his study.[100]

The next day, October 2, 1973, Alice Roe was brought to the saline unit for her scheduled abortion. Dr. Edelin looked at the varying estimates of gestational age on her medical record, examined her yet again, and noted on her chart his estimate of gestational age to be twenty weeks. He began the saline infusion, but when several "bloody taps" indicated that the needle was not directly entering the amniotic sac, he concluded that the anterior placenta was connected to the front of the uterine wall, thus making it impossible to get a completely clean injection. He consulted with his supervisor, Dr. James F. Penza, and they agreed that if Penza was unable to do the saline procedure the next morning, Edelin would perform a hysterotomy, a procedure in which the uterus is opened through an abdominal incision and the fetus is removed.[101] Because it is major surgery requiring general anesthesia, a hysterotomy is used for abortions only when less invasive procedures have failed or are not advisable. After Penza made one last unsuccessful effort to perform the saline abortion, Edelin, assisted by fourth-year medical student Steve Teisch, went ahead with the surgical hysterotomy. After making his first incision, Edelin swept his fingers through the uterine cavity, carefully detaching the anterior placenta from the uterine wall. He then began peeling the amniotic sac away from the placenta, intending to extract the intact sac through the incision, but the sac ruptured while he was easing it through the incision. Edelin took hold of the lower extremity of the fetus to ease it through the incision, leaving it detached from the placenta and removed from the sac, but physically inside the uterine cavity.

Finding no heartbeat or other signs of life, Edelin removed the fetus from the uterine cavity, placed it in a stainless steel basin, and completed the surgical procedure on Alice Roe, who recovered without incident. According to usual practice, the fetus and the placenta were transferred to the pathology laboratory, where second-year resident pathologist Dr. Frank Juliano Fallico weighed the fetus, recorded its weight of 600 grams, placed it in a 10 percent solution of formaldehyde and, following regulations requiring pathology residents to notify their supervisors about fetuses older than twenty weeks gestational age, set it aside for his supervisor's inspection. Two days later, the fetus was transferred to the morgue, where it would stay for two months, until the state medical examiner Dr. George Curtis discovered it during his investigations that followed the council hearings on fetal research.

Every detail leading up to, including, and subsequent to the abortion procedure would come under intense scrutiny during the trial. It was not, however, entirely clear that there would be a trial, because it was still not entirely clear that there was a victim. On October 9, 1974, Edelin's lawyer, the noted civil libertarian and trial lawyer William Homans, submitted a motion for dismissal. He argued that Massachusetts law required that a fetus be born alive in order to be subject to the protection of criminal and civil law, and that because the autopsy showed "no evidence of respiration or of independent circulation outside the body of the mother," there was no legal victim subject to those protections.[102] Opposing dismissal, ADA Newman Flanagan insisted that the fetus was a "victim, a viable child... genotypically, actually, and legally a human being and had a right not to be killed. The defendant unlawfully caused the death of this human being and is now answerable to manslaughter."[103] Flanagan's language picked up on all the key words used to establish fetal personhood, Homan's motion to dismiss was rejected, and the trial was scheduled for January 6, 1975.

Homans made two key strategic decisions at the onset of the trial, both of which he would come to regret. The first decision was to ask for a jury trial. Edelin's case had been assigned to Judge James P. McGuire, a graduate of Catholic University and Boston University Law School. McGuire volunteered and contributed to the Catholic Charities Appeal and the United Way, attended church at St. Joseph's, and was a member of the Knights of Columbus.[104] Homans concluded that "there would be enormous pressure put on him [McGuire] by the Catholic community" and that a jury might be less susceptible to those pressures.[105]

The second decision was not to request a change of venue. The city was awaiting Judge Arthur Garrity's decision in the school segregation case, and tensions between the Irish-Catholic and African-American populations in general and in the South Boston and Roxbury communities in particular were extremely high. Aware of the ways in which the politics of busing had infused the O'Neil hearings and concerned that Edelin's case would become swept up in this drama, the defense commissioned jury consultant Irwin "Tubby" Harrison of Decision Research Corp. to determine whether or not Edelin should take his chances in Suffolk County or request a change of venue. Harrison's research indicated that Suffolk County was not likely to be significantly more biased against Edelin than any other in Massachusetts, and the defense decided not to request a change of venue. Instead, they planned to use their peremptory challenges to eliminate the jurors Harrison had identified as likely to be biased against Edelin—low-income Catholics older than fifty, who had attended parochial school and subscribed to the official newspaper of the Boston Archdiocese, the Pilot.[106] Edelin's defense team had not realized how difficult eliminating that type of juror would be.

In 1974, Boston, like many other cities, selected juries through a computer programmed to form panels with twice as many men as women. Citing childcare responsibilities, a disproportionate number of women requested and were granted exemptions from jury duty, making the jury pool even more imbalanced. The grand jury that had indicted Edelin, for example, had fourteen men and four women, and the jury pool for Edelin's criminal case had ninety-nine men and thirty-two women. The day the trial was supposed to begin, Homans submitted a motion to dismiss on the basis that the jury selection process discriminated on the basis of sex and constituted a violation of Edelin's right to be tried by a jury of his peers. Harrison, the jury consultant, testified that nearly 11 percent of Boston residents would automatically find a doctor guilty of manslaughter for performing an abortion in the second or third trimester of pregnancy, and that men were more likely than women to fall into that 11 percent. Flanagan argued that it would still be possible to get an unbiased group of sixteen jurors from the existing panel, and after conducting a *voir dire* of the jury pool, McGuire agreed and rejected Homans' motion to dismiss.[107] When the final jury of thirteen men and three women had been selected, the *Boston Globe* commented on the fact that "the members of the jury are Dr. Edelin's peers only in the legal sense. None is black, twelve are Catholic, none is a doctor."[108]

At its most basic level, the charge of manslaughter requires the prosecution to establish that a person had died, the very question raised by Homans in his pretrial motion to dismiss. Before the jury could even consider whether or not Edelin was guilty of manslaughter, which McGuire defined for them as "the unlawful killing of another without malice," they had to be persuaded that, according to McGuire's instructions that the word "person has applicability only post-natally," the aborted fetus was a legal person when it died.[109] The prosecution then had to convince the jury that at some point after being born alive, this person had died as a direct consequence of Edelin's actions. In contrast, the defense had to create reasonable doubt by convincing the jury that the fetus had died prenatally, that no legal person had been "born alive," and that Edelin had done nothing but perform a legally and medically sanctioned abortion. The jury would need to weigh the prosecution's claim that Edelin had smothered a baby against the defense's claim that the fetus had died *in utero,* either as a result of the failed saline infusions or as a result of Edelin's medically reasonable actions during the hysterotomy.

The trial quickly became a competition between these two narratives, each of which relied upon entirely different vocabularies. Was the alleged victim a fetus? A male child? A baby boy? Was the victim smothered, suffocated, murdered, as the prosecution claimed? Or did the fetus die *in utero* of anoxia and asphyxiation, as the defense claimed? McGuire had a pretrial meeting with the prosecution and defense to establish a list of words each could use in their opening and closing statements. The first problem was what to call the alleged victim of manslaughter:

Flanagan: "Baby boy" is the term that is actually used in the indictment. The jury is going to read the indictment. The Commonwealth will introduce evidence, or hopefully will do so, that the deceased is a baby boy. The medical examiner described it as a baby boy in his autopsy report and the Commonwealth will introduce evidence to that effect.

Homans: I would object to the use of any word except "fetus," your Honor.... Considering the baby boy as the earliest kind of male human being, I would suggest, your Honor, that there is no evidence, and that there will be no evidence that this fetus ever breathed, and that therefore it never became a human being, ergo, not a baby boy, and I would object to the use of those words.

McGuire ruled that Flanagan could not use the words "baby boy" but could use the words "human being" or "male human being" or "male child."[110] A similar exchange revolved around Homan's objections to allowing the words "suffocate," "smother," or "murder" to be used as synonyms for "anoxia" or "asphyxia" in describing the manner of death of the fetus. McGuire's ruling: "in view of counsel's [Flanagan] statement that he intends and expects to introduce evidence as to the generally accepted meaning of the word anoxia as including suffocation, I will allow him to use that word. I will not allow you to use the word 'smother' or 'murder.'"[111]

The struggle over language continued throughout the trial. An analysis of the transcript identifies at least forty terms used to describe the alleged victim during the trial: fetus, live fetus, black fetus, child, unborn child, male child, deceased male child, living child, newborn child, products of conception, result of pregnancy, subject, specimen, baby, baby boy, very immature baby, young one, the deceased, person, body, independent person, human being, independent human being, premature human being, offspring, unborn offspring, newly developed young one, embryo, infant, liveborn infant, infant male, victim, blob, big bunch of mucus, neonate, neonatal life, individual, member of the human race, survivor, loved one.[112] Other pairs of terms—viable versus alive, womb versus uterus, patient versus mother—were similarly defined, redefined, contested, and negotiated throughout the testimony and cross-examination of the witnesses.

Homans, who referred only to the "fetus" or "products of conception" in his opening statement, carefully alerted the jurors to the performative and politicized role of language in the trial:

I suggest to you that, as I said at the outset, that it is important that you keep your eye on the ball concerning the meaning of the words you hear.... We will show, we suggest, to your satisfaction, that although the indictment refers to the killing of a "baby boy," that in fact no "baby boy" ever existed and certainly no "baby boy" was ever killed. You heard in the indictment, and you heard my brother [Flanagan] refer to a person. We will demonstrate, we suggest, to your satisfaction, that no person ever existed and no person was ever killed.[113]

The testimony of the first witness for the prosecution, Dr. Mildred Jefferson, offers a particularly revealing example of this verbal contest.

The same Dr. Jefferson who had testified at Dapper O'Neil's hearings about fetal research was, in addition to being vice president of MCL, the first African-American woman to graduate from Harvard Medical School and a general surgeon on the staff of Boston University Medical Center.[114] Jefferson was not, however, an expert in obstetrics, embryology, or perinatology, and despite the fact that she had never performed an abortion and had not delivered a baby since 1951, the prosecution called her as an expert witness to testify on matters relating to those very specialties.[115] Under direct examination, Jefferson repeatedly referred to the "developing baby" and the "newly developing young one," until the judge finally upheld one of Homans' repeated objections. "Disregard at this time the use of the word baby," McGuire told the jury. "It has been substituted by the witness, I think inadvertently, for the word fetus. So you will consider the word fetus."[116] Newspaper coverage of the first day of the trial generally used Jefferson's language without including the judge's admonition, suggesting that Jefferson had succeeded in resetting the terms of the debate outside of the courtroom, if not inside it.

While the prosecution deployed evocative language to frame the case as a moral drama, the defense deployed medical expertise to expose it as a political witch hunt. Intent on contrasting the objectivity of his witnesses to the biases of the prosecution's, Homans' cross-examination of Jefferson emphasized the fact that her definition of a premature fetus delivered by hysterotomy as a "live birth" differed from standard medical and legal definitions, and was based upon her pro-life beliefs rather than any familiarity with the current literature and practice of obstetrics.

> Homans: During the time at which the fetus is within the uterus of the person you call the mother, it is unborn, is it not?
>
> Jefferson: Until it is delivered, it may be considered unborn.
>
> Homans: The fetus inside the body of the patient carrying the fetus is unborn, is it not?
>
> Jefferson: No, not in my personal opinion, if that is what you are asking for…my understanding, based on my own knowledge of physiology, apart from the observations made by obstetrical textbooks, is that once the placenta is completely separated, and the offspring is no longer attached to the mother, then, although it has not been removed from the mother's womb, it has been born.[117]
>
> Homans: May I ask you to assume, then, that the placenta had been detached, separated, that the fetus never breathed, that the fetus was inside

the uterus of the mother, or excuse me, of the patient who eventually becomes a mother. I ask you, then, considering the fact that the fetus never breathed, do you persist in your definition that this fetus was born?

Jefferson: I do.

Homans: Will you tell us the name of one textbook by a recognized medical authority that supports the definition you just gave?

Jefferson: I am referring to other sources.

Homans: What?

Jefferson: The handbook on pediatrics which carried the recommendations of the Committee on Internal Health and the Child, of the American Medical Association, which defined both "stillborn infant" and "live birth."

Homans: Nowhere in any of these textbooks is there any definition of "being born" as being the result of the condition which we have discussed— that is the separation of the placenta, the failure of the fetus to breathe, the remaining of the fetus inside the uterus, whether or not the uterus was open. Is that correct?

Jefferson: Not in that wording, but that qualifies for the definition of still-born infant.

Homans: Would you tell us whether the conditions to which you refer are defined as "born" or "stillborn"?

Jefferson: The conditions to which I referred, if there is no proof that there was no evidence of vital activity, would qualify as "stillborn."[118]

The prosecution followed up that line of inquiry on redirect examination:

Joseph Mulligan, ADA: Doctor, after the placenta is detached in the course of an operation, do you have an opinion as to whether or not at that time a member of the human race is born or not?

Jefferson: I do....My opinion is that, at that point, when to continue living it must depend on its own systems, it indeed is born.

Mulligan: What do you mean, Doctor, by "continue on its own systems"?

Jefferson: In order to get oxygen to continue living, it must breathe in and out either air or oxygen supplied by someone in a resuscitation effort.[119]

These exchanges highlight strategic differences between the prosecution, which was relying on the jury's empathy for the fetus as being a "member of the human race," and the defense, which was relying on the jury's ability to interpret and evaluate complicated medical definitions and procedures.

In creating a scenario requiring the prosecution to provide evidence of some sort of postnatal "vital activity" as proof that the fetus was born alive and had subsequently died as a result of Edelin's actions, the defense was hampered by its inability to provide counterevidence supporting their argument that the fetus had died *in utero*. Homans had planned to have Holtrap, the admitting physician who had originally examined Alice Roe, testify that the repeated "bloody taps" raised the significant possibility that the fetus had died the day before the procedure, but McGuire excluded Holtrap's testimony, finding that Holtrap could not offer "reasonable certainty" that the fetus sustained any damage from the attempted saline infusions.[120] Absent Holtrap's testimony, there was no proof that the fetus had died as a result of the saline because neither Edelin nor the attending physician Dr. Penza had attempted to take a fetal heartbeat before beginning the surgical hysterotomy. Despite the fact that the entire burden of proof was on the prosecution, the defense's inability to prove a time of death prior to the hysterotomy allowed the prosecution to suggest that the fetus, alive after the hysterotomy, had subsequently died because of Edelin's conduct.

The defense confronted a different problem when their witnesses unintentionally undermined their credibility by refusing to speak in colloquial language familiar to the jurors. In his direct examination of Penza, Flanagan showed how easy it was to skewer the scientific and legal precision of the defense as wordplay:

Flanagan: My question is whether or not the fetus was alive prior to the commencement of the hysterotomy. When I say alive, I mean alive in the mother's womb. Did you understand my question?

Penza: I don't understand your question unless you are going to define the word "alive."

Flanagan: I see. Well, when a particular fetus is in its mother's womb, and is attached to the umbilical cord, which is attached to the placenta, and there is a 140 fetal heartbeat, would you consider the fetus a live fetus in the mother's womb?

Penza: The fetus is viable in that circumstance.

Flanagan: Is it alive in the mother's womb?

Penza: We don't speak of fetuses as being alive or dead. They are either viable or not viable.

Flanagan: Doctor, assume if you would, that there is a fetus within the mother with a fetal heartbeat of 140, would you describe that the fetus in that particular case was viable at the time that examination was made?

Penza: Yes.

Flanagan: And, Doctor, I would ask you if you would look through that particular hospital record to determine whether or not there is anything in that hospital record that you can base on reasonable medical certainty that prior to the commencement of the hysterotomy that that fetus which you've described was viable if it had 140 fetal heartbeats became nonviable?

Penza: It would be very difficult to answer it with a yes or no answer.

Court: Can you answer it with reasonable medical certainty?

Penza: The answer would be no, then.[121]

And in trying to get Penza to define as precisely as possible the meaning of the word *viable,* Homan's cross-examination highlighted exactly the kind of legalistic parsing that Flanagan had just exposed:

Homans: You've earlier in your examination by Mr. Flanagan, Dr. Penza, used the word "viable" in response to my brother's use of the word "alive." With respect to a fetus inside the mother's uterus, at what point, adopting your use of the word "viable" in these circumstances—at what point does the fetus first show signs of viability?

Penza: The detectable viability by fetal heart sounds, with present-day techniques is as early as twelve weeks' gestation.

Homans: So that in a sense you have used the word "viable" it could be used as early as twelve weeks' gestation, is that correct?

Penza: It could be clinically perceived as early as twelve weeks, yes sir.

Homans: And you do not, as I understand it, use the word "viable" the way you've used it here in response to Mr. Flanagan's questions to connote to mean the ability of the fetus to survive for any period of time after removal from the uterus of the mother, do you?

Penza: No, I do not mean that.[122]

In emphasizing the difference between medical and colloquial uses of the term *viable,* Homans's point was that even if the fetus was viable at the time of the hysterotomy, that did not necessarily mean that it had been born alive, or that it could have survived.[123] But although technically accurate, this exchange between Homans and Penza skirted the question that most concerned the jurors.

The contradictory estimates of gestational age and competing opinions of expert witnesses further complicated the question of viability. The jury heard hours of testimony debating the definitions of life, embryo, fetus, viable birth, born, abortion, and death. Despite medical student Alan Silberman's repeated insistence that he had no experience and had noted his estimate only as a reminder to ask for help, Flanagan argued that gestational age could have been twenty-four weeks, as Silberman had first estimated. Homans argued that gestational age was more likely to have been twenty weeks, as the more experienced Holtrap had estimated.

The defense worked to highlight the pro-life politics of the prosecution's witnesses, all of whom readily admitted that they were members of organizations opposed to abortion or that they refused to perform abortions themselves. The defense also tried to emphasize the ways in which the opinions of the prosecution's doctors fell outside of the mainstream of the medical profession.[124] But rather than clarify the issue, these arguments seemed to convince the jury that doctors who were unable to define basic terms like *born* and *unborn* were not likely to be able to determine with any precision a fetus's gestational age or assess with any certainty whether or not a fetus was viable.

After making the case that the fetus was a legal person, the prosecution needed to convince the jury that the timing and location of Edelin's actions made this a case not of abortion but of manslaughter. Flanagan had told the jury in his opening statement that "Edelin remained motionless with his hand in the woman after he detached the placenta from the uterine wall, thereby cutting the fetus off from its oxygen supply" as part of his contention that but for the defendant's deliberate delay in removing the fetus from the uterus, the fetus would have lived outside its mother.[125] Flanagan called his only eyewitness, Dr. Gimenez-Jimeno, the resident who had examined Roe on September 30, and who was in the operating room when Edelin performed the hysterotomy, to the stand, to support that claim.[126] Edelin explains in his memoir that Gimenez-Jimeno had a long-standing grudge against him for personal and professional reasons—Edelin had dated Gimenez-Jimeno's ex-girlfriend, and Edelin had given Gimenez-Jimeno several negative job evaluations.[127] The jury, of course, did not know this when they listened to Gimenez-Jimeno's damaging testimony:

> Flanagan: And how long did it take, Doctor, to insert his hand, and detach the placenta?
> Gimenez-Jimeno: It didn't take more than one minute.
> Flanagan: All right. After that, Doctor, what did he do?
> Gimenez-Jimeno: He left his hand in the uterus and looked at the clock in the operating room.
> Flanagan: Could you see the hand itself?
> Gimenez-Jimeno: No.
> Flanagan: What, if anything, did you observe in connection with his hand?
> Gimenez-Jimeno: At the time he was looking at the clock, nothing.
> Flanagan: And where is the clock?
> Gimenez-Jimeno: It was on the operating room wall.
> Flanagan: All right. And how long did he look at the clock?
> Gimenez-Jimeno: At least three minutes.[128]

As the only witness to offer any incriminating testimony about Edelin's actions, Gimenez-Jimeno's testimony describing the three minutes during which Edelin may have caused the death of the fetus was crucial to the prosecution's case that Edelin had affirmatively caused the death of the fetus.

Testimony from Dr. George Curtis, the medical examiner for Suffolk County, was equally crucial in supporting the other key claim of prosecution's case, the claim that the fetus was born alive. Before Curtis testified, Homans and Flanagan met in McGuire's chambers to debate whether the prosecution would be allowed to introduce as evidence photographs of the fetus taken before the autopsy. At a time when fetal images were becoming increasingly familiar to the public, first through Lennart Nilsson's photographs and then through increasingly common use of sonograms beginning in the late 1960s, it was clear that the photographs would have an enormous impact.[129] Arguing that the photograph should be excluded, Homans claimed that having been stored in formalin for more than four months before the picture was taken, the fetus looked very different than it had when Edelin performed the abortion. The prejudicial value of the photograph, Homans argued, would be overwhelming:

> Obviously none of us is a physician other than the defendant and the various witnesses who have testified.... None of us is exposed on a day-to-day basis, or even for that matter, one day in our life to this kind of material. We do not have the background, nor does the jury have the background, to be able to assess what they see in these photographs in light of the rather narrow, rather complex issues in this case.[130]

McGuire disagreed, allowing the photograph to be used in court. He did, however, give the jury the following caveat before they saw the photograph:

> You must not view this in any way, in fairness to the defendant, from any emotional point of view. Your emotions are not to enter into this case in any way. Nor is this picture intended, nor could it be properly introduced for any inflammatory reasons. You are not to view it in that sense. You are to view it to determine whether it offers any assistance to you, that is whether it has any evidential value on the material in this case. That's the only purpose for which it this picture is intended.[131]

Journalist Diane White was covering the trial for the *Boston Globe*, and noted the reactions of the jurors as they passed the photo around. "Each of the 13 men and three women examined the photograph quickly and passed it on to the next juror. None looked at it for more than 10 seconds.... If the photograph affected them, their faces didn't betray their feelings."[132] Posttrial interviews with the jurors indicated that the photograph played a much larger role in their decision than White had detected.

The picture had little to do with Curtis's testimony, which would hinge on his claim that the fetus had breathed air into its lungs while it was still alive, and after the photograph had made its rounds, Flanagan began with the autopsy report. Flanagan asked Curtis to explain what he meant when he said that although most of the alveoli were collapsed, some were only partially collapsed and some were expanded:

Flanagan: What, if anything, does that indicate?
Curtis: Well, the expansion indicates that there was respiratory activity.
Flanagan: And respiratory activity is what, doctor?
Curtis: It means that there was inhalation and expiration of the lungs taking place.[133]

Dr. John Ward, a pathologist from Pittsburgh, corroborated Curtis's testimony. His reading of the microscopic analysis of lung tissue indicated to him that "the subject did breathe outside the uterus."[134] And with that, the prosecution rested its case.

Arguing that the prosecution had not met their burden of proof, Homans immediately filed for a directed verdict of not guilty: "The Commonwealth's proof shows, at most, that the defendant's conduct was conduct wholly protected by the decision of the Supreme Court of the United States in *Roe v. Wade*, 410 U.S. 113 (1973)…and the defendant is not shown by the Commonwealth's proof to have been responsible for the death of a person."[135] The Commonwealth rebutted those claims by returning to Gimenez-Jimeno's testimony: "Dr. Gimenez described the defendant as detaching the placenta in the mother's uterus and remaining motionless with his hand inside the uterus for at least three minutes. These actions caused the death of a viable infant either born or in the process of being born. The death was caused by anoxia and was manslaughter."[136] McGuire dismissed the motion for a directed verdict, and the defense began to put on their case.[137]

The first obligation of the defense was to challenge the most damaging attacks made by the prosecution, particularly Gimenez-Jimeno's claim that Edelin had deprived the live fetus of air for up to three minutes. Steve Teich, the medical student who had assisted Edelin in the operating room, was the first witness. Homans asked Teisch if he had observed Dr. Edelin standing still looking at a clock for three minutes or any other significant period. Teich's answer was an unambiguous "no." Two BCH nurses similarly challenged Gimenez-Jimeno's testimony. Ellyn Curtis, who had assisted during the abortion procedure, insisted that there was no clock in the operating room that day, that it had been removed to be repaired. "There was no clock on the wall in operating room 2 at that time," she said. "The clock was missing from the wall from the time of my employment in the operating room until this past June." Ruth Cox, the head nurse of the gynecology operating room, was not in the room at the time of the procedure, but confirmed that the clock had been missing from that room for most of the fall of 1973.[138]

The defense challenged interpretations as well as facts. Perinatal pathologist Kurt Benirschke was called to analyze the autopsy and to challenge the prosecution's claims that the fetus had breathed *ex utero*. Benirschke testified that the red blood vessels Curtis and Ward had interpreted as evidence of *ex utero* respiration were "not a result of the separation of the placenta," but were more likely evidence that the lungs had been immersed in amniotic fluid. "In other words, Doctor," Homans asked, "was the fetus alive *in utero* prior to the hysterotomy?" "No," said Benirschke. "It is my opinion that the fetus did not respire air after removal from the uterus."[139] Benirshke's testimony gave strong support to Homans's claim in his opening statement that "the fetus never drew a single breath outside the body of the mother."

Having undermined the prosecution's two central witnesses and two main arguments, the defense focused on convincing the jury that Edelin's actions were no more and no less than standard protocol in a legally protected medical procedure. Homans opened his direct examination of Dr. Jack Pritchard, the editor of the most respected and widely used obstetrics textbook, by asking if Pritchard had an opinion, based upon a reasonable medical certainty, as to whether the fetus was alive or dead at the time immediately after the performance of the last attempts at amniocentesis:[140]

Pritchard: Yes, sir.
Homans: What is that opinion?
Pritchard: That the fetus was dead.
Homans: What is the basis of your opinion, sir?
Pritchard: The presence of debris in the lungs that you describe, the presence of red cells that look to be old red cells, would indicate to me that there had been a hemorrhage previously as a consequence of the attempts at saline abortion.[141]

Homans knew that the prosecution needed to prove the existence of actual life rather than the capacity for future life, and his priority was to challenge any implication that postnatal respiration, indicating the actual existence of *ex utero* life, had taken place. But he also knew he had to address the issue of viability in order to persuade the jury that this was essentially a political trial about abortion dressed up as a legal trial about manslaughter. He called up a series of expert witnesses to make those arguments. Benirschke had testified that fetal lungs are not developed enough to sustain life outside the mother until the twenty-eighth week of gestation.[142] Pritchard estimated the gestational life of the fetus to be between "18 and a fraction weeks and no older than 24 weeks," and testified that the chances for survival of a fetus at twenty-four weeks were "essentially zero."[143] Dr. Arthur Hertig, who had worked with John Rock in the 1930s and 1940s and was now a professor emeritus of pathology at Harvard Medical School, made a similar argument that, even if it had not died a result of the saline infusions, a fetus between 600 and 693 grams would have almost certainly died almost immediately after delivery. "In my opinion," he said, "a fetus becomes viable around the 28th week of gestation when it should weigh 1000 grams."[144] Dr. Charles Hendricks, chairman of the department of obstetrics and gynecology at the University of North Carolina, went even further. Even in the unlikely event that the fetus was still alive after the hysterotomy, he testified, "since the decision had already been made to terminate the pregnancy, there was no need to determine whether the fetus was dead or alive."[145] These witnesses were central to the defense's claim that the prosecution was really trying Edelin for performing a legal abortion, a process intended to end a pregnancy, not to save a fetus.

The courtroom had, of course, been waiting to hear from Edelin, and Homans called him as the defense's final witness. Under direct examination, Edelin detailed his every move in the treatment of Alice Roe, beginning with the failed attempts at saline infusions and concluding with the hysterotomy. Edelin described his actions after making the first abdominal incision and the second uterine incision, when he began to separate the placenta from the uterine wall this way:

Edelin: It doesn't take extremely long to separate the placenta and the amniotic sac from the uterine wall, I would say maybe fifteen or twenty seconds. Then I attempted to ease the products of conception out of the incision, and I would say that the rupture of the amniotic sac occurred very shortly thereafter.
Homans: And what did you do when the amniotic sac ruptured?
Edelin: With my two fingers I attempted to grasp one of the lower extremities of the fetus to extract it from the uterus....I attempted to extract the fetus from the uterus. I had some difficulty and it was a difficult extraction.
Homans: Describe the difficulty you had.
Edelin: Well, the problem was that making the incision in the lower uterine segment, or the area of the lower portion of the uterus, a very thick muscle, that it doesn't give. And given the incision was small. That is because the portion of the uterus is small and narrow. It was difficult getting the fingers out of that incision.
Homans: And whether or not you eventually got the fetus out of the incision?
Edelin: Yes, sir....After the fetus was removed, I observed it and in the process of passing it from the operative field to a stainless steel basin, which my scrub tech was handing me, I also checked it for a heartbeat by touching the anterior chest wall.

Homans: Looking for a sign of life, is that correct sir?

Edelin: Yes, sir.

Homans: And what did you do after you had examined by touching the chest, sir?

Edelin: I placed the fetus in the stainless steel container that the operating room tech had handed me....I turned my attention back to the patient and I removed the rest of the placenta, took a sponge, wiped out the inside of the uterus to remove any remaining membranes, because the membranes had ruptured from the uterine cavity. Took an instrument, passed it down through the cervix from the inside to open up the cervix so it would have proper drainage and proceeded to repair the incision in the uterus.

Homans: Was there any time, sir, when you looked at the clock in the operating room while holding your finger or hand in the uterus for a pro-longed period of time, sir?

Edelin: Absolutely not.[146]

Edelin was the only witness who talked about the pregnant woman as the central patient in this entire event. Flanagan picked up Edelin's emphasis on his care for Alice Roe, and began his cross-examination by exploring how his commitment to her affected his care for the fetus:

Flanagan: Doctor, in an abortion, do you consider whether you owe any duty to the fetus?

Edelin: Not at the outset, no.

Flanagan: So that your only duty at the outset is concerning the mother?

Edelin: Yes, sir.

Flanagan: So that just prior to the commencement of your hysterotomy in this case you felt you had no duty to the fetus, is that correct?

Edelin: That's correct.

Flanagan: And you also felt that whether the fetus was alive or not was not important, is that correct?

Edelin: At the start of the hysterotomy?

Flanagan: Prior to the commencement of this specific hysterotomy?

Edelin: Yes, sir.

Flanagan: And therefore, Doctor, your only concern at that time was with the mother?

Edelin: Yes, sir.

Flanagan: And as a matter of fact you weren't sure if this particular subject was alive or dead at the commencement of the hysterotomy?

Edelin: That's correct.

Flanagan: And it would have made no difference to you?

Edelin: No, sir.

Flanagan: Well, let me ask you this, Doctor. Assume that the fetus was alive. Would you have a pediatrician there in the O.R. with you?

Edelin: No.

Flanagan: Why?

Edelin: Because this was an abortion.

Flanagan: So what does that mean to you, Doctor?

Edelin: This was an abortion being performed before viability, and I thought that would be, number one, contrary to the patient's wishes, and number two, contrary to good medical practice.[147]

This exchange makes clear the defense's point that this case was a referendum on abortion, not a referendum on Edelin's specific actions. The closing statements by each side illustrate this even more explicitly. Homans went first and began by laying the groundwork for his argument that the death of the fetus is implicit in abortion and that Edelin had followed standard medical procedure. "This case, whatever you may hear, whatever you have heard, is about the abortion process," he said. He reiterated the credibility of the expert testimony on behalf of Edelin, referred dismissively to the testimony of Gimenez-Jimeno, and emphasized the larger implications of this case:

> This is a case about facts. And this is a case about the judgments that physicians can make on the basis of the facts that are available to them.... The question is, can thousands of physicians, can your physician, embark on a medical procedure using his or her best judgment on the basis of the information that they have at hand and after consultation?[148]

Homans argued that for the jury to find Edelin guilty, they needed to find him guilty of gross misconduct:

> Unless you find that Dr. Edelin was some kind of ogre who was going out to terminate the existence of babies, to kill babies with some kind of malicious intention, instead of a physician performing a medical task, however pleasant or unpleasant it may seem to you, I suggest that you will find that Dr. Edelin acted in accordance with his best judgment and in accordance with the best of medical practice as he understood it.[149]

He concluded with a clear direction to the jurors:

> I ask you to go into the jury room and think about what the hard evidence is here. Don't speculate. Don't say to yourself, "well, it might have happened." I suggest to you that when you have done that, you will find that without question, this defendant engaged in a procedure which in his best judgment

as a physician was sanctioned, not only by medicine, but by the law, and that under the circumstances, under all the circumstances you have heard, that you will find him without question, "not guilty."[150]

In defending Edelin, Homans gave the jury the power to uphold the rights of the medical and legal professions and of the Supreme Court. Given the declining public confidence in doctors, and the even more precipitous decline in public confidence in lawyers and politicians that the recent Harris Poll had documented, as well as the increasing intensity of the pro-life movement and the particular demographics of this jury, it was a risky strategy.

In his closing statement, Flanagan gave the jury the power to protect the rights of the unborn citizens of Massachusetts. Urging the jurors to study the photograph of the fetus, he asked,

> Is this just a subject? Is this just a specimen? Look at the picture, who is it to anybody? What would you tell you it was? Use your common sense when you go to your jury deliberation room and humanize that. Are you speaking about a blob, a big bunch of mucus, or what are we talking about here? I respectfully submit that we're talking about an independent human being that the commonwealth of Massachusetts must protect as well as anybody in the courtroom, including the defendant.[151]

The fetus, said Flanagan, was no different than any other person, both under the law and under the microscope: "Do you remember the verbiage that was used in the autopsy as to what part of the anatomies that were examined? Ask yourself, 'is there any difference in the verbiage that is used or the parts of the anatomy that were examined in this subject, its heart and lungs, than there is in any other individual, whether it be you or your loved ones?"[152] This emphasis on the personhood, the individuality of the fetus, was central to Flanagan's argument that abortion was not about the right of physicians to practice medicine, or about recognizing women's right to control their bodies, but was about protecting "the right of an individual, one that's independent and on its own system, once it's separated from its mother, once it is no longer dependent upon his mother but upon society." His instructions to the jury reiterated that argument:

> Mr. Foreman and ladies and gentlemen of the jury, when you go into your jury deliberations and ask yourself in our society, although a woman has her rights and we have our rights, so does an independent human being, and in this case the baby boy, the male child, as indicated in this particular indictment—he has those rights once he is on his own and no one has the right to take it away from him.[153]

The next day, February 14, 1975, the jury received their instructions from McGuire before beginning their deliberations. The instructions emphasized the high burden of proof necessary for a conviction and seemed to support the defense's case. In order to render a guilty verdict, McGuire emphasized, they needed to find that the fetus had been born alive, not that the fetus might have lived had Edelin acted differently. McGuire reminded them that manslaughter was the death of a person, defined as an infant born alive and able to exist outside the uterus, caused by "wanton or reckless conduct," rather than merely "negligence or carelessness."[154] Shortly after one o'clock on Saturday afternoon, February 15, 1975, the jury returned to the courtroom and the foreman Vincent B. Shea announced the verdict: guilty.[155]

The verdict produced shock waves that rippled through Boston and the nation. Edelin issued the following statement:

> I have done nothing that is illegal, immoral, or bad medical practice. Everything I did was in accordance with the law and with good medical practice. . . . People have tried to make me into a hero and a martyr, but I think the real heroes and martyrs are the women who before January 22, 1973 had to put their lives on the line. I hope this verdict won't throw us back so they'll have to put their lives on the line again.[156]

Homans echoed these concerns. Asked how he thought the decision might affect women seeking abortions in Massachusetts, he replied, "I think the answer to that question is obvious." He went on to say that the verdict "was a decision about abortion, not manslaughter. It is a decision responsive to and reflective of a certain part of the community and not responsive to or reflective of the legal burden of proof and medical standards of care."[157] Boston City Hospital issued a statement of support of Edelin, calling him "an outstanding physician whose professional performance has been and continues to be at the highest level. . . . We strongly reaffirm his continuing staff appointment."[158]

Mainstream media immediately attacked the conviction. The *Boston Globe* described Edelin as "a victim of judicial inadequacy that no society should tolerate."[159] The *Washington Post* editorialized that the Edelin conviction brought "disgrace and shame" to the State of Massachusetts and the entire judicial system. Criticizing the judge for allowing the case to go to the jury and attacking the ways in which the "prosecutors used the process of the law to harass those whose views they would not tolerate," the editorial predicted that the impact of the decision "on the practice of medicine and on medical research in Boston, and elsewhere is likely to be enormous."[160] The *New York Times* called the decision "unbelievable," opining that "it will now become more difficult than ever for women to obtain abortions when they are in the second trimester after conception."[161]

Many in the local and national medical communities echoed Edelin's fears that the conviction would inspire the legislature to impose even more restrictions on second-trimester abortions and would scare hospitals and doctors away from offering abortions. The medical house officers of New England Deaconess Hospital issued this statement: "It is distressing that a physician of exemplary character in performing his legal function (as defined by the Supreme Court and his peers) should be made the victim of an ideological warfare between religious groups and aspiring politicians."[162] Dr. Louis Burke, head of the obstetrics and gynecology department at Beth Israel Hospital, declared the decision "a travesty of justice. This man was working in the context of the Supreme Court guidelines."[163] Obstetrician Frederick Ostermann expressed more personal concerns: "It gives me Kafkaesque nightmares to think it could happen, to think I might convicted of a crime when I think I'm doing my best to help people."[164] The American College of Obstetricians and Gynecologists issued a statement reaffirming their support for "unhindered access by women to abortion services.... It is the hope of the college that the Edelin decision does not conflict with this concept." The ACOG also warned that the profession "must guard against local jurisdictions or vocal minorities imposing their ethical positions for medical care on family planning and abortion on patients or doctors who do not hold those positions."[165]

Advocates for women's rights expressed similar concerns. Planned Parenthood worried that the decision will "make doctors fearful of performing second trimester abortions," and that it could "drive women back to dangerous illegal abortions." The National Abortion Rights Action League (NARAL) worried that "women most affected were going to be women with no financial means or alternative options."[166] There was a strong feminist community in Boston in the 1970s, and groups including the National Black Feminist Organization, which had been raising money for Edelin's defense fund, and the Boston-based Combahee River Collective, a black feminist group that had been attending the trial in support of him, organized a crowd of approximately 1,500 women on the State House steps to protest the verdict.[167] Combahee worked on issues including sterilization abuse, reproductive rights, employment discrimination, domestic violence, and prison reform—and the Edelin case, which involved the intersection between race, sex, and class, captured their attention.[168] The Edelin case also provided an opportunity for disparate feminist groups to come together. At the 1975 Conference on Women and Health, held in Boston, from April 4 to 7, sponsored by a wide range of feminist organizations, the keynote address highlighted the significance of the Edelin decision. Dr. Dorothy Brown, in a talked titled "History of Abortion Laws in the United States," called for a national mandate to set aside the verdict in the Edelin case, which is a *national disgrace* that was apparently used deliberately by the National Right to Life Organization as a landmark decision to kick off their national campaign to repeal the Supreme Court decision of 1973. The tragic import of the Edelin decision taken to the ultimate interpretation means that *any* physician doing an abortion is within his or her legal right to *do* the abortion but can be held guilty of manslaughter if every measure to preserve the life of the developing fetus has not been exhausted from the day of conception to zygote to developing fetus to the date of separation by birth.[169]

Another group concerned about the implications of the Edelin decision was the Boston medical research community, still anxiously awaiting the grave-robbing trial scheduled for June. The National Commission for the Protection of Human Subjects of Biomedical and Behavioral Research, putting together their recommendations and report on fetal research, acknowledged that the conviction was an example of the public's resistance to accepting medical authority as the last word on controversial issues.[170] Dr. Frank Falker of the Samuel S. Fels Research Institute cited the Edelin decision in a letter decrying what he saw as a dangerous trend: "Lay groups of citizens are starting to be required to make decisions...without understanding the key issues involved....Unless the public comes to learn about, understand, and trust the biomedical profession, controversies over abortion will continue to push downhill the course of progress in medical research."[171] Dr. Kenneth Ryan, chair of the National Commission, compared the Edelin case to the 1925 Scopes Trial, explaining that Edelin and Scopes were both found guilty on the basis of emotion rather than evidence; both trials were about the clash between religion and science. Perhaps, Ryan said, like the uproar over the Scopes trial, "the uproar over the Edelin verdict will help eventually to bring a reasonable accommodation among those who back abortion and those who oppose it."[172]

In contrast to the variety of groups disturbed by the decision, pro-life activists were elated, seeing this decision as their first successful effort in their struggle to reverse *Roe v. Wade.* Between June 1973 when Senator James Buckley (I-NY) introduced a bill calling for a "Human Life Amendment" and September of 1974, eighteen bills sponsoring constitutional amendments had been introduced into Congress. In 1974, subcommittees of the House and Senate Judiciary Committees began to conduct hearings on all proposed amendments, but none had passed by February 1975, and the Edelin conviction offered the movement its first real victory.[173] "This verdict starts America back on the road to respect for the dignity of human life," said Nellie J. Gray, for the Washington, D.C. Right to Life Committee.[174] Rabbi Samuel Fox, a member of MCL, said that "the fact that he

[Edelin] was convicted, even if he later wins an appeal, indicates a moral consciousness of humanity that the Supreme Court cannot legislate away."[175] Kenneth VanDerHoef, president of the National Right to Life Committee, praised the decision as showing the "sensitivity that people have, that they will not tolerate the taking of life." Dr. William Lynch, a Boston obstetrician and founder of the National Commission for Human Life, criticized the reaction of doctors as evidence that "the only thing that will deter them from abortions is not the threat to human life, but the threat of a malpractice suit."[176] A member of the Illinois Right to Life Committee was encouraged by the decision, saying that "a year ago, I would have said that we didn't have a chance [to overturn *Roe*] but today I think we're making progress."[177]

Pro-life activists' enthusiasm for the conviction was slightly undermined when Judge McGuire sentenced Edelin. Edelin's conviction carried with it a maximum sentence of twenty years, but on February 18, 1975, McGuire sentenced him to one year of probation and stayed the execution of sentence until the determination of the anticipated appeal.[178] Jay W. Bowman of the Georgia Right to Life Committee was attending a pro-life rally when he was informed of the Edelin sentence. He took to the podium to tell the crowd, who, according to *Newsweek*, "gasped."[179] Most physicians and medical organizations interpreted the sentence as a vindication of Edelin and an indictment of the jury. The medical staff of BCH praised the sentence and affirmed their belief that Edelin should immediately return to work. "We consider it imperative," they said, "to allow Dr. Edelin to continue his dedication and service."[180] Dr. Ernest W. Lowe, BCH chair of obstetrics and gynecology stated, "There's nothing to prevent him from returning today." Edelin returned to work the day after his sentencing, greeted by "cheering staff members, a 'Welcome Home Dr. Edelin' banner, and the prospect of delivering a baby."[181]

Homans submitted a motion asking McGuire to set aside the conviction or order a new trial. He cited the 1944 Supreme Court decision in *Commonwealth v. Gricus*, which found that a judge had "a right and duty to set aside a verdict when in his judgment it is so greatly against the weight of the evidence as to induce in his mind the strong belief that it was not due to a careful consideration of the evidence, but that it was the product of bias, misapprehension, or prejudice."[182] McGuire dismissed the motion, whereupon Homans appealed to the Supreme Judicial Court of Massachusetts. On December 17, 1976, in a unanimous ruling, that court overturned Edelin's conviction.[183] This ruling supported the argument made by legal and medical professionals, feminist and civil rights activists, and the mainstream media that the case against Edelin should never have made it to the courtroom and, once it had, should have resulted in an easy acquittal.

How, then, to explain Flanagan's commitment to the case, and the jury's unanimous conviction? The fact that Flanagan announced his candidacy for district attorney the day after the conviction suggests that he may have been politically motivated, or at least that his personal beliefs happily coincided with his political goals. But the jury was not motivated by such transparent political ambition. Why, then, did they see this case so differently from much of the public and from the Supreme Judicial Court of Massachusetts?

Jurors were unusually vocal in discussing how they reached their verdict, and the reason most frequently cited in explaining their decision was the visual impact of seeing the fetus. The controversial photograph went a long way toward convincing the jury that, despite the lack of legal precedent and despite the lack of medical evidence of wrongdoing, the fetus was a person who had been killed. Anthony Alessi of Roxbury, father of three and a foreman for New England Telephone Company, placed significant weight on the inflammatory picture. "We passed all the evidence around the table and everyone looked at each piece, but we paid a lot of attention to that picture," he said. "None of us had ever seen a fetus before. For all we knew, a fetus looked like a kidney. The picture was obviously of a well-formed baby, over 13 inches long."[184] Other jurors concurred, telling Diane White that "the picture of the dead fetus had disturbed them deeply."[185] Paul Holland, a Boston Edison customer service representative and father of four from Dorchester, emphasized the impact of the photograph as well. "Everyone had to decide whether or not they believed that the fetus was a person because it couldn't be manslaughter unless the fetus was a person," he said. "I personally don't believe it's a person from conception but maybe the picture helped people make up their minds that the fetus was a person."[186] Liberty Ann Conlin, a self-described homemaker from West Roxbury and mother of two, told reporters that she had been disturbed by the picture. "It looked like a baby," she said. "I'm not speaking for the rest of the jurors, but it definitely had an effect on me."[187] An unidentified woman interviewed in the *Globe* derided the decision, saying, "It is probably the first time in courtroom history that a defendant was found guilty because his alleged victim looked like a person!"[188]

The emphasis on the photograph supports Homans's claim that abortion, not Edelin, was on trial. Because there was no question of the legality of the abortion procedure, the jurors had to be convinced beyond a reasonable doubt that Dr. Edelin had been guilty of "wanton or reckless conduct" at some point after the abortion. It is hard to imagine how a photograph of a preserved fetus could be evidence of this kind of conduct, but Alessi explained that the jury had reached a guilty verdict based on a standard of negligence lower than the definition given by the judge. "We felt the doctor didn't give the baby enough of an opportunity," Alessi said. "He [Edelin] said he placed his hand on the baby's chest for three to five seconds. We didn't weigh this as a real attempt to see if the baby was alive."[189] Francis E. McLaughlin echoed those sentiments. "I don't think he [Edelin] did his job once it [the fetus] was removed," he said.[190] Conlin was one of the last jurors to vote to convict and had ultimately been convinced, she said, by this argument that Edelin was guilty of not acting to save the fetus, rather than of acting to kill the fetus, as Gimenez-Jimeno had testified.[191] "We thought the fetus was alive when he [Edelin] went in [the uterus] and he neglected to do his duty to save life," Conlin said. "We all thought that was negligence."[192] These two reasons—the photograph and the belief that Edelin had been guilty of negligence by not proactively trying to save the fetus—would be at the heart of the appeal's claim that the photograph should have been excluded as evidence and that the finding of negligence did not meet the standard of "wanton and reckless conduct" demanded by the indictment.[193]

Another less explicitly acknowledged reason for the conviction reflected the dynamics of the deliberation process itself. After the closing statements, four of the sixteen original jurors were chosen to be alternates and were not part of the deliberation process. As it turned out, three out those four later told a reporter they were convinced of Edelin's innocence.[194] In a straw poll taken before beginning deliberations, four jurors voted "not guilty." One by one, they changed their minds. John Kelley was the last to switch his vote. "It's very difficult to feel confident when eleven other people feel the other way," he said. "I will never be sure I made the right decision."[195] Also persuaded to change her vote, Conlin expressed similar reservations. After the sentence was passed, she told a reporter that she was pleased that it was a light one. "I wish Edelin could be exonerated completely," she said. "I wish I'd had the strength to stick to my not guilty vote. I regret my guilty vote but I was sick and tired and couldn't fight."[196]

Inside the courtroom, the jurors were asked to evaluate contested definitions of medical terms, incompatible sets of facts, and competing versions of events. They were asked to do this while ignoring what was going on outside of the courtroom, in the cities of Boston and Washington, D.C., and in their own lives. And although both prosecution and defense assiduously avoided alluding to race or religion during the trial, these issues immediately moved to the center of controversy after the conviction. Kenneth Edelin was black, Alice Roe was black, and the alleged victim was black; all twelve deliberating jurors were white, ten were Catholic, ten were men, none had graduated from college; Homans was the Harvard-educated scion of an elite Boston Yankee family; Flanagan was an Irish-Catholic father of seven who had worked his way through Boston College Law School as a longshoreman. Did any of this matter?

The prosecution and the jurors rejected any implication that race factored into their decisions to prosecute or convict. Flanagan even denied knowing that

Edelin was black. "I was shocked when I learned, long after I'd first seen him, that he was black," Newman Flanagan said, referring to the fact that Edelin was extremely light-skinned. "I don't remember exactly how I found out—I think it was from a newspaper story—but I do remember going to Garrett [Byrne] and saying, 'Damn it, Garrett, Edelin is black.' He wasn't any happier than I was. We knew that, with the busing issue so hot here in Boston, we'd run into cries of 'racism' before the trial was over."[197] Jurors Alessi and Conlin similarly dismissed the notion that race played any role in their deliberations. "Tell me this," Alessi said. "If we were such racists and saw that it was a black baby, what the hell would we have cared?" Conlin agreed. "I don't know anyone on the jury who was influenced by color or religion," she said. "I can't remember either subject coming up even once."[198] Alternate juror Michael Ciano was not in the deliberation room, but when he was interviewed after the verdict, he charged that at least two jurors had repeatedly referred to Edelin with racial slurs. He quoted one juror as saying, "That black nigger is as guilty as sin."[199] When he was told about Ciano's comment, Homans responded, "I was defending a black man who was defending a black woman's right to an abortion. In this city. You decide if race was a factor."[200]

Edelin himself referred to the trial as a "witch hunt" and called the motives of the jury and the city of Boston into question. "I don't think this jury was fair," he said. "I don't think it would have been possible to get a fair trial in Suffolk County no matter how many challenges we had."[201] Edelin's ex-wife, Ramona Hoage Edelin, chair of the African-American studies department at Northeastern University, agreed. After attacking the jurors for relying on Catholic doctrine rather than legal authority to reach their decision, she went on to highlight the hypocrisy of their verdict. "What, realistically," she asked, "do they care about a black fetus? These same people are spitting and throwing rocks at black children going to school on a bus. What they perceive now as a right to life would in six years be a right to be called names."[202] Thomas Atkins, former Boston city councilman, president of the Boston chapter of the NAACP, and leader of the pro-busing movement, condemned the Edelin verdict as "insupportable by the evidence and tainted by impermissible racial or religious motivation."[203] Atkins saw the Edelin conviction and busing riots as "proof positive that ours has become a state in which racists feel comfortable."[204]

But if the African-American community in Boston felt victimized by the verdict, the Irish-Catholic community in Boston felt victimized by these reactions. MCL issued a statement in which they said although they had "scrupulously refrained from commenting on the manslaughter trial" they could not be silent in the face of "efforts to discredit the character of the jurors." They dismissed the accusations of racism, saying they "cannot be taken very seriously when made only after the issuance of an unfavorable verdict."[205] Some charged that these reactions to the verdict illustrated a kind of reverse discrimination. When Charles J. Dunn, who had been a consultant to Flanagan throughout the trial, lost his job as legal counsel to the Massachusetts Association of Hospitals, his lawyers described the situation as "part and parcel of the whole recent effort to color judicial proceedings with overtones of racial and religious bigotry directed particularly at Catholics and persons of Irish-Catholic descent."[206] The *Pilot*, the official paper of the Boston Archdiocese, published an editorial saying much the same thing. While deploring the role "any racial prejudice...might have played in the trial," the editorial expressed concern about the "shoddy, lightly-veiled anti-Catholic slurs that came from the defense spokesmen during and after the trial."[207] William Buckley, conservative commentator and founder of the *National Review*, put it this way:

> One must ask, why Edelin? On the face of it, he is a dubious hero for the Champions of permissive abortion. He killed a well-formed child, whether with technical legality being a secondary point. Prudence would seem to recommend that the pro-abortionists keep a discreet distance from such a case, and take refuge in the usual banalities about the "complexities" and "sensitivity" of the issue. But Edelin, like his client and his victim, is a Negro. The case can be presented as the lynching of a black Marcus Welby by a bigoted community.[208]

The best way to make sense of these contradictory interpretations of the racial and religious overtones of the Edelin trial may be to accept them at face value, to acknowledge that historical truth resides in their simultaneity and coexistence, rather than in any false reconciliation of them. In deciding the *Roe* case, the Supreme Court explained the complexities that inform people's beliefs about abortion:

> One's philosophy, one's experiences, one's exposure to the raw edges of human existence, one's religious training, one's attitudes toward life and family and their values, and the moral standards one establishes and seeks to observe, are all likely to influence and to color one's thinking and conclusions about abortion. In addition, population growth, pollution, poverty, and racial overtones tend to complicate and not to simplify the problem.[209]

The particular dynamics of Boston perfectly capture this complex of factors shaping the process by which people come to a position about abortion. The trial was held in the context of people's actual lives, lives in which race, religion, ethnicity, neighborhood, class, gender, and countless other identities and experiences are always at play. It is not necessary to identify racism as the smoking gun behind the prosecution and conviction of Edelin, or to point to anti-Catholicism as the smoking gun behind the attacks on the verdict and the jury, in order to believe that no one involved in the BCH cases could have been unaffected by the political climate of Boston in 1974 and 1975.

As Ramona Hoage Edelin and Thomas Atkins suggested, that climate was charged by the busing controversy. In June 1974 Judge W. Arthur Garrity issued his decision mandating that the Boston School Committee remedy the racial imbalance of the public schools through busing.[210] The first phase of the plan required busing children between Roxbury and South Boston, and the 1974–1975 school year at South Boston High School was full of stone throwing, name calling, white flight, nonattendance, and riots. Hoping to avoid riots following a stabbing incident, SBHS closed early for Christmas vacation, on December 11, reopening on January 8, 1975, two days into jury selection for the Edelin trial. That trial would take place—geographically, chronologically, and politically—at the center of the busing crisis.

As Homans and Flanagan were delivering their closing statements and as members of the jury were deliberating and delivering their verdict, more than two thousand students from all over the country were meeting at Boston University for the founding of the National Student Conference Against Racism (NSCAR). The weekend was full of workshops and panels about race relations in Boston, most of which focused on affirmative action, busing, bilingual education, and community control. On Friday, February 14, the panel about racially motivated political "frame-ups" included a discussion of the Edelin trial. One speaker listed the multiple connections between the antiabortion and antibusing movements: Raymond Flynn, South Boston's state representative and leader of the antibusing movement, was the person who notified "Dapper" O'Neil about the goings-on at BCH; O'Neil's council window was festooned with ROAR (Restore Our Alienated Rights) and MCL (Massachusetts Citizens for Life) posters; D.A. Gabriel Byrne had only narrowly beaten ROAR leader Louise Day Hicks in his last election, and ADA Newman Flanagan was planning to run against Byrne; and Patrick McDonough, city council president, had a brother on the Boston School Committee and a sister who was a member of MCL.[211] When the verdict came down the next day, the students were shocked. Jon Hill, a member of NSCAR and reporter for the *Militant*, described their reaction:

> The news traveled through the conference like electricity. A hung jury was the least that many activists felt was in store. For the women at the gathering, the verdict was doubly stunning. Here they were, mapping out a campaign to defeat the anti-Black bigots, and Edelin had been railroaded by anti-busing

officials who had no love for women's liberation.... The connection between the foes of Black rights *and* women's rights was clear. That Edelin was a target of a mentality spurred by the segregationist campaign was unmistakable.... Code words like "forced busing" and "neighborhood schools" were being used to mask racism, just as the bogus concept of "the right to life" was a cover for denying women their democratic rights.[212]

Like the women of NSCAR, the women of ROAR had also recognized the link between busing and abortion, albeit from a different perspective. In January 1975, they announced that they would be sending representatives to Boston women's groups' meetings to "press the issue of forced busing as a woman's issue."[213] Hicks, who had been one of the first members of NOW and a supporter of the ERA, had also always opposed legalized abortion. In 1975, in addition to leading ROAR, Hicks was also the sponsor of a Massachusetts resolution urging the state supreme court to declare abortion on demand unconstitutional. For her, her opposition to busing and abortion reflected her Irish-Catholic identity, her status as a mother, and her definition of feminism, which stood in stark contrast to mainstream second-wave feminism or the more radical visions of women's liberation.

On April 10, three hundred supporters of the Equal Rights Amendment were at Faneuil Hall, attending a rally sponsored by the Governor's Commission on the Status of Women. ROAR members showed up at the event, wearing their antibusing buttons and shirts, and holding signs proclaiming "Abortion Is Murder," and placards with pictures of aborted fetuses, including the one that was shown to the Edelin jurors.[214] For Hicks, a supporter of the ERA and opponent of abortion, these competing rallies must have highlighted the ways that feminism was becoming a movement that increasingly excluded women like her. And on May 3, when hundreds of women rallied on the Massachusetts State House steps in a show of their support for Edelin, ROAR was there. The signs that each side carried with them capture the conflict. The women for Edelin carried signs declaring "Defend Dr. Edelin, defend abortion rights," and the women of ROAR carried signs declaring "Protect the Unborn Children of Boston."[215] Both groups of women were carrying signs proclaiming "Protect Our Right to Choose." The Edelin supporters wanted the right to choose whether or not to have an abortion; the ROAR activists wanted the right to choose where to send their children to school. Their use of the rhetoric of choice captures ROAR's strategic acumen in recognizing that the pro-choice rhetoric was resonating with America, and exploiting it. The fact that such competing beliefs invoked that rhetoric captures the ambivalence about rights that continues to muddy the political left and right.

Covering the Edelin trial for the *Boston Phoenix*, Connie Paige noted that from early in 1973, the "right-to-lifers in Boston had begun establishing ties with the city's primary anti-busing organizations."[216] She explains their effort this way: "The Irish-Catholic community of Boston was growing increasingly insecure as newcomers were encroaching on their see....With their hegemony slipping, some of the Irish started to shore up their ethnic pride by opposing busing. Others chose abortion as their target."[217] According to Paige, the antibusing and antiabortion movements both emerged, at least in part, out of a new kind of populist politics based on Irish-Catholic efforts to maintain their political and cultural dominance in a city that was growing increasingly diverse. William Safire, who after working as President Nixon's speechwriter had recently become a columnist for the *New York Times,* was similarly struck by the connections between the busing and pro-life movements. "A political connection also exists between abortion and busing," he acknowledged. "A challenge to the local District Attorney was mounted late last year by one of the fiercest anti-busing school board members and the D.A.—who draws his primary support from the same constituency—needed an issue of his own to shore up his strength."[218] But although political interests were certainly part of the explanation, Safire concluded that the "most pervasive connection between the two issues is the resistance of most people at the local level to rapid social change demanded at the national level."[219]

The local response to the two BCH cases portended the political future in which working-class white ethnics, particularly Catholics, would leave the Democratic Party despite their historic commitment to the liberalism of the New Deal and the Great Society. As part of the Democratic Party's stronghold in Massachusetts, Charlestown and South Boston were proud of producing "Honey Fitz" Fitzgerald, James Michael Curley, Jack Kennedy, Thomas P. "Tip" O'Neill, and Joe Moakley. Democratic politicians had a hard time imagining this tradition changing. Asked if he was concerned about his constituents leaving him because of his support for busing and abortion, Moakley dismissed the question with his famous quote that "as soon as we're born, we're baptized into the Catholic Church, we're sworn into the Democratic Party, and we're given union cards."[220]

In the 1976 Massachusetts presidential primary, Democrat George Wallace put that dictum to the test, pushing his pro-life and antibusing positions in a state he had written off in the past but now felt he could win. He came in third place in the Democratic primary, but carried Charlestown and South Boston, white ethnic enclaves where unemployment was close to 15 percent, and where working people resented the fact that their taxes were paying for social programs like Medicaid, AFDC, and food stamps that were going disproportionately to the growing number of welfare recipients in Roxbury and the South End.[221] Comments like one from a blue-collar worker in South Boston, who complained that he was "working his ass off and I'm supposed to bleed for a bunch of people on relief?" indicate the increasing fracturing of the Democratic Party's coalition of immigrants and white ethnic workers, and blacks.[222]

When Jimmy Carter won the 1976 Democratic nomination, he knew that he had to work hard to regain the votes Wallace had taken from him in the primary without losing the other wing of his support: the educated, middle-class liberals. He did it by straddling the issues that had worked for Wallace. Although opposing the four versions of the Human Life Amendment proposed between 1973 and 1976, each of which would have had the effect of overturning *Roe v. Wade*, Carter repeatedly told crowds that he was "personally opposed to abortion, and personally opposed to government spending for abortion services." On the busing issue, he had this to say: "I'm not in favor of mandatory busing, also I do not favor a constitutional amendment to prohibit busing."[223] This strategy worked in 1976, but it was a short-lived victory. In 1980, with the support of "Reagan Democrats," Reagan carried both Charlestown and South Boston, winning a landslide victory based on the electoral shift that began with the busing and abortion controversies.[224]

In contrast to this slow and incremental political realignment was the more immediate legacy of the Edelin trial—the accumulating restrictions limiting availability of and access to abortions. A few days after Edelin's conviction, the Long Island Coalition for Life notified the Nassau County district attorney that a fetus aborted at the Nassau Medical Center had been denied life support and was thus a victim of infanticide. The D.A. had no plans to pursue the case, but nonetheless the Nassau County Medical Center announced that they would no longer provide abortions after the twelfth week of pregnancy except to save the mother's life.[225] Hospitals in Nashville, Los Angeles, Hartford, Detroit, and Pittsburgh imposed similar bans against performing abortions after anywhere between twelve and sixteen weeks. These policies would be felt most acutely by women who were not able to travel far, or who were unable to pay for the higher priced abortions in hospitals that charged more in order to pay for life-support equipment. Less than one month after the conviction, a director of a Planned Parenthood clinic in Pittsburgh said the case was creating a "severe burden on a great many women, some of whom are really strapped for funds," and reported a 10 percent increase in women coming to them for abortions after being turned away by doctors and hospitals in their seventeenth and eighteenth weeks of pregnancy.[226]

Other hospitals did not ban later-term abortions, but instead passed policies that made them prohibitively expensive. Beth Israel Hospital of New York, for example, began mandating that lifesaving equipment be on hand during any second-trimester abortion, even while acknowledging that "this new policy would add hundreds of dollars a day to the cost of an abortion."[227] Hospital superintendent Donald H. Eisenberg explained this policy by saying that "doctors who perform abortions want assurances that their best medical efforts will not end in criminal charges. We can't guarantee that so we have to protect them in other ways."[228] For Dr. William J. Curran, professor of legal medicine at Harvard, this policy, soon adopted by hospitals across the country, raised troubling questions: "What about the mother who thinking she was having an abortion was later handed a child, one with a substantial risk of being brain-damaged? Who will pay the bills that can reach $500 per day in the limited number of intensive care units to keep premature infants alive? The mother? The hospital? The state?"[229]

Stymied not at all by these kinds of question, or by the Supreme Judicial Court of Massachusetts's reversal, but aware of the growing national consensus in support of *Roe,* pro-life activists took heart from hospitals' self-imposed restrictions and began focusing their attention on limiting access to and availability of abortions as a more achievable strategy than overturning the Supreme Court decision. Their first success was the passage in 1977 of the "Hyde Amendment," named for Illinois Republican Congressman Henry Hyde, which banned the use of federal funds for abortions and therefore targeted low-income women receiving Medicaid.[230] Similar restrictions on using federal funds to provide abortion services subsequently targeted Native-American women, federal employees and their dependents, Peace Corps volunteers, residents of Washington, D.C., federal prisoners, and military personnel and their dependents.[231]

From the very beginning, Edelin feared these kinds of restrictions on women's options. In 1996, Edelin reviewed Stephen Maynard-Moody's *The Dilemma of the Fetus* for the *New England Journal of Medicine.* He praised it as "thoroughly researched," "accurate," and "important reading," but offered the following caveat:

> As may be expected, since this is a book about the fetus, there is very little discussion of the other important persons in the abortion debate—women. Maynard-Moody believes that "abortion is always a tragedy." There are many who would disagree. Many women choose abortion because of tragedies in their lives and in the circumstances surrounding their pregnancies. For these women, abortion itself is not a tragedy; instead, it liberates them from tragic circumstances. Women must never be left out of the abortion debate or the debate about fetal research, medical progress, and moral politics.[232]

It had been more than twenty years since his trial when Edelin wrote this review. During those twenty years, Edelin has been an activist and practicing physician at Boston University Medical School. As a chairman of Planned Parenthood Federation of America, Edelin has remained committed to ensuring that women's voices are heard and has continued to fight for women's reproductive rights.[233] Although the conviction against Edelin was overturned and the charges against the researchers were dropped, the issues that erupted at Boston City Hospital and the fractures exposed and exacerbated by that eruption have not gone away so quietly. Although the prosecution's basic argument that obstetricians were obligated to treat the fetus as their second and equally important patient did not withstand the scrutiny of the Massachusetts Supreme Court, it contributed to a perceived equivalence between fetuses and babies, and generated efforts to regulate, legislate, and litigate expectant women's obligations and responsibilities toward fetuses in contexts other than abortion.

CHAPTER 4

DEFENDING FETAL RIGHTS: 1970S–1990S

In 1991, a bartender in Seattle tried to dissuade a pregnant customer from ordering a rum daiquiri by showing her the surgeon general's warning label describing the dangers posed to a fetus by drinking during pregnancy. The customer complained to the manager, and the bartender was fired. The next month, the bartender appeared on the *Oprah Winfrey Show* with his lawyer, who defended his client by asking this rhetorical question:

> What if the woman had come in a month from now with her newborn child and ordered two drinks, one for her and one to put in the baby's bottle.... [W]ould the waiter have been justified in refusing service to the baby because it is underage? Of course. Then what's the difference between wanting to protect a child that is newly born and one that is about to be born?[1]

Phrased to elicit the only possible response that "of course," there was no difference between wanting to protect a child who is newly born and one who is about to be born, the lawyer's question illustrates the antiabortion movement's success in erasing the distinction between fetuses and children, an effort illustrated dramatically in the Edelin trial and one that quickly expanded beyond the single issue of abortion. In the 1980s and 1990s, increasing media attention to the problem of expectant mothers who put their interests and needs and rights over the interests, needs, and rights of their unborn children testified to the success of that strategy.[2] Headlines like "Protecting the Unborn: The Problem of Expectant Mothers on Drugs," "Drug Babies Push Issue of Fetal Rights," "Stillbirth Is Called Murder: Mother Admitted She Used Cocaine," and "Court Acting to Force Care of the Unborn" plastered the front pages of national newspapers, portraying expectant mothers as irrational and irresponsible.[3] Using more measured language, legal and medical journals examined similar conflicts in articles like "Fetal versus Maternal Rights: Medical and Legal Perspectives," "Maternal versus Fetal Rights: A Clinical Dilemma," "Fetal Patients and Conflicts with Their Mothers," "Mother versus Her Unborn Child," "Should Mom Be Constrained in the Best Interests of the Fetus?" and "Keeping Baby Safe From Mom."[4] Identifying fetuses as babies threatened by mentally incompetent, misguided, or malevolent mothers, antiabortion activists, physicians, employers, and politicians argued, in a variety of different situations and for a variety of different reasons, that a fetus's "right to life" should outweigh a woman's "right to choose."

Beginning in the 1970s, Americans were increasingly confronted by the possibility that the postwar economic expansion that had once seemed unbounded was approaching its limits. At a metaphorical level, the late-twentieth-century confrontation with the boundaries of economic expansion created a kind of "frontier anxiety" similar to the one created through the late nineteenth-century confrontation with the boundaries of geographic expansion. In the face of this new frontier, rights were no longer conceptualized as an infinitely available resource to be discovered, but as a fixed commodity to be distributed.[5] The fetus, whose body could be protected only by invading the impregnable frontier of pregnant women's bodies, and whose rights could be recognized only by taking them from women, became a symbol encoding those anxieties. Those displaced, discomfited, and dismayed by the social, cultural, political, and economic changes wrought by the social movements of the 1960s and 1970s fought back in the name of "fetal rights."

Beginning in the 1970s, conflicts between this new category of "fetal rights" and women's rights as patients, workers, and citizens erupted. The practice of fetal medicine and court-ordered medical interventions, the implementation of fetal protection policies in the workplace, and the prosecution of crimes of fetal abuse triggered a series of conflicts. These conflicts revolved around competing interpretations of medical and scientific evidence; conflicting narratives of risk, etiology, and protection; contradictory interpretations of women's behavior; and contested struggles between women and authorities, including physicians, employers, and the state. The construction of conflicts between fetal rights and women's rights also transformed the antiabortion movement from a single-issue campaign to a referendum on motherhood, feminism, and liberalism.

Fetal medicine was born in tandem with abortion politics. In 1973, the same year as the *Roe v. Wade* decision, the American College of Obstetricians and Gynecologists, recognizing what they described as the "advances in fetal medicine made over the past ten years," formally designated "fetology" as a separate specialty.[6] The relationship between fetal medicine and abortion politics was not inevitable, and certainly many fetologists neither opposed abortion nor connected their political positions to their medical practice, but fetal medicine did contribute to a fundamental reimagining of the maternal-fetal relationship as one involving two individuated patients.[7]

Dr. William Liley, a New Zealand obstetrician responsible for many of the advances that had facilitated physicians' understanding of the fetus as a patient separate from the pregnant woman, was also active in the antiabortion movement. In 1965, Liley left his chairmanship in perinatal physiology at the Postgraduate School of Obstetrics and Gynaecology at the University of Auckland to go to Columbia Presbyterian Hospital in New York City, where he worked to develop procedures and techniques for *in utero* diagnosis, treatment, and surgery.[8] A founding member of the Society for the Protection of Unborn Children (SPUC) in New Zealand, Liley continued his activism in the United States by testifying before Congress in support of the Human Life Amendment.[9] Central to his research and his politics was Liley's belief that the fetus is a being independent of the pregnant woman. He describes women who "speak of *their* waters breaking and *their* membranes rupturing" as speaking "so much nonsense.... These structures belong to the fetus. At no stage can we subscribe to the view that the fetus is a mere appendage of the mother."[10] And he calls the fetus "our new individual...very much in charge of the pregnancy" while calling the pregnant woman a "suitable host," "a pregnant uterus," and "a plastic, reactive structure."[11] Politics notwithstanding, separating the medical needs of the pregnant woman from those of the fetus, and identifying the fetus as a patient to be diagnosed and treated while still *in utero,* raised the possibility that the rights and interests of the fetus might conflict with the rights and interests of the pregnant woman.

This potential conflict offered some physicians a vehicle through which they could assert their authority in the face of challenges made by feminist health activists since the 1970s.[12] Historian William Arney described this possible function of the "fetal patient": "Obstetricians found in the fetus not just a new point for intervening in pregnancy but also a way to blunt the critical edge of women's concerns about the way obstetricians treated them.... Obstetricians became fetal advocates and women were left to mount their struggle against an adversary who had acquired a potent ally in the fetus."[13] Legal scholar Janet Gallagher similarly interpreted physicians' requests for court-ordered cesarean sections as efforts to reinforce their authority "after a decade of 'consumer' rebellion against the medicalization of birth and of movement toward alternatives like midwives, birthing centers, and homebirth."[14] Obstetricians did not articulate, and perhaps did not recognize, this struggle for authority and control with pregnant women. But they did challenge women's competence to make medical decisions and insisted that they knew better than the patient herself what she "really wants." Efforts to resolve those "maternal-fetal" conflicts through court-ordered medical interventions made on behalf of "fetal rights" explicitly called into question the rationality of pregnant women's minds and the integrity of pregnant women's rights.

Three particular cases highlight how women's status as pregnant or as mothers delimited their rights as patients. In 1964, the perceived obligations of a mother intersected with the perceived interests of fetal patients to produce the first in what would become a pattern of conflicts over the question of whether and when physicians could require a pregnant woman to undergo medical procedures without her consent. That year, the New Jersey Supreme Court granted Raleigh-Fitkin-Paul Morgan Memorial Hospital's request for a court order allowing them to override the wishes of Willimina Anderson, who was five months pregnant at the time, and give her a blood transfusion.[15] The precedent for this decision was a 1963 court order allowing Georgetown University Hospital to give a blood transfusion to Jessie Jones, the mother of a seven-month-old baby, against her wishes.[16] In 1976, a New York judge denied a hospital's request for a court order allowing a blood transfusion to be given against the wishes of Kathleen Melideo.[17] All three of these women were Jehovah's Witnesses, trying to adhere to their religion's dictates against blood transfusions. But they were different in one crucial respect: Jessie Jones was a mother, Willimina Anderson was pregnant, and Kathleen Melideo was not pregnant and had no children.

Although not relevant to their medical situations, the parental status of these three women was a significant factor in determining the court's response to the conflict. The judge found that Jones, the mother of the seven-month-old baby, was "not in a mental condition to make a decision," and concluded that "the state, as *parens patriae*, will not allow a parent to abandon a child, and so it should not allow this most ultimate of voluntary abandonments."[18] The only evidence offered to challenge Jones's mental competence was the fact that she rejected her doctor's recommendation on the basis of her religious beliefs. A mentally competent mother would, in the court's logic, presumably not make that decision.

In the case of Anderson, who was pregnant, the judge cited her "inability to recognize her best interests," agreed with the hospital that "the welfare of the child and the mother were so intertwined and inseparable that it would be impracticable to attempt to distinguish between them," and concluded that "the unborn child is entitled to the law's protection."[19] If the decision in Jones's case depended upon the state's role in ensuring a mother meet her obligations to her child, the decision in Anderson's case imputed those same obligations to an unborn child. These decisions diverged significantly from the long-established precedent protecting patients' rights to refuse medical treatments.[20] In contrast, the court determined that Melideo was "fully competent" to refuse treatment, a finding based at least in part on the fact that "she is not pregnant, and has no children."[21] That the decision to refuse treatment in the cases of Jones and Anderson was deemed irrational and incompetent, while that same decision in Melideo's case was interpreted as reasonable and legitimate, suggests that the rationality and legitimacy of these three women's decisions was determined primarily by their parental status.

Throughout the 1970s and 1980s, courts repeatedly granted court orders mandating transfusions for pregnant women who refused to give consent. One judge explained his decision by saying that "the decisive nature of the interests of the unborn fetus" outweighs the woman's "important and protected interest in the exercise of her religious beliefs."[22] Another judge chastised the woman for putting "the hospital and her doctors in an untenable position" by refusing to have a blood transfusion.[23] Precedents established in these cases would be used to justify court-ordered cesarean sections, a surgical procedure far more invasive and risky than a blood transfusion, and one far more likely to create a potential disagreement between women and their doctors.

As the increasingly common use of electronic fetal monitoring (EFM) made detecting symptoms of fetal distress easier, the frequency of cesarean deliveries sharply increased.[24] At the same time, increasing numbers of pregnant women began resisting their obstetricians' recommendations for cesarean sections. Analyzing this pattern in 1979, Dr. J. R. Lieberman concluded that a woman's decision to reject her obstetrician's advice reflected, at best, "medical ignorance," and at worst, the "*mens rea*" (guilty mind) of a woman who does not want to be pregnant:

> It is probable that the patient hopes to be freed in this way of an undesired pregnancy and in no case will the patient share her secret thoughts with the physician. It may be undesired because it is an unwanted pregnancy, the woman is divorced or widowed, the pregnancy is an extramarital one, there are inheritance problems, etc.[25]

Other physicians explained the seemingly inexplicable pattern of pregnant women who refuse to follow physicians' advice by arguing that pregnant women are, by definition, not rational. "Pregnancy," Dr. Stuart Asch wrote in 1985, "will shake the most mentally healthy person, and some manifestation of anxiety is always present during pregnancy. In the most serious reactions, this can take the form of any possible psychiatric picture, including phobias, depressions, and psychoses."[26] To identify pregnant patients suffering from these mental disorders, Asch instructed doctors to look for the telltale symptoms of "assertiveness and a desire to experience vaginal childbirth, ideally natural childbirth."[27] The most dangerous patient, in Asch's estimation, was a woman who is "fanatic in her zeal for vaginal delivery childbirth. The intensity of her demands and her uncompromising attitude on the subject are danger signals, frequently indicating severe psychopathology.... A patient of this sort...requires close and constant psychiatric support."[28] Although they ascribed irrational, selfish, and patholog-ical motives to women refusing to agree to have a cesarean section, neither Lieberman or Asch supported forcing invasive and potentially dangerous med-ical procedures upon patients against their will. Lieberman, for example, described performing a cesarean section without a patient's consent tantamount to "assault and battery."[29] Other physicians and courts, however, saw it differently.

In 1981, Jessie Mae Jefferson became the first American woman ordered by a court to have a cesarean section against her wishes. Married to a minister and mother of three children, Jefferson had sought and received prenatal care throughout her pregnancy. She also believed in faith healing. At an appoint-ment a few days before her due date, Jefferson had an ultrasound at the Spaulding County Hospital in Griffin, Georgia, which indicated that her pla-centa was blocking her cervix. An attending physician explained to Jefferson that a vaginal delivery could pose serious risks to her life and health, and to the health and life of her fetus, and recommended a cesarean section. Jefferson rejected his recommendation, preferring, she said, to leave her future and her unborn child's future up to "the Lord's will."[30] The hospital took Jefferson to court, where the Supreme Court of Georgia determined that Jefferson was "not competent to make decisions about her labor and delivery or about anything else," and granted temporary custody of the "unborn child" to the Department of Human Resources, which consented to the surgery on behalf of their new charge. When Jefferson delivered a healthy baby vaginally a few days before the scheduled surgery, she believed that her prayers had moved the placenta blocking the birth canal. Whether or not one accepts that inter-pretation, it is true that many of the court orders were based on incomplete or inaccurate diagnoses and prognoses. Although the Georgia court's decision in this case was never implemented, it did establish a troubling precedent and pattern.

A study published in the *New England Journal of Medicine* in 1987 found that 46 percent of obstetricians advocated the use of court orders and hospital detention to enforce compliance from pregnant women.[31] This study analyzed court-ordered obstetrical interventions between 1981 and 1986 and concluded that courts had granted 86 percent of hospitals' requests to perform involuntary cesarean sections, to compel pregnant women to have blood transfusions, or to detain in custody pregnant women who refused medical treatment.[32] Political scientist Cynthia Daniels put these statistics in stark relief by describing exam-ples where enforced medical interventions and procedures were strictly prohibited:

Robbery suspects cannot be forced to undergo surgery in order to remove critical evidence, such as a bullet from their bodies. Persons suspected of drug dealing cannot be forced to have their stomachs pumped if they swallow evidence. Suspected rapists cannot be forced to undergo involuntary blood tests for AIDS. Parents cannot be forced to donate bone marrow to a child who is dying of bone cancer. Organs cannot even be taken from a cadaver without the prior consent of the dying.[33]

It would seem that a pregnant woman refusing treatment deemed to be in the best interests of the fetus has fewer rights than a rapist, drug dealer, robbery suspect, or cadaver; and that a pregnant woman has a greater obligation to the fetus than a parent does to a child. These conclusions could be justified only by the belief that a pregnant woman was so irrational as to no longer be competent.

Putting aside Asch's position that pregnancy rendered all women mentally unstable, certain characteristics made some women particularly susceptible to being categorized as irrational, incompetent, or dangerous. As Jessie Mae Jefferson's experience suggests, religion was one of those characteristics. In 1984, Dr. Harold Brody reported to a conference on medical ethics that "in almost all cases that have arisen to date, the woman refusing C-section is a member of some religious group or subculture which holds beliefs at variance with the majority in our country."[34] Women were also singled out by their race and socio-economic status. According to the *NEJM* study, 81 percent of the pregnant women subjected to court-ordered intervention were black, Asian, or Hispanic; 44 percent of them were unmarried; 24 percent of them did not speak English as their primary language; and none of them were privately insured.[35]

Some physicians insisted that their pregnant patients were grateful to have complex decisions made for them. For example, obstetrician Mary Jo O'Sullivan described one case in which she had to obtain a court order allowing her to perform a cesarean section on an unwilling patient. "To my surprise, when I showed the patient the court order, she seemed relieved that the decision was out of her hands."[36] The extent to which some women went in trying to avoid coerced procedures—Daniels describes, for example, the story of a Detroit woman who went into hiding "after being informed that she would be picked up by police and forcibly transported to the hospital if she didn't report by a specified date and time for a cesarean section"—suggests that relief was not the dominant emotion experienced by many of these women.[37] Pitting the fetus's well-being, framed as a public issue of social concern, against the mother's rights, framed as a private issue of personal preference, courts repeatedly found the interests of the fetus sufficiently compelling to override a woman's decision. The increase of court-ordered medical interventions on behalf of the fetus reflected the greater deference given to a physician's concern about the fetus's health—or to a hospital's concerns about potential litigation—than to a pregnant woman's right to refuse medical treatment, a right that had previously been interpreted to include "the right to refuse medical treatment even if refusing leads to death."[38] On at least one occasion, however, it was the medical treatment itself that contributed to, or hastened, death.

In 1987, Angela Carder, a twenty-seven-year-old woman, who was twenty-five weeks pregnant, was diagnosed with an inoperable brain tumor. She went to her Washington, D.C. hospital complaining of back pain and shortness of breath.[39] Carder and her doctors decided that, despite the great risks, she would deliver by cesarean section at twenty-eight weeks, the point at which her fetus would have a reasonably good chance of survival. Carder's condition deteriorated quickly in the days following this decision, and it became questionable that she would live until her twenty-eighth week of pregnancy. Against the wishes of Carder, her family, her oncologist, and her obstetrician, hospital administrators appointed a lawyer to represent the fetus, and the lawyer went to court to ask for permission to perform an emergency cesarean section. The court granted his request, and, hours later, Carder underwent the court-ordered operation.[40] Her twenty-six-week old fetus died two hours after delivery; Carder died two days later.[41] Carder's family, with the help of lawyers from the ACLU Reproductive Freedom Project, sought to vacate the original order, thus limiting its use as a precedent. In 1990, in its opinion *In re A.C.*, the D.C. Court of Appeals became the highest court in the land to rule against forced cesarean sections, finding that they drive "women at high risk of complications during pregnancy and childbirth out of the health care system to avoid coerced treatment," and that they violate women's constitutionally protected rights.[42]

In a reversal of the pattern in which pregnant women (disproportionately African-American women with few resources) were condemned for refusing medical treatment that might benefit their fetus, other pregnant women (disproportionately white women with relatively substantial resources) were honored for pursuing it. Fetologists repeatedly championed the heroism and courage of women who pursued experimental treatments that posed not-insubstantial risks to themselves and promised less-than-definite benefits to their fetuses. In her analysis of pregnant women deciding whether or not to pursue particular procedures, Nancy Rhoden quotes one fetal surgeon as saying that the "vast majority of these heroic women accept significant risk, pain, and inconvenience to give their babies the best chance possible."[43] A second surgeon speaks with respect of the women he sees who "would cut off their heads to save their babies."[44] Dr. Michael Harrison, Dr. Mitchell Golbus, and Dr. Roy Filly dedicated their textbook on fetal medicine entitled *The Unborn Patient* to the "courageous mothers, who by pursuing treatment for their unborn babies, enfranchised the fetal patient."[45] Suggesting with the word *enfranchised* that the fetus is a citizen with rights, and with the word *courageous* an implicit critique of mothers who made different choices, these physicians posited a relationship between the physiological and political status of the fetus, and a conceptualization of the maternal-fetal relationship that made explicit ideas that had been central to fetal medicine since its inception.

As prenatal diagnostic screening, reproductive technologies, fetal monitoring, and fetal therapies offered women more opportunities to take "heroic" measures to save the life and enhance the health of their future babies, the question became what to do about women not ready to "cut off their heads" to save their babies.[46] When medical communities, courts, and the public focus on the personal choices women make under extremely difficult circumstances, they can obscure the political, economic, and cultural factors that shape those choices, and position mothers who pursue treatment against those who do not. This demarcation underlines already existing judgments about good and bad mothers, but it also pretends that these treatments are available to any and all pregnant women, just for the asking. The reality, of course, is that opting for prohibitively expensive fetal surgery may have less to do with one's heroism and more to do with one's resources. And even for those who can afford these interventions, questions remain. In July, 2001, for a *New York Times* article exploring advances making possible the treatment of spina bifida *in utero*, journalist Maggie Jones interviewed doctors who championed the potential benefits of the procedure to the fetus as well as those who emphasized the potential risks of the procedure to the mother. Jones concluded that one of the dangers of fetal surgery is that "while women may never be forced to submit to these procedures, they may certainly feel pressured to undergo surgery to get the best baby medicine has to offer."[47] She may be right that women would never be forced to submit to cutting-edge procedures like the ones she described in her article, but the history of pregnant women subjected to medical treatment against their will suggests that could change.

At the same time that fetal medicine defined good mothers as those who would pursue any means necessary to protect the health of the fetus and defined bad mothers as those who made irrational or selfish decisions by putting their own interests ahead of the purported interests of the fetus, a similar dichotomy was being articulated in an entirely different context—the workplace. Beginning in the early 1970s, some U.S companies began passing policies—called "fetal protection policies," "fetal vulnerability policies," or "fetal exclusion policies"— that excluded pregnant women, fertile women, and sometimes all women from jobs in relatively lucrative, if potentially dangerous, industries.[48] In 1974, the

Lead Industries Association issued a policy statement opposing the employment of fertile women in jobs where they would be exposed to lead. A 1975 study of the occupational health problems of pregnant women in the workplace conducted by the U.S. Department of Health, Education, and Welfare found "growing scientific evidence that occupational exposure to some chemicals and substances can affect a worker's capacity to produce normal children," and identified lead as the most dangerous of these substances.[49] By 1979, approximately 100,000 jobs had been closed to women on grounds of reproductive hazards; in 1985, the Office of Technological Assessment (OTA) estimated that at least fifteen Fortune 500 companies had implemented fetal protection policies; and in 1989, 20 percent of chemical and electronic firms in the United States had some kind of policy that restricted women's role in the workplace by invoking the right of the fetus to be protected from dangerous toxins, chemicals, and environmental hazards.[50]

These policies identified yet another category of women—those taking relatively high-paying, historically male jobs in factories and industrial workplaces—as putting their unborn children at risk. Court-ordered obstetrical interventions raised the question of whether a physician could, on behalf of the fetus, override a pregnant woman's decisions about her medical treatment, and hinged on the assumption that physicians were more capable of making medical decisions than were irrational or incompetent mothers. Corporate-sponsored fetal protection policies raised the question of whether an employer could, "on behalf of the fetus," delimit women's employment or reproductive rights, and hinged on the assumption that a company was more concerned about the health and safety of the fetus than ambitious or avaricious mothers. Claiming that they needed to protect fetuses from women who insisted on taking jobs that would expose them to substances that could damage fetuses and embryos, while assuming that a well-paying job with health benefits was less beneficial to the health of the fetus than exposure to these teratogenic substances was harmful, companies implemented fetal protection policies that ignored any corporate responsibility to provide safe working environments (mandated in 1970 by the Occupational Safety and Health Act), and abrogated women's rights protected under Title VII of the Civil Rights Act of 1964, which prohibited discrimination by employers on the basis of race, color, religion, national origin, or sex.[51]

The idea that women's reproductive capacity justified their differential treatment in the industrial workplace had been legally enshrined in the 1908 Supreme Court decision of *Muller v. Oregon*.[52] An Oregon statute prohibiting the employment of any women "in any mechanical establishment, or factory, or laundry" for more than ten hours a day was legal, according to the court, because "healthy mothers are essential to vigorous offspring...the physical well-being of woman becomes an object of public interest and care in order to preserve the strength and vigor of the race."[53] Following the *Muller* decision, states passed countless "protective" labor laws restricting women's employment.[54] These laws were rendered illegal in 1964, by Title VII of the Civil Rights Act.[55] Some historians and legal scholars have argued that fetal protection policies are essentially protective labor laws rewritten to comply with Title VII.[56] Fetal protection policies are undoubtedly part of the historical effort to regulate women's participation in the paid workforce, but although the historical and legal relationships between fetal protection policies and protective labor legislation are clear, the differences between the two are equally significant.[57] The *Muller* decision was made at a time when approximately 22 percent of women worked, comprising approximately 19 percent of the paid workforce, whereas the fetal protection policies of the 1970s were implemented at a time when approximately 42 percent of women worked, comprising 38 percent of the paid workforce.[58] *Muller* explicitly identified protecting the health of mothers as the linchpin to the future health of society, whereas fetal protection policies target the health of the fetus *qua* fetus as their concern.

This last difference might be attributed to a growing awareness of *in utero* transmissions of environmental hazards from mother to fetus, except for the fact that such awareness was hardly new.[59] Dr. Alice Hamilton, Progressive Era reformer, Harvard Medical School professor, and founder of the occupational health movement, spent a lifetime trying to convince the public of the dangers industrial toxins posed to all workers, particularly to pregnant women workers.[60] Primarily interested in the impact of lead on pregnant women, she argued in 1919 the following:

> The most disastrous effect that lead has upon women is the effect on the generative organs. Women who suffer from lead poisoning are more likely to be sterile or to have miscarriages and stillbirths than are women not exposed to lead. If they bear living children, these are more likely to die during the first year of life than are the children of women who have never been exposed to lead. This means that lead is a race poison, and that lead poisoning in women affects not only one generation but two generations.[61]

Female susceptibility to lead was not an inherent defect of biology, Hamilton insisted, but a social defect of culture, explained "by the fact that they [women] are usually more poverty stricken than the men, are under-nourished and obliged to do work for their families in addition to their factory work."[62] Although she clearly understood the social and economic conditions that made women uniquely vulnerable to lead, Hamilton advocated banning women from working in the lead industries, rather than working to transform those social and economic conditions, as most effective way to mitigate the dangers of lead.[63] The Women's Bureau of the Department of Labor agreed, although they recognized that excluding women from the lead industries presented a dangerous possibility:

> Under the guise of 'protection' women may be shut out from occupations which are really less harmful to ... them than much of the tedious heavy work both in the home and in the factory which has long been considered their special province. Safe standards of work for women must come to be safe standards of work for men also if women are to have an equal chance in industry.[64]

Despite these concerns, the bureau ultimately concluded that protecting women from the dangers of lead or from overly long hours was preferable to insisting that men and women workers be treated identically. Members of the National Woman's Party and supporters of the Equal Rights Amendment in the 1920s did not agree with this assessment.[65] Believing that this kind of legislation confirmed the stereotype of women as weak and reified the identification of all women as mothers or potential mothers, these "equality" feminists argued unsuccessfully that women and workers should fight to make companies provide safe working conditions for all workers, not just women workers.

Political coalitions, ideological assumptions, and economic imperatives combined to reshape the regulation of male and female workers in the dramatically changing workforce and political economy of the 1930s and 1940s. The New Deal shifted the terms of what had been a strategic and ideological debate between fighting for women's rights in the workplace on the basis of their equality to or difference from men, to one that weighed the costs and benefits of federal regulations to protect all workers.[66] The culmination of that debate was the putatively race- and gender-neutral Fair Labor Standards Act of 1938.[67] As World War II heightened demand for women workers in the industrial labor force, distinctions between men and women workers that had been exaggerated in the *Muller* era were minimized.[68] So in 1942, when the U.S. Department of Labor recommended that pregnant women avoid workplace exposure to certain known toxic substances, including lead, benzene, and radium, the high demand for women workers in war industries precluded industry from acting upon that recommendation and government from enforcing it.[69] The case of the Bunker Hill Mining Company is a particularly good example of how the demand for labor was the crucial factor in determining the treatment of women working in historically male industries.

Founded in the late 1890s in Kellogg, Idaho, Bunker Hill was one of the nation's largest producers of lead and zinc.[70] Women had not been allowed to work in the lead smelter until 1943 when, one year after Department of Labor's recommendation, Bunker Hill lifted that prohibition, citing a recent textbook on industrial medicine to justify gender-neutral workplace policies: "Women, like men, can safely work with any material if the engineering and medical controls are adequate. The susceptibility of women, if such does exist, should imply more extensive medical and engineering control measures, not exclusion from the job."[71] Bunker Hill did not, however, offer "more extensive medical and engineering control measures." And women workers would soon see this briefly opened door closed again. In 1946, as the men who had gone to war returned to their jobs, women were again banned from jobs in the lead smelter, a prohibition that would last for more than twenty-five years.[72] Almost ten years after the passage of Title VII, under pressure from the Equal Employment Opportunity Commission, Bunker Hill reopened these high-paying jobs to women in 1973.

Over the next two years, forty-five women took jobs in the lead smelter and zinc plant. In April 1975, however, Bunker Hill enacted an "exclusionary policy" prohibiting fertile women from working in lead-exposed environments.[73] Referring to the newly released D-HEW report on the dangers of lead exposure to pregnant women, and citing their concern for potential damage to the "unborn children of our female workers," the company issued a new policy requiring any woman wanting to keep her job in a lead-exposed area to provide a physician's letter verifying that she was sterilized, postmenopausal, or infertile.[74] All women without this letter would, within six months, be transferred to "safe" work areas. Twenty-nine women transferred to the maintenance crew, taking a substantial pay cut, and OSHA estimated that "at least three women obtained sterilization procedures within the next two to three months solely to be allowed by the company to return to their former jobs."[75]

Forced to choose between sterilization and demotion, the women of Bunker Hill sought help from their union, the United Steelworkers Association of America. Claiming that it would be prohibitively expensive to fight the policy, the USWA turned down the women's request. The union also argued that fighting and losing would create more problems for women workers in the steel industry as a whole than this one policy presented for the women at Bunker Hill. In ways that union officials did not explicitly acknowledge, growing concerns about how the changing political economy was impacting the steel industry were likely factors contributing to their unwillingness to challenge the Bunker Hill policy.

Economic indicators signaling the approaching limits of postwar economic growth were becoming increasingly obvious. Productivity and employment were declining as global competition and inflation were rising, and the combination of deindustrialization and stagflation imposed enormous pressures upon American industry and industrial workers.[76] The steel industry and steelworkers were particularly subject to those pressures, which were exacerbated by the oil embargo of 1973–1974 and the subsequent energy crisis.[77] In the early 1970s, sales of American cars dropped by more than 10 million cars a year, the United States became an importer rather than exporter of steel, and Japan surpassed the United States as the leading producer of steel. In 1973, joining forces to ward off the consequences of these economic conditions, the USWA and the steel industry signed the Experimental Negotiating Agreement, in which the union promised not to strike in exchange for the industry's promise to increase wages by 3 percent annually regardless of declining profits and rising inflation.[78]

The steel industry was not the only struggling sector of the economy. In 1974, the unemployment rate of 7.2 percent was the highest since 1960.[79] During that period, the percentage of women in the workforce had grown from 35 percent to 44 percent.[80] Although many of these women were joining the "pink-collar" sector, others obtained unionized industrial factory jobs from which, until very recently, they had been excluded, if by custom rather than by law.[81] Charged with enforcing the provisions of Title VII, the Equal Employment Opportunity Commission was the regulatory impetus behind that trend, one that the steel industry could not avoid. In 1973, the EEOC, the Department of Labor, and the Department of Justice filed a suit against the nine largest steel producers in the country and the USWA, charging them with discriminatory hiring, promotion, assignment, and wage policies. After five and a half months of negotiations, the companies and the union made two key concessions that led to settlement. They agreed to distribute $31 million in back pay to about 40,000 minority and women employees, and they agreed to establish a set of hiring goals requiring 25 percent of supervisory jobs and 50 percent of trade and craft jobs be filled with women and minority workers.[82]

When their union had refused to back them, the women at Bunker Hill had turned to the Idaho Human Rights Commission. The IHRC devised a compromise solution that required the women to transfer to different jobs, and required the company to pay those women the same wages they had earned while working in the lead and zinc smelters. Both the company and the women rejected this plan. Bunker Hill's vice president of environmental affairs Dennis Brendel defended the company's policy to the EEOC, saying, "Bunker Hill is willing to be criticized for not employing some women—but we are not willing to cause birth defects to unborn children."[83] Brendel knew, of course, that there were no "unborn children" in lead-exposed areas of Bunker Hill, as none of the women in question were pregnant.

In January of 1976, the women filed a complaint with the Equal Employment Opportunity Commission, and when the EEOC endorsed the same compromise recommended by the IHRC, the women were forced to accept a plan that required them to concede that lead posed a danger to the health of any potential unborn children, and to agree that they could not work around lead whether or not they were pregnant or intended to become pregnant. The company was required to reimburse the women who had transferred to lower paying positions for lost wages, to guarantee their current jobs, and to promise that women involved in the controversy would not be punished by the company and would be transferred to "safe" jobs at comparable pay. Future women hired by the company would be placed in "safe jobs," at a lower rate of pay.[84] This decision was, in effect, a complete victory for the company. It was not forced to provide universally safe working conditions, and was obligated to pay higher wages only to the twenty-nine women who, under the fetal protection policy, had been forced to change departments. Following this EEOC decision, companies including Eastman Kodak, Union Carbide, Dow Chemical, Firestone Tire, General Motors, and AT&T soon implemented some version of a policy that restricted or prohibited women from working in positions where they would be exposed to dangerous chemicals.[85] Whereas the events at Bunker Hill had remained essentially a local story, the proliferation of fetal protection policies aroused the anger of environmentalists, feminists, and labor activists. The case of American Cyanamid, a chemical manufacturer, was the first to generate national attention.

Like Bunker Hill, American Cyanamid had started hiring women at its Willow Island, West Virginia, plant in 1973 in response to the threat of sanctions from the EEOC.[86] As one of the highest paying local employers, the company was flooded with applications from women in the area.[87] Women going to work at the plant faced powerful resistance and resentment from their fellow workers. The foreman opposed hiring women, protesting, among other things, that women's breasts would get caught in the equipment. One female worker, Betty Riggs, described showing up at work and seeing "graffiti on the plant walls, written by male coworkers: 'Shoot a woman, save a job.' I was made to feel ashamed, when it was the company that should have been ashamed. The almighty dollar was more important than a human being."[88]

Almost immediately after they began hiring women, the board of American Cyanamid asked the corporate medical director Dr. Robert Klyne to develop a policy banning fertile women from jobs exposing them to toxic substances. Considering teratogenic effects transmitted by the pregnant woman to the fetus *in utero,* while ignoring mutagenic effects transmitted through the reproductive genes of both men and women, Klyne identified through "an educated guess" twenty-nine toxic substances.[89] He acknowledged that "the ideal is that the workplace has to be safe for everyone—the man, the woman, and the child," but dismissed that possibility as "totally unachievable without emasculating the chemical industry." Rather than risk the "emasculating" effect of providing safe working conditions, and rather than trust women who "neither knew when they were pregnant nor planned their pregnancies," Klyne recommended that the company exclude all women between the ages of fifteen and fifty from jobs exposing them to these twenty-nine substances.[90] On February 1, 1978, the Willow Island plant implemented his recommendations. After hearing complaints from female employees, the company reduced the list of dangerous substances from twenty-nine to one. Ironically, that single substance, lead, was the only one of the twenty-nine for which there was clear evidence of reproductive hazards for men as well as women.[91]

In October of 1978, fewer than 30 of the 560 Willow Island employees were women. Only 7 of these women worked in jobs that did not expose them to lead. The company presented the remaining women with two options. They could transfer to another job within the company where, after ninety days of receiving the same rate of pay they had in the lead-exposed jobs, their pay would be reduced to the standard rate for that new job. Alternatively, if they wanted to stay in their higher-paying jobs, they could opt for surgical sterilization, a procedure that the company's medical insurance would cover.[92] At least five of the women, none of whom were pregnant or planned to become pregnant, chose to undergo surgical sterilization. One of those women was Betty Riggs, then twenty-six years old, divorced, supporting her aging parents, and a mother of a twelve-year-old son.[93] Another woman explained her decision this way: "They don't have to hold a hammer to your head—all they have to do is tell you that it's the only way you can keep your job."[94] Another woman explained that this job paid six times as much as her previous job as a cashier in a market, allowing her to take her son and leave her abusive husband.[95] Two of the women took lower paying jobs in the janitorial department, some women quit, and thirteen of them turned to the American Civil Liberties Union (ACLU) for help.[96]

The ACLU filed a sex discrimination complaint with the EEOC, and also successfully encouraged the Oil, Chemical, and Atomic Workers Union (OCAW) to file a complaint with OSHA. After conducting an investigation, OSHA came to the following conclusions:

> Exclusionary policies such as those imposed against pregnant women undermine the principle that the workplace should be a safe environment for all

persons....High risk industries should not be able to reduce their liability for damage awards by excluding classes of workers....No worker should be forced to sacrifice her reproductive right to privacy to hold her job.[97]

OSHA charged American Cyanamid with violating federal regulations. By "adopting and implementing a policy which required women employees to be sterilized in order to be eligible to work in areas of the plant where they would be exposed to certain toxic substances," American Cyanamid was violating the federal requirement to provide "employment and a place of employment which are free from recognized hazards that are causing or are likely to cause death or serious physical harm."[98] President Carter's secretary of labor Ray Marshall demanded that American Cyanamid comply immediately with health and safety standards, repeal their policy, and pay a fine of $10,000.[99] Rather than meet these conditions, American Cyanamid closed its Willow Island paint production facility—dismissing, in the process, the five women who had been sterilized in order to keep their jobs—and appealed the fine to the Occupational Health and Safety Review Commission (OHSRC). The OHSRC agreed with American Cyanamid that the labor secretary's citation did not fall under any existing category of violation, and they repealed the fine.

The OCAW Union appealed this decision, but in 1984, the District of Columbia Circuit Court unanimously upheld the ruling of the OHSRC.[100] Judge Robert Bork wrote the court's opinion, which began by saying that the company was faced with choosing between the "unattractive" alternatives of firing the women or letting them get sterilized; and that on the other hand, the women were faced with the "distressing...most unhappy choice" between losing their high-paying jobs or being sterilized.[101] Because American Cyanamid could not "reduce lead concentrations to a level that posed an acceptable risk to fetuses," the fetal protection policy should be understood as a solution to a dilemma arising from forces beyond the company's control. Bork added that "[a]n employee's decision to undergo sterilization in order to gain or retain employment grows out of economic and social factors which operate primarily outside of the workplace. The employer neither controls nor creates those factors."[102] According to Bork, the company could neither control the lead in the workplace, nor could it control the circumstances of workers' lives outside the workplace. So although the company had no control, the women did have a choice. After President Reagan nominated Bork to the Supreme Court, this decision would haunt him in his confirmation hearings. Bork defended the decision, explaining that some women agreed to be sterilized because "some of them, I guess, didn't want to have children."[103] One of the plaintiffs in the American Cyanamid case sent a telegram to the committee, saying that she was horrified by Bork's comments.

"This was the most awful thing that happened to me," she said. "I cannot believe that Judge Bork thinks we were glad to have the choice of getting sterilized or getting fired."[104] This issue was only one of many that led the Senate to vote against Bork's confirmation, but it does suggest that fetal protection policies were not uncritically accepted by the general public and in political debate.

Despite repeated references to "unavoidable physiological facts" and "legal precedent," the court's decision was shaped, it would seem, as much by ideological assumptions about the maternal-fetal relationship as by those more concrete reasons. OSHA's general duty clause required that employers eliminate any workplace hazard that posed a "substantial risk of serious bodily harm or death to employees." To find the policy in compliance with the general duty clause, it had to find that lead exposure did not constitute a hazard to the health and safety of the women workers themselves, but a hazard transmitted through the pregnant woman's body to her fetus. Further, the court had to find that sterilization did not constitute a "hazard" to the health and safety of women, but constituted a "choice" that the women made in response to social and economic conditions outside of the company's control. The ruling did this by erasing one boundary and accentuating another. By treating the fetus as a tiny visitor to the factory floor, the court's ruling accepted the erasure of the boundary between fetuses and babies. In the words of an American Cyanamid executive, "We don't allow children in the workplace and we shouldn't allow the fetus in the workplace."[105] And by treating the pregnant woman's body as a mere conduit of danger, the ruling highlighted the boundary between fetuses and pregnant women, and implied that American Cyanamid cared more about their unborn children than did the women themselves.

The pending sex discrimination suit that the ACLU had filed against American Cyanamid on behalf of thirteen of the women was unaffected by the district court's ruling. The company, which had fought strenuously to avoid paying the $10,000 fine for violating OSHA regulations, settled the sex discrimination case for $200,000 to be divided among the remaining eleven plaintiffs.[106] Acknowledging the sex discrimination charge while rejecting the charge that they had implemented exclusionary policies as a way to circumvent their obligation to provide a safe and healthy workplace, American Cyanamid created what political scientist Sally Kenney calls the "false impression that, in bringing cases on exclusionary policies, women seek the right to poison themselves and their children."[107]

If anyone might be less sympathetic than a corporation exposing its workers to toxic chemicals, it might be a pregnant woman exposing her fetus to those same conditions. In forcing the women to oppose fetal protection policies on the basis of sex discrimination rather than on the basis of workplace safety, the company was also banking on the idea that settling charges of sex discrimination in the short term was cheaper than ensuring safe working conditions in the long term. The Bunker Hill and American Cyanamid cases ended in unhappy compromises for the women workers. They also established precedents encouraging companies to maintain or implement similar exclusionary policies.

Another consequence of the proliferation of fetal protection policies was the coming together of union activists, environmental activists, and feminist activists. In 1979, labor unions, women's groups, legal organizations, health organizations, environmental groups, and individuals joined together to form the Coalition for the Reproductive Rights of Workers. Citing the American Cyanamid case as their catalyst, the CRROW issued a statement declaring its mission to "defend the employment rights and reproductive freedom of workers who are exposed to toxic chemicals and other hazards; to combat exclusionary employer policies; and to fight for the reproductive health of male and female workers exposed to hazardous substances."[108] The American Public Health Association explained their membership in CRROW this way:

> Noting that this so-called corporate concern for fetuses, has focused on women in better paying jobs in industries in which they have not traditionally worked and little concern has been shown for the fetuses of women in traditional, lower paying jobs; Noting that men are the victims of this corporate policy as much as are their women co-workers because if they remain in plants where they are exposed to toxic substances, they face the possibility of impotency, sterility or genetic mutations which cause birth defects in their children;...therefore [we] join with other concerned groups and individuals in the Coalition for the Reproductive Rights of Workers.[109]

The Coalition of Labor Union Women, another CRROW member, argued that fetal protection policies discriminated against both men and women workers, and attacked American Cyanamid for "focusing on dangers of the workforce, not dangers of the workplace."[110]

The CRROW initiated an educational campaign to parallel their legal and political fight against fetal protection policies. Their newsletters and promotional literature worked to expose the hypocrisy of fetal protection policies that ignored the dangers of industrial toxins transmitted through sperm and those in occupations in which women would be difficult to replace; ignored the dangers of industrial toxins that seep through factory walls; ignored the dangers of industrial toxins to the health of the workers themselves. It also criticized policies that inflated the dangers of industrial toxins to the health of fetuses as compared to the dangers of maternal poverty.[111] Cartoonists soon picked up these arguments, skewering the purported motivations behind corporate fetal protection policies with a reminder that profits, not concern for the health of unborn fetuses, drive corporate decision making. One cartoon depicts a talking-head corporate spokesman holding a press conference. As he is telling reporters, "Our chief corporate concern is health," a worker is shown walking past the crowd, heading into work at an unidentified factory, gasping for breath. The next panel shows the worker collapsing on the ground, while the spokesman remains oblivious. In the final panel, as the worker is being carted away by an ambulance, the spokesman concludes, "Healthy profits that is."[112]

Other cartoons argued that fetal protection policies posed serious health risks to all workers, not just to fertile women. Cartoonist Nicole Hollander depicts a conversation between two corporate executives. One says to the other, "The team has come up with an elegant solution to our health and safety problem in the plant." "How much will it cost?" the other asks. "Nothing," the first replies. "That's the beauty of it. We just fire all the women of childbearing age and all other workers who breathe deeply" (figure 4.1).[113] Signe Wilkinson makes a similar point in her cartoon showing the dangers of allowing companies to shift attention away from larger issues of industrial health and safety for all workers to the much narrower issue of workplace dangers for fetuses. Two women are walking to work. As they enter the factory gates, one woman says, "I'm certainly glad I'm past childbearing age so I can continue to work in this vile, polluted atmosphere." "Yes," the other woman responds. "We are indeed privileged to have the opportunity to develop many debilitating illnesses that a less greedy management would have deprived us of."[114] This fictional exchange offers a clear reminder that the hope of Alice Hamilton and the Woman's Bureau that protecting women workers would be the first of many steps toward protecting the health of all workers remained unmet in the 1970s and 1980s.

Other cartoons focused on how these policies obscured the problem of industrial toxins to unborn children for male workers and to unsuspecting mothers and their children. One depicts two men walking into "The All Male Lead Factory." Black smoke is coming out of the factory and blowing into an adjacent neighborhood of small houses and a playground. Mothers are pushing their strollers through the smoke. The caption reads, "Thank God! The women and children are safe from lead poisoning."[115] This cartoon reminds readers that industrial toxins pose risks to male workers, risks that may be transmitted by sperm to as-yet-unconceived-children, and that these risks inevitably affect surrounding communities. This cartoon resonated with the increasing number of citizens concerned about health problems and birth defects caused by toxic chemicals in places as far apart as Love Canal and Vietnam.[116]

These cartoons highlight the ways in which corporate concern for the health of fetuses masked less altruistic agendas. Claims that fetal protection policies

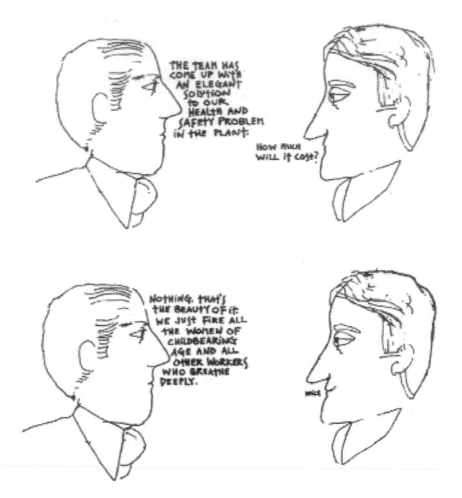

Figure. 4.1 @ 1980 by Nicole Hollander

reflected corporate concern for the health of their workers' potential children were undercut by the fact that substances posing mutagenic risks to men did not generate similarly "protective" policies for men, and by the fact that industries dependent upon female workers, particularly low-wage female workers, did not implement any sort of fetal protection policies, even if those female workers were exposed to dangerous substances. Operating room nurses, for example, are regularly exposed to a variety of chemicals, including anesthetics shown to triple rates of miscarriage; all nurses are exposed to infections, including rubella, that endanger fetal development; daycare workers are exposed to viruses, including the cytomegalovirus, which has been shown to cause severe mental retardation in a developing fetus; office workers are exposed to a variety of toxic chemicals from photocopying fluids, including ozone shown to be cytotoxic and mutagenic; and cleaning women are exposed to cytotoxic and teratogenic cleaning chemicals. None of these jobs are subject to any fetal protection policies.[117] And in what political scientist Rachel Roth calls "the most incriminating example of the fetal protection double standard," women have been banned from working with pesticides as high-paid factory workers although they have not been banned from working with those same chemicals as low-paid agricultural workers.[118] Arguments about the transparency of corporate motivations and about the discriminatory nature of these policies, like the ones made in public discourse and in courtrooms by ACLU, the OCAW, and CRROW, would not successfully persuade the courts to overturn fetal protection policies until 1991, when the United States Supreme Court heard the case of Johnson Controls, the nation's largest manufacturer of automobile batteries.[119]

In 1973, Johnson Controls had, like Bunker Hill and American Cyanamid, responded to EEOC pressure to begin hiring women in their battery production plants in Bennington, Vermont. In 1977, the company implemented a "voluntary fetal protection policy," in which they advised women planning on having children against applying for a job at the battery plant, and required any woman taking a job there to sign a consent waiver acknowledging that she had been informed of the dangers of lead exposure.[120] Despite this discouragement, many women applied for the jobs and signed the waivers. In 1982, after what the corporate spokesperson described as a process of "carefully weighing" the goal of "gender equality...against threats to the health and safety of unborn children from toxic manufacturing operations," Johnson Controls changed their policy to one excluding all "women who are pregnant or who are capable of bearing children" from jobs "involving lead exposure or which could expose them to lead." The company announced the policy change with the following statement: "A child born with lead poisoning is tragic. To knowingly poison unborn children is morally reprehensible. Johnson Controls will do everything within its power to avoid having that happen at our manufacturing plants."[121] The women workers and their union, the United Auto Workers of America, were not persuaded that the policy shift reflected the company's concern about the health of their workers' possible future children, much less the health of the workers themselves, but reflected a more pragmatic response to the hypothetical fear that children born with birth defects caused by *in utero* exposure to lead might sue the company.

On behalf of seven workers, the UAW sued the company for sex discrimination. The plaintiffs included four women in their fifties who were premenopausal but had no plans to become pregnant; a woman in her thirties who underwent sterilization in order to keep her job; a woman whose husband had had a vasectomy; and a man whose request for a transfer from the lead-exposed area while he and his wife attempted to have a child had been denied.[122] One of the plaintiffs testified that she thought her husband's vasectomy would exempt her from the company's policy. "However the plant manager told me that even though my husband had been sterilized, I could still 'screw around.'" Rather than get sterilized, she took a job at a fast-food restaurant "at a substantial cut in pay." Another plaintiff described a similar exchange, in which she asked whether her husband's vasectomy was sufficient to comply with the policy, and was told that "I could still fool around and get pregnant. I decided to have the sterilization because I needed to keep my job."[123]

To make their case, Johnson Controls had to prove that lead posed substantial and irremediable risks to fetal development that could be transmitted only by the mother, but that lead posed no such dangers to workers themselves. They also had to prove that their decision was made not to discriminate against women, or to protect themselves from liability, but to protect fetuses. The strategy for making these arguments involved blurring the lines between fetuses and children, treating all women as potentially pregnant, and condemning the women as making selfish choices. A company executive put it this way: "Johnson Controls wants to employ women. We have many in good-paying, responsible jobs. What we do not want is to put their children in jeopardy."[124] To emphasize the selfish behavior of the women, the company cited women's response to the company's "voluntary" fetal protection policy: "For years, Johnson Controls encouraged women capable of bearing children to voluntarily transfer out of high lead exposure jobs. This effort was ineffective as several women failed to do so and became pregnant while their blood levels exceeded the safety point for their children."[125] Therefore, because "the employer is not able to determine which employees will become pregnant," Johnson Controls argued that they had the right, perhaps the obligation, to exclude all "employees in the excluded class [who] possess the trait that creates the safety problem."[126] The trait that creates the safety problem, according to this logic, is the reproductive capacity of women workers, not the lead itself.

In 1989, adopting the company's framing of the issue as one that emphasized the women's decisions rather than the company's obligations, the Seventh Circuit Court of Appeals determined the women's "interests in financial reward" does not sufficiently outweigh "a medically established risk of the birth of a medically or physically deprived baby."[127] In the words of Judge John L. Coffey, who authored the court's decision, this case was "about women who want to hurt their fetuses for a slightly higher wage."[128] This logic ignored the fact that the plaintiffs were not pregnant, and the fact that one of the plaintiffs was a man. And in an unusual twist, it defined the women working in a battery plant as the party motivated by profits and the company for whom they worked as the party motivated by concern for her unborn child. The UAW appealed the decision, and on March 20, 1991, in the case of *International Union, UAW v. Johnson Controls, Inc.,* the United States Supreme Court unanimously found that fetal protection policies constituted a violation of Title VII. Writing for the majority, Justice Harry Blackmun, author of the *Roe v. Wade* decision, argued that "being potentially pregnant does not render women incapable of making batteries" and that "the threat of tort liability of injured children [could not] justify the exclusion of fertile women." He concluded that "decisions about the welfare of future children must be left to the parents who conceive, bear, support, and raise them rather than to the employers who hire those parents."[129] This decision put an end to fetal protection policies.

But at the same time that Blackmun argued that parents are the best judges and keepers of their children's well-being, others were making the opposite claim, making pregnant women criminally liable for damages transmitted *in utero.* The practices of performing medical procedures on pregnant women against their will, and of excluding some or all women from jobs exposing them to toxins dangerous to fetal development, took shape in the context of the 1970s and 1980s, but grew out of a much longer history of circumscribing and regulating women's rights as patients and as workers. In contrast, although the belief that drug and alcohol use by pregnant women posed risks to fetal health can also be traced back to the late nineteenth century, the practice of criminally prosecuting pregnant women for fetal neglect and abuse was a phenomenon unknown before the 1980s.

In 1973, investigative reporter Geraldo Rivera hosted a special report on WABC-TV entitled *The Littlest Junkie,* in which he explored the problem of heroin addiction in infants born to addicted mothers. As the show began, the following statistic scrolled down the screen: "In 1966, about 300 addicted babies were born here [New York City]. By 1972, it was around 1,500. Right now, 1 out of every 40 babies born in city hospitals is born a heroin addict. And in some hospitals it is as high as 1 in 25."[130] Displayed behind that text, images of a heroin-addicted baby experiencing withdrawal convulsions alternated with images of the by-now-familiar Lennart Nilsson image of the *in utero* fetus (figure 4.2). In one segment, Rivera took to the streets of Harlem, interviewing pregnant women who were either high on heroin or looking to get high, and interviewed the doctors and nurses who treat the addicted babies. He interviewed a social worker who told him about a mother who "shoots up her baby" to keep it quiet. Although Rivera told the viewers that the problem of heroin addiction crosses

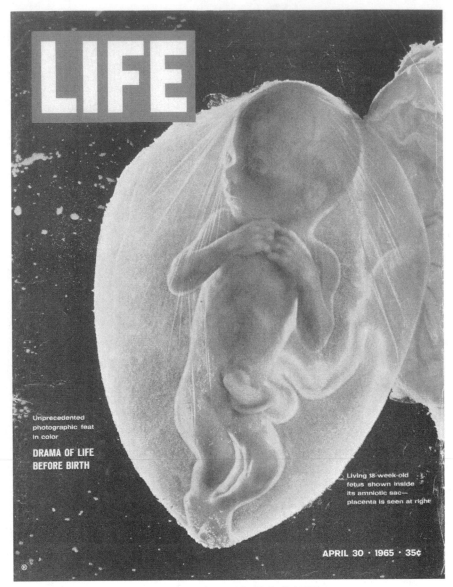

Figure. 4.2 Lennard Nilsson, *Life*, Vol. 58, no. 17, 30 April 1965.

racial, social, and economic lines, every one of the pregnant women addicts he interviewed was African-American.[131]

The racial iconography embedded in Rivera's program had very real consequences. A 1990 *New England Journal of Medicine* study concluded that although 15 percent of white women and 14 percent of African-American women used illegal drugs during pregnancy, African-American women were ten times more likely than white women to be reported to authorities.[132] Although a 1998 Department of Health and Human Services report on substance abuse founded that the "common stereotype, fostered by the media...that some 'racial' or ethnic groups use drugs more than others...is not borne out by the data," women of color were consistently represented disproportionately in the numbers of pregnant women arrested for drug use.[133] In 1990, the Reproductive Freedom Project of the American Civil Liberties Union estimated that 70 percent of the prosecutions for prenatal abuse were targeted at women of color, a statistic that Dr. Ira Chasnoff explains more anecdotally: "When a woman walks into a hospital in Pinellas County, and this is not, I can guarantee you, only in Pinellas County, if she walks into a hospital and has just used drugs, a black woman has a ten times higher chance of being reported into the [child protection] system than a white woman."[134] Legal scholar Dorothy E. Roberts questions the motives behind these patterns. "If the government were truly concerned about the health of Black infants," she asked, "why hasn't there been a material commitment to ensuring that pregnant women in poor communities receive high quality pre-natal care?"[135] In distinguishing between pointing a cultural spotlight on black fetuses and demonstrating a "material commitment" to them, Roberts demanded an accounting of the relationship between cultural politics and the political economy.

One way to begin that accounting process is to examine what purpose the ideology of fetal rights served in late-twentieth-century American political culture. Beginning in the 1980s, the Republican party exploited images of neglectful mothers and innocent fetuses to create a sense of crisis about "crack mothers" and "crack babies." Blaming individual mothers for social problems created a perceived crisis that fed into an ascendant political culture of conservatism, a culture committed to exposing the dangerous consequences of unrestrained liberalism.

"Crack mothers" were not the first women to have their drug use or addiction condemned on the grounds that it undermined their ability to fulfill their maternal destiny, but interpretations of the dangers of maternal drug use changed along with changing cultural anxieties about motherhood. Physicians in the 1880s adopted a eugenic discourse, in which they attacked "ignorant," "lazy," and "backward" women who indulged in opiates during their pregnancies, and blamed them for causing qualities of "restlessness" and "moral and mental weakness" in their offspring.[136] These physicians expressed relief that most of those infants would die because "the moral and mental strength of these children is so far below par as to make them liable to much subsequent suffering."[137]

In the 1920s, concerns about the decadence of the New Woman inflected condemnations of "opium vampires," pregnant women "rich in idleness and money…ambitious and well-born…[who] under the influence of the drug they stop at nothing in their adventures in opium…even drugging their unborn babies for the sake of a night on the town."[138] In her 1926 exposé of heroin addiction, *Opium: The Demon Flower*, Sara Graham-Mulhall concluded that "no addict mother [should] be allowed to care for her addict baby…. [Their] cells and nerves are so impregnated with the poison of the narcotic…that it is impossible for them to beget a healthy child."[139]

In the 1950s, experts blamed addicted women for giving birth to "monstrous neonates," but also blamed overprotective and neurotic mothers for the "frightening wave" of heroin addiction.[140] In 1960, Dr. Robert J. Chessick relied on contemporary psychoanalytic theories to explain that "to the addict, the drug has become equivalent to the milk and love he received as an infant." Addiction, he explained, was an "oral fixation," an "ongoing search for the breast" that resulted from "a frustrating, denying, seductive mother."[141] *The Road to H*, a 1964 analysis of the causes and consequences of this crisis, argued that mothers of addicts were "usually insecure women, concealing their conflicts and insecurities behind a facade of efficiency, responsibility, and excessive mothering; they were usually religious and prone to preaching; they were opinionated, judgmental, rigid, authoritarian, and dictatorial."[142]

Experts throughout the twentieth century targeted women as dangerous producers and reproducers of addiction and its consequences, but changing ideas about race, class, and gender shaped those discourses of blame in particular ways. When analyzing the heroin crisis of the 1950s, for example, physicians identified race as a contributory factor, but only in the context of urban poverty, rather than as a biological or cultural category. Between 1950 and 1959, obstetrician Dr. Roy Stern compiled a study of pregnant women addicted to narcotics at Metropolitan Hospital of New York Medical College, in which he concluded that 40.9 percent of the sixty-six subjects of his study showed obstetrical complications as compared to 15.6 percent of the rest of pregnant patients at the hospital.[143] But for Stern, the disease and consequences of addiction could not be extracted from the social and economic context in which these women lived. Addiction went hand-in-hand with poor nutrition and minimal prenatal care. Attributing these obstetrical complications to addiction, rather than to nutrition and health care, missed the point:

> Because the factor of addiction is combined in our sample with poor prenatal care…we have no way of knowing whether the obstetrical complications which occur during these pregnancies are due in any way to the drug

use or whether they are due to the poor prenatal care which they receive.... The best approach would be for an intensive and immediate program to be started with the addict should she present herself to the clinic at any time during her pregnancy.[144]

Stern's emphasis on treatment, rather than on punishment, reflected the contemporary understanding of drug addiction as a disease, rather than as a crime. The U.S. Supreme Court embraced this understanding in its 1962 decision in the case of *Robinson v. California,* which found that California could not "criminalize the condition, status, or affliction of addiction, even if an addicted person engaged in illegal acts such as narcotics purchase, sale, use, or antisocial or disorderly behavior."[145] Addicts, Justice William O. Douglas argued, were in the grip of a power beyond their control and should be considered no guiltier than "babies who get the drug while in the womb from their mothers who are addicts."[146] Neither the baby nor its mother, he argued, would be better served by imprisonment than treatment.

In the 1970s, as U.S. drug policy reconceptualized addiction as a crime to be punished rather than as a disease to be treated, addicted pregnant women became treated as perpetrators of a crime, rather than as victims of a disease.[147] Between 1977 and 1998, at least two hundred women in thirty states were prosecuted for crimes of "fetal abuse."[148] Some of the earliest cases were preemptive efforts to regulate the behavior of pregnant women in the name of protecting their fetuses. In 1981, for example, a Louisiana juvenile court had, in response to a welfare agency's report that a pregnant teenager was neglecting herself and thus harming her fetus, taken jurisdiction of a woman's fetus by confining the teenager to a hospital for the last two months of her pregnancy.[149] In 1984, an Illinois judge made a fetus a ward of the state, finding a pregnant woman addicted to heroin was in violation of state child abuse statutes.[150]

More frequent than detaining women during their pregnancies were prosecutors' efforts to punish women after they gave birth for crimes—including child neglect, child abuse, delivering drugs to minors, corrupting a minor, and assault with a deadly weapon—perpetrated against their fetuses while they were pregnant.[151] In 1977, after giving birth to twins exhibiting heroin withdrawal symptoms, Margaret Reyes was accused by the district attorney of San Bernardino County of felony child endangerment, making California the first state to charge a woman for a crime against her fetus.[152] In 1985, after she had given birth to a baby who tested positive for amphetamines immediately after delivery, Pamela Rae Stewart was accused by the district attorney of San Diego

County of "willfully failing to provide necessary care for a child."[153] In 1987, Jennifer Clarise Johnson, after giving birth to a baby who tested positive for cocaine, was accused by the district attorney of Sanford, Florida, of delivering a controlled substance to a minor through her umbilical cord.[154] Each of these cases was overturned on appeal or dismissed. Reyes' conviction was overturned by an appellate court, which found that the relevant child abuse statute applied to harm done to a child, not a fetus.[155] Stewart's case was dismissed on the same grounds in 1986 by municipal court Judge E. MacAmos, who suggested that the state could pass a different law "protecting the unborn from abuse by its mother."[156] Johnson's conviction was overturned in 1992 by the Supreme Court of Florida, which found that "prosecuting women for using drugs and 'delivering' them to their newborns appears to be the least effective response to this crisis. Rather than face the possibility of prosecution, pregnant women who are substance abusers may simply avoid prenatal care for fear of being detected."[157]

In light of these and similar decisions, states began following MacAmos's suggestion that the problem needed to be addressed legislatively. Between 1986 and 1998, thirty-five states passed laws dealing with prenatal narcotics exposure.[158] Some states required that hospitals notify social service agencies of evidence of prenatal drug exposure, some required pregnant women receiving state assistance to undergo drug-screening tests at their prenatal visits, some treated evidence of prenatal drug exposure as *prima facie* evidence of child abuse, and some required pregnant women with substance abuse problems to participate in drug treatment programs.[159]

This last policy seems reasonable until one takes into account the fact that federal funding for government health programs had been eroding during the 1980s, and that women—particularly pregnant women, more particularly pregnant women with substance abuse problems, and most particularly low-income pregnant women with substance abuse problems—were disproportionately affected by these budget cuts. Public health experts Rae Banks and Assata Zerai found that between 1977 and 1984, maternal and child health block grants were reduced by one-third, leading to cutbacks on well-baby, prenatal, and immunization clinics, and that between 1981 and 1991, the budget for the National Health Services Corps was reduced by 64 percent, leading to a reduction in physicians working in low-income neighborhoods.[160] In 1990, Dr. Wendy Chavkin found that that 54 percent of drug treatment programs in New York City did not accept pregnant women, 67 percent of them did not accept women who relied on Medicaid for payment, and 84 percent of them did not accept pregnant women addicted to crack.[161] In 1991, in Florida, there were an estimated 135 residential treatment beds available for pregnant women, and an estimated 4,500

pregnant women who needed them. In 1989, the year Jennifer Johnson was prosecuted for fetal abuse, there was a waiting list of 2,000 women for those 135
beds.[162] In addition to the shortage of treatment options, few available programs
provided childcare, requiring women already at odds with social service agencies
to leave their children in foster care in order to get treatment.[163]

Two stories—one about a woman in Virginia and one about a hospital in New
York City—illustrate the hurdles and risks facing pregnant women trying to get
help for their addiction. When Britta Smith realized that she was pregnant in 1991,
she began calling as many drug treatment programs in the Roanoke, Virginia area
as she could find, hoping that one could help her with her cocaine problem. After
finding that none of the programs accepted Medicaid, Smith went to her local
emergency room for advice. In accordance with Virginia law, the nurse there called
in child protective services, whereupon Smith was charged with child abuse, and
placed under probation, but not given any treatment.[164] In 1993, ACLU attorney
Joan Bertin represented a group of women in a sex discrimination suit against
Harlem's Joint Disease and North General Hospital. The public hospital had a
fifty-bed, in-patient detoxification program, a program that automatically
excluded pregnant women, including the plaintiffs in this case. The hospital
argued that its policy was not discriminatory because it was based on the fact that
the hospital "lacks the equipment to treat them [pregnant women] safely, it has no
obstetricians on its staff and it is not licensed to render obstetrical care." The ACLU
contended that "the blanket exclusion of all pregnant women is medically unwarranted, that each woman must be assessed individually to determine whether she
can be treated safely for substance abuse." A lower court agreed with the hospital
that excluding pregnant substance abusers did not constitute gender-based
discrimination but, rather, was "a medical determination based on appropriate
treatment for its patients." Even though the court of appeals overturned that
decision, it did not require the hospital to increase its services.[165]

Although Congress enacted no federal laws similar to those passed at the
state level, a series of congressional hearings in 1989 and 1990—luridly titled
"Falling Through the Crack," "Born Hooked," and "Addicted Babies"—illustrate
the national mobilization around the issue of prenatal drug exposure. The hearings, which detailed the dangers posed by pregnant women addicted to drugs to
the "generation of citizens as yet unborn" and "our most vulnerable unborn citizens," were part of a national obsession with the crack epidemic.[166] In the late
1980s and 1990s, newspapers, magazines, and television were full of stories doc-
umenting the devastating effects of cocaine and predicting a lost generation
irredeemably damaged by the effects of their mother's cocaine use. In its May 13,
1991, cover story on "Crack Kids," *Time* magazine ran photographs of hospital-
ized babies—all African-American—born addicted to crack. The photographs

had captions reading, "[T]heir mothers used drugs, and now their children suffer," and "[A] mother's sad legacy: Can the innocent legacies of drug use be rescued?"[167] Earlier that year, a *New York Times* article on crack babies quoted a teacher from the Bronx saying, "I can't say for sure it's crack, but I can say that in all my years of teaching I've never seen so many functioning at low levels."[168]

The congressional hearings linked this national obsession with the "crack babies," characterized as a "biologic underclass" constituting a "threat to national security," with anxieties about changing gender roles and about the changing role of the United States in a post-Cold War global economy.[169] According to this scenario, crack babies were caused by women's rejection of their natural biological roles and, in turn, caused the decline of the nation's political and economic security. California Governor Pete Wilson (R) described this phenomenon in the following way:

> One of the most tragic and insidious aspects of crack use by a pregnant woman is that it seems to almost destroy the maternal instinct....The long-term implications for America are truly staggering in terms of who will be the earning members of a society in a social security system and whether or not...America can remain competitive in the global marketplace.[170]

Witnesses repeatedly testified that crack addiction was undermining women's natural "maternal instincts," contributing to the belief that pregnant addicts were producing, as social scientist Nancy Campbell put it in her 2000 book *Using Women: Gender, Drug Policy, and Social Justice,* "a lost generation of untouchable newborns who would become the horrifying crack addicts who weighted not just our heart strings but also our purse strings, and the kite strings that draw our national ambitions aloft."[171]

In her analysis of these hearings, Campbell argued that, "the deflection of responsibility for social problems...onto figures that embody them is a consistent pattern in the policy-making apparatus of liberal democratic capitalism. In the governing mentalities of drug policy makers, women who lack maternal instincts produce the structural effects of economic erosion and neighborhood disintegration."[172] This process was, Campbell argued, part of the efforts by conservative think tanks and legislators to:

> [d]einsitutionalize U.S. government responsibility for social provision. By deflecting "responsibility" onto the individualized figure of the "parent," they detached social from individual responsibility; thus employers and the government were not responsible for providing individuals with the means to meet their responsibilities. Individual "parents" are assumed already to possess the ways and means to reproduce society in a vacuum of support.[173]

Campbell characterized this process as "postmodern Progressivism," a term she coined to explain how the "expansive Progressivism of the early twentieth century" was transfigured "in the context of the ideological contraction of the state's responsibility for social provision."[174] This transfigured progressivism was expressed in rhetoric and policies that attributed social problems to individuals' behavior, demanded solutions based on personal responsibility, and were championed by a new movement within the Democratic Party, led by the Democratic Leadership Council.

Recognizing that one of the triumphs of Reaganism was the discrediting, even demonization of, traditional liberalism, Al From founded the Democratic Leadership Council in 1985, an organization that recognized the changed political landscape and hoped to stake a new claim in it by developing policies, championing candidates, and gaining a voice in the Democratic Party and the public sphere.[175] An advisor to Ed Muskie and Jimmy Carter in the 1970s, From was the executive director of the House Democratic Caucus from 1981 to 1985, which gave him a front-seat view of the successes of the Republicans and failures of the Democrats to capture the public imagination and shape public policy. The DLC worked to define a governing philosophy based on a "third way" that rejected the existing paradigms of right/left and conservatism/liberalism by trying to redefine the center of the Democratic Party. The central principles of the DLC included the beliefs that the government should promote equal opportunity, but not special privileges; that the best generator of economic growth is the private sector; and that government programs should be "grounded in the values most Americans share: work, family, personal responsibility, individual liberty, tolerance, faith, and inclusion."[176] These values were associated with policies like charter schools, free trade, and welfare reform, and with commitments to privatization and devolution; programs and commitments that challenged some of the basic beliefs and interests of traditional Democratic constituencies and that overlapped with some of the basic beliefs and interests of the Republican Party. The valorization of individuality that included the fetus, and the backlash against women's rights and reproductive rights that was expressed in language about protecting the fetus combined to generate an ideology of fetal rights that fit into this more conservative political culture.

Only seven years after its founding, the DLC saw the presidency of the United States go to its own former chairman. In 1992, Bill Clinton led his realigned Democratic Party to victory with the principles of the DLC, including the position that abortion should be "safe, legal, and rare."[177] In his first State of the Union address, he promised the "end of welfare as we know it," and few offered a defense of the welfare system that had, in the words of Representative Charles Rangel (D-NY), created a "new class of one in five Americans who had no stake in the civic culture and conventional values that bind us together as one nation...[and] threaten to unspool the basic tenets of our economic and social infrastructure." Rangel did not, however, blame individual women for this phenomenon, but saw the "crack baby" crisis as a "symptom of a wholesale disintegration of essential social and economic infrastructures, which once created opportunity, assured public health, provided affordable housing, put food on the table, and extended to all our citizens the hope that they could share in the American dream."[178] Senator Daniel Patrick Moynihan (D-NY), whose 1965 report "The Negro Family: The Case for National Action" had sparked decades of controversial debate about the causes and solutions to what he described as the "deterioration of the Negro family" and the resulting "tangle of pathology" in the African-American population, offered a different analysis. He suggested that the "concentration of crack babies in the inner city," resulted from "teen pregnancy rates, high illegitimacy rates, and welfare receipt."[179] In short, for Moynihan, crack babies represented the dangers of the welfare state; for Rangel, they represented the dangers of an absent welfare state. For Clinton, they represented an opportunity to test out his new vision of government.

Three months after the 1994 Congressional elections put the Republicans in charge for the first time since 1954, in his second State of the Union address, Clinton declared that the "era of big government was over."[180] Clinton's speech represented an accommodation to the ideology of the new Republican Party, led by Newt Gingrich. The newly elected Republican Congress had put forth what they called a Contract with America, in which they called for, among other things, lower taxes and welfare reform. Eighteen months later, President Clinton signed into law the Personal Responsibility and Work Opportunity Reconciliation Act of 1996, better known as the Welfare Reform Act.[181] Written by a Republican Congress, it passed the Senate by a vote of 74 to 24, and although it more accurately reflected the ideas and ideals of the Republicans than the Democrats, it also grew out of Clinton's original promise and political philosophy. The main goal of the act was to replace welfare with work, and it included work participation requirements, established a cumulative lifetime limit of five years of benefits paid by federal dollars, cut food stamps, and made legal immigrants ineligible for food stamps or Supplemental Security Income.[182] Senator Edward Kennedy (D-MA) voted against the bill and characterized it as "legislative child abuse." Harris Wofford, former Democratic senator of Pennsylvania and head of the National Service Corps, responded to the passage of the bill by saying that "if the era of big government is over, the era of the big citizen had better begin."[183] Kennedy was talking about the children of legal immigrants and welfare recipients who would suffer as a result of cutbacks, and Wofford was talking about the need for voluntarism and community activism to fill the void of federally funded programs. But from another perspective, the big citizen still seen as deserving of state protection was the fetus.

South Carolina was in the vanguard of the movement to establish and protect this unborn citizen, a movement led by Charles Condon, first as the solicitor of Charleston and then as the attorney general of the state. Born in Charleston to an Irish-Catholic Democratic family, Condon had always been a staunch opponent of abortion and of the death penalty. When he ran for solicitor of Charleston County in 1980, the local party leaders persuaded him to change his position on the death penalty to make him more electable. He won, becoming the youngest solicitor in South Carolina history at the age of twenty-seven. In 1990, he changed parties because he no longer felt "at home" in the Democratic Party, and in 1994, he was elected attorney general as a Republican. His opponent in that race, Dick Harpootlian, criticized Condon's political opportunism, saying that "he has the ability to disabuse himself of any beliefs he had and to adopt the beliefs that 51 percent of the people have at that moment."[184] University of South Carolina political scientist David Lublin describes Condon as "willing to do anything to court the Republican right-wing electorate" and ready to "take clever political advantage of the backlash against the 'moral looseness.'"[185] Whatever his true beliefs might have been, Condon represented a larger trend of populist conservative politicians, the southern version of Reagan Democrats, who depended upon social issues and cultural symbols to build an electoral majority.

In 1989, as Charleston County solicitor, Condon worked with the Charleston Police Department and the Medical University of South Carolina (MUSC) to develop and implement what they called the "Interagency Policy on Cocaine Abuse in Pregnancy." This policy allowed MUSC to surreptitiously test for cocaine any pregnant woman who showed indications of poor prenatal care, preterm labor, poor fetal growth, prenatal birth defects, drug or alcohol use, or intrauterine fetal death. Any positive cocaine results were then sent from the hospital to law enforcement officers, who would come to the hospital to arrest the woman who tested positive. The policy held that if the woman was less than twenty-seven weeks pregnant, she would be charged with possession; if she was twenty-eight or more weeks pregnant, she would be charged with delivering drugs to a minor; and if she gave birth while testing positive, she would also be charged with child neglect. In 1990, the prosecutor's office added an "amnesty" incentive, allowing women who tested positive the option of drug treatment to avoid arrest. Those who failed to follow through on treatment or who tested positive a second time would be arrested.[186] The hospital described this policy as intended to encourage these women to seek out and stay in treatment, rather than go to jail.

Other hospitals tested the babies rather than the women, a policy with similar goals and similar results. Cornelia Whitner, a twenty-eight-year-old woman from Pickens County, South Carolina, gave birth February 22, 1992, to her third child, a healthy baby boy, at the Easley Baptist Medical Center. Tevin Whitner showed no symptoms of damage, but when traces of cocaine were found in his urine, the hospital notified child welfare services, and Whitner was charged with criminal child neglect for using an illicit drug during the third trimester of her pregnancy. She pled guilty to child neglect charges, hoping to get into a drug treatment program. Her court-appointed lawyer explained to the court that Whitner was in a counseling program, had been clean since giving birth to Tevin, and requested that Whitner be placed in a residential treatment center. Judge Frank Eppes rejected the request, saying, "I think I'll just let her go to jail," and sentenced her to eight years in prison. The ACLU challenged her conviction, arguing that a fetus was not a child under the child neglect statute and that Whitner had had inadequate counsel who had not advised her that the statute might not apply to prenatal drug use. The court of appeals agreed, finding that the child neglect law did not apply to prenatal drug use, issuing an order for post-conviction relief, and releasing Whitner from prison after nineteen months. The state appealed that decision, and in October of 1997, when the South Carolina Supreme Court upheld the original conviction, it became the highest court in the land to uphold a conviction for delivering drugs to a minor *in utero*. The court had set itself the task of determining whether or not it had been the legislature's intent to include the fetus in the child endangerment statute and found that "the plain meaning of 'child' as used in the statute includes a viable fetus":

> The abuse or neglect of a child at any time during childhood can exact a profound toll on the child herself as well as on society as a whole, however the consequences of abuse or neglect which takes place after birth often pale in comparison to those resulting from abuse suffered by the viable fetus before birth. This policy of prevention supports a reading of the word "person" to include viable fetuses.[187]

The U.S. Supreme Court refused to hear Whitner's appeal, so the South Carolina Supreme Court's decision stands as of 2008, leaving pregnant women in South Carolina liable for behavior—even legal behavior such as drinking and smoking—deemed potentially harmful to the fetus.

The decision also meant that Cornelia Whitner was sent back to prison to fulfill her sentence. In a 1999 letter she wrote to the governor of South Carolina, she described her situation:

> I know that I did wrong by smoking crack while pregnant but I was sick with the worst addiction anyone could ever have.... I feel like I am being wrong-

fully punished. And it's not fair to me or my children.... I just want you to see how bad I have been treated because I was sick with a crack cocaine addiction. It wasn't like I refused treatment. I could not even get help from the sentencing judge and I did ask.... I feel like I was made an example of because I am poor and black.[188]

Although acknowledging her personal responsibility for her situation, Whitner also made clear that she saw the entire process as unfair. The governor did not respond to Whitner's letter, and she remained in prison until 2001.

Condon praised the decision, calling it a "landmark decision for protecting children" and claiming that "a viable fetus is a citizen and a fellow South Carolinian," deserving of the state's protection. "If you can't protect babies," he asked, "who can you protect?"[189] He described the U.S. Supreme Court's refusal to hear the case a "big, big victory for the babies of South Carolina."[190] In Condon's office was a photograph of Patrick J. Buchanan with an inscription reading, "To Charlie Condon, who is saving lives while others prattle on about the rights of drug addicts."[191] For Condon, the Whitner decision was part of much larger cultural struggle. "This decision is much more in line with American culture," he said. "A fetus has inalienable rights that come from God."[192]

Although Condon advocated "fetal rights" as part of his struggle to push back against what he saw as the dangerous excesses of liberalism, people like Wyndi Anderson, the director of the South Carolina Advocates for Pregnant Women, saw that connection quite differently, as part of a historic effort to oppress and demonize African Americans. Noting that Condon was both the "greatest advocate" of policies criminalizing pregnant women's behavior and someone who "staunchly defends the state's policy of flying the Confederate flag," Anderson said that she and her organization "believe that it is no coincidence that the only state that continues to fly the Confederate flag is also the only state that jails African-American women who continue their pregnancies despite drug problems." She went on to explain that what she calls Condon's "uniquely punitive" policy was "first introduced and applied to African-American women who were taken out of their hospital beds in chains and shackles." The evocative language pitting the chains and shackles of slavery against the Confederate flag makes clear how closely entwined racial politics were with reproductive politics, and set the stage for the next legal challenge to South Carolina's policy, a challenge that was as much about race as it was about women's rights.

At the same time that Whitner's case was making its way through the legal system, MUSC was confronted with a lawsuit challenging the constitutionality of their testing policy. In October 1993, ten African-American women filed a civil suit against the hospital, claiming that the policy was racially discrimina-tory. It violated the Equal Protection Clause of the Fourteenth Amendment, they argued, as well as their Fourth Amendment right to be free of "unreason-able searches" and their constitutional right to privacy. The women described their ordeal in graphic language. Lori Griffin went to the MUSC for prenatal care, and without her consent, her urine was tested for cocaine. "After I got dressed three policeman came in, put handcuffs and shackles on me and told me I was under arrest for distribution of cocaine to a minor," she said. Sandra Powell describes an even more dramatic scenario. Immediately after giving birth at MUSC, she was told that her urine tested positive for cocaine and that she would be immediately arrested for unlawful neglect of a child. "I just had a baby, I was still bleeding, I was still in pain.... Before that day was over I was in jail.... I felt so ashamed because I [didn't] know what I had done for them to treat me like that." After testing positive for cocaine, Crystal Ferguson explained her eager-ness to enter an outpatient drug program. "I had no problem with getting treatment, my problem was I couldn't go inpatient because I had two other chil-dren," she said. Because there were no places in outpatient programs available, she was arrested.[193] Other women had similar experiences of being misled, coerced, and misinformed, but nonetheless, a federal judge rejected their request for an injunction requiring the hospital to suspend drug testing.

Three months later, the women, represented by the Center for Reproductive Law and Policy (CLRP), filed a complaint with the National Institutes of Health (NIH), claiming that MUSC was "engaging in research on human subjects without obtaining the necessary institutional review and patient consent." Under the direction of Secretary of Health and Human Services Donna Shalala, the Office for Civil Rights (OCR) of the Department of Health and Human Services initiated an investigation into MUSC for possible violations of Title VI, the federal law that prohibits discrimination in federally funded programs. Marie Chretien, regional manager of OCR, investigated the women's charges and reported back to Shalala that the policy "results in an adverse dispropor-tionate impact on African-American women." All but one of the women arrested were African-American, and Shirley Brown, the obstetrics nurse running the program, noted on the one white woman's chart that she "lives with her boy-friend who is a Negro."[194] The OCR notified the MUSC of this finding, reminded hospital administrators that federal funding could be not be used to support a discriminatory program and warned them that if they did not voluntarily comply with government requirements, the NIH would initiate "administrative proceedings to terminate federal financial assistance."[195]

Rather than lose government funding, the hospital abandoned its policy of drug testing, a decision that angered Condon, who attacked the "liberal sensibilities of Donna Shalala and Bill Clinton," the "liberal, feminist, New-York based" CRLP, and the "politically correct resolutions" from the American Medical Association and the American Pediatrics Association, for putting "a gun to the hospital's head."[196] He characterized Clinton and Shalala as being "ideologically driven by the absurd notion that a woman's privacy rights overrule a mother's most basic responsibility to her own child," and he defended the program against charges of racism, arguing that "the hospital serves a primarily indigent population, and most of the patient population is black."[197] But the women convicted of child endangerment before the hospital discontinued its drug-testing policy did not stop when their case had forced the hospital to stop the program; they appealed their case to the U.S. Supreme Court.

The Supreme Court agreed to hear the case, and on March 21, 2001, in the case of *Crystal Ferguson et al v. City of Charleston,* six justices agreed with the women, finding that the hospital's policy was discriminatory and an unconstitutional violation of women's fourth amendment privacy rights.[198] Writing for the majority, Justice John Paul Stevens dismissed the state's argument that drug testing pregnant women falls under the "special needs" exception of the Fourth Amendment's protection against unreasonable searches and seizures, and emphasized the importance of confidentiality in the medical context. Pregnant women, he wrote, should rely upon "the reasonable expectation of privacy enjoyed by the typical patient undergoing diagnostic tests in a hospital [which] is that the results of those tests will not be shared with nonmedical personnel without her consent."[199]

The court also agreed with the plaintiff's argument that MUSC's policy disproportionately targeted low-income women of color, whose reliance on public medical services made them far more likely to have their drug use detected and reported than were middle-class white women using private medical facilities with higher standards of privacy and confidentiality. Additionally, the court held that a number of the criteria used to trigger testing under the MUSC policy had little to do with drug use per se and had much more to do with poverty. For example, the hospital tested women who had received little or no prenatal care. Yet, with fewer resources and less access to medical services than middle-class women, poor women were more likely to delay seeking prenatal care until relatively late in pregnancy or to obtain no prenatal care at all. Inadequate prenatal care contributes to conditions such as unexplained preterm labor, birth defects or poor fetal growth, separation of the placenta from the uterine wall, or intrauterine fetal death, all conditions that the MUSC policy also identified as grounds for testing pregnant patients.

The *Ferguson* decision suggested that fetal rights were going to have a limited legal life. Reproductive rights activists praised the *Ferguson* decision for its general protection of the integrity of women's rights. Catherine Weiss, director of the ACLU's Reproductive Freedom Project, lauded Steven's opinion for underscoring the fact that "pregnant women have as great a right to privacy, bodily integrity, and autonomy as other free adults" and for recognizing that "women do not become wards of the state or forfeit their constitutional rights when they become pregnant." Julie Sternberg, an attorney with the Reproductive Freedom Project and the author of the ACLU's legal brief in the case, commended the decision as being "especially important to low-income women who disproportionately use public hospitals where the risk of collaboration with law enforcement is greatest."[200]

Public health experts also championed the decision, as most agreed that prosecuting for fetal abuse pregnant women taking illegal drugs was bad medicine and bad public policy. Studies on drug use during pregnancy consistently show that the abuse of other substances, both legal and illegal, can harm fetal development as much as or more than cocaine, making it clear that singling out cocaine was not scientifically justifiable.[201] Deborah Frank, a public health and pediatric expert at Boston University and author of the 1992 comprehensive study analyzing the impact of maternal cocaine use on fetal and child development, argued that the law distorts the effect cocaine has on unborn children. Although prenatal illegal drug use by women does have negative effects on infants, she found that its effects are no more severe than if the woman smoked or drank alcohol during pregnancy. Frank concluded that poverty remained the overwhelming cause of most of the infants' problems. Medical associations and public health organizations repeatedly emphasized the fact that the policy did more harm than good. Sternberg's brief argued that "intertwining medical care with law enforcement not only violates pregnant women's constitutional rights and the confidentiality of the doctor-patient relationship, it also deters them from seeking prenatal care."[202]

Amici curiae briefs submitted by, among others, the American Medical Association, the American College of Obstetricians and Gynecologists, the March of Dimes, and the American Public Health Association argued that prosecuting women for their behavior during pregnancy was more likely to prevent pregnant women using drugs from seeking prenatal care or drug treatment than it was to deter them from taking drugs in the first place.[203] Susan Dunn, counsel for South Carolina Advocates for Pregnant Women, put it this way: "The word on the street is that it is much more likely that your kids will be taken away from you if you go for help."[204] A 1997 study of two drug treatment programs in Columbia, South Carolina, indicate a precipitous drop in the number of pregnant women entering their facilities, a finding that supports these fears. Between 1996 and 1997, one clinic admitted 80 percent fewer pregnant women than it had the previous year; the other clinic saw 54 percent fewer pregnant women during the same time period.[205]

Although the Supreme Court decision in the *Ferguson* case ruled against the MUSC policy, it did not overrule the *Whitner* decision upholding the state statute defining a viable fetus as a person. Only two months after the *Ferguson* decision, on May 15, 2001, a South Carolina jury in Horry County deliberated for fifteen minutes before finding Regina McKnight, a twenty-four-year-old African-American woman with an IQ of 72, guilty of homicide. McKnight had dropped out of high school in 1992, after completing tenth grade, and she lived with her mother until her mother was killed in a car accident in 1998. Since then, McKnight had lived on the streets. In May of 1999, McKnight was eight and a half months pregnant and had received no medical care throughout her pregnancy. Feeling ill, she went to the emergency room at her local county hospital, Conway Hospital. Several hours later, McKnight gave birth to a stillborn girl. Both she and her baby tested positive for cocaine, and McKnight was subsequently arrested and charged with homicide by child abuse.

Her defense lawyer called upon a Charleston pathologist, who testified that it was impossible to determine the cause of nearly 40 percent of stillbirths, but the prosecution called upon two others who attributed the death of the baby to maternal cocaine use. Perhaps the jury was convinced by the prosecution's witnesses, or perhaps they agreed with prosecutor Bert Von Hermann's assessment of McKnight's behavior as "callous," an assessment he explained this way: "she only cried when she was sentenced...she slept through a lot of the trial. I don't think she showed that she really cared."[206] Whatever their reasons, McKnight was convicted, becoming the first woman in the country convicted of homicide for killing an unborn child through drug abuse. She was given a twenty-year sentence, suspended to twelve years in prison with no chance of parole. Condon praised the verdict as a "landmark case" illustrating South Carolina's position "on the cutting edge of protecting the innocent life of the unborn as well as the born.... Today, South Carolina's unborn children have a much better chance at a long, happy life than they did yesterday."[207]

Critics of the decision suggest that, as a black homeless woman, McKnight was an easy target for prosecutors looking for a test case. Out of the thirty women prosecuted for similar crimes, twenty-nine of them were black and none of them had private health insurance.[208] Despite these statistics, prosecutor Greg Hembree dismissed questions about whether McKnight's personal situation and identity affected his decision to prosecute. "When you don't have anything else to argue about, you argue about race and poverty," he said. "It didn't matter to me. It could've been a doctor's wife."[209] Be that as it may, McKnight and the vast majority of pregnant women prosecuted in South Carolina for crimes of fetal abuse were not the wives of doctors. On May 12, 2008, the South Carolina Supreme Court ruled that McKnight did not receive a fair trial, concluding that her counsel was "ineffective in her preparation of McKnight's defense through expert testimony and cross examination." Accepting a causal link between McKnight's cocaine use and the stillbirth was determined to be factual error, and failing to call medical experts as witnesses who could refute that link or using the most updated scientific studies were determined to a legal error. Regina McKnight was be released after nine years in prison, but the *Whitner* decision upholding the South Carolina statute that defines a fetus as a child or person in the child abuse and endangerment statute stands in the South Carolina Children's Code.[210]

Efforts to regulate and punish the behavior of pregnant women on behalf of the fetus have been, for the most part, technically unsuccessful in that higher courts have thus far overturned them. These efforts have succeeded, however, in contributing to a larger phenomenon of blaming social problems on individuals—particularly on relatively powerless individuals without resources—and thereby exempting from responsibility the more structural forces underpinning poverty, substance abuse, and inequality. It is in this sense, then, that the phenomenon of "fetal rights" can be understood as a referendum on the weakened liberalism of the late twentieth century.[211]

Using the fetus to demonize particular kinds of mothers impinges upon the rights of all women, but it also jeopardizes the inviolability of the rights of all citizens, and ignores the obligations of the state to protect those rights. The premise of an inevitable conflict between women's rights and fetal rights, a conflict resolvable only through privileging one set of rights over the other ignores the ways in which everyone's rights are called into question when one group's rights are made contingent, and obscures the social costs of fetal rights. Fetal rights may provide an inexpensive tool for corporations trying to skirt their responsibilities for creating workplaces safe for all workers, or for states trying to avoid treating substance abuse as a public health crisis, but they impose high costs on the rest of society. Fetal rights are paid for in the erosion of privacy, medical research, environmental protection, industrial safety, public health, and racial and economic justice. Accepting those costs as inevitable or making them invisible are the consequences of a liberalism premised upon the recognition of individual rights without a concomitant obligation of the state to ensure political, social, and economic justice for all its citizens.

CHAPTER 5
DEBATING FETAL PAIN,
1984–2007

On November 6, 2006, South Dakotans voted on the Women's Health and Human Life Protection Act, a bill that prohibited all abortions except those intended "to prevent the death of a pregnant mother," and claiming to "fully protect the rights, interests, and health of the pregnant mother; the rights, interest, and life of her unborn child, and the mother's fundamental natural intrinsic right to a relationship with her child."[1] One month later, on December 5, 2006, the Republican-controlled House of Representatives of the 109th Congress voted on the Unborn Child Pain Awareness Act, which, invoking notions of "informed consent" and a women's "right to know," required physicians to tell women seeking abortions after the twentieth week of pregnancy that "Congress finds that there is substantial evidence that the process of being killed in an abortion will cause the unborn child pain, even though you receive a pain-reducing drug or drugs."[2] Two days later, in the joined cases of *Gonzales v. Planned Parenthood of America* and *Gonzales v. Carhart,* the U.S. Supreme Court heard arguments about the constitutionality of the 2003 Partial Birth Abortion Ban Act, an act that described the procedure as one that "is not only unnecessary to preserve the health of the mother, but in fact poses serious risks to the long-term health of women and in some circumstances their lives."[3] Although the details and outcomes of these efforts differ—South Dakotans voted down the ban; Congress sent the bill back to committee; and the Supreme Court upheld the act—collectively, their shared assumption that abortions were dangerous and damaging to women, and their shared argument that these restrictions and regulations were intended to protect women, reconceptualized the maternal-fetal relationship in ways radically different from the one dominant in the post-*Roe* era while eerily similar to the one dominant in the late nineteenth-century movement to criminalize abortion.

Beginning in the 1980s, two new claims—that women were psychologically traumatized by abortion and that the fetus experienced pain during an abortion—were woven together by some antiabortion activists into a new rhetorical strategy that emphasized the ways that abortion hurt women and fetuses. In 1984, Dr. Bernard Nathanson used that strategy in his film *The Silent Scream,* in which he videotaped and narrated an abortion procedure performed on a twelve-week-old fetus.[4] In the 1990s, it emerged in a series of congressional debates about banning partial-birth abortions. By 2006, the South Dakota ban, the Unborn Child Pain Awareness Act, and the arguments for the constitutionality of the Partial Birth Abortion Ban, explicitly linked the interests of the woman with the interests of the fetus. And in 2007, in the *Gonzales v. Carhart* and *Gonzales v. Planned Parenthood Federation of America, Inc., et al.* decision, the Supreme Court gave their imprimatur to that link.[5] This rhetorical strategy was developed and deployed within a new political context—the growing influence of the religious right on the Republican Party, as reflected first in the 1980 election of Ronald Reagan, and subsequently in the 1994 election of a Republican majority in Congress, the increasing number of Republican-controlled state legislatures, and the 2000 and 2004 election of George W. Bush. It was also shaped by a new cultural context, represented by the increasing public presence of and pressure from the "family values" movement, as championed by organizations like the Moral Majority, the Christian Coalition, the Family Research Council, the Eagle Forum, and Focus on the Family. This strategy also operated within a new legal context, illustrated by the fact that Republican appointees constituted the majority of judges on ten out of thirteen federal appeals courts, and the replacement of the liberal Supreme Court Justice Thurgood Marshall with a conservative one, Clarence Thomas in 1991; and the replacement of the moderate defender of *Roe,* Sandra Day O'Connor with a conservative and vocal opponent of *Roe,* Samuel Alito in 2006.[6] Debates about fetal pain and partial birth abortion between 1984 and 2007 are best understood as a commentary on those changing circumstances, conflicting visions of motherhood and gender roles, and politicized struggles over the relative authority of scientific evidence and religious values, as well as a referendum on the sixties liberalism that had produced them.

Fetal politics subsequent to the *Roe* decision typically posited the interests of pregnant women and fetuses as distinct from one another, with opponents of legalized abortion emphasizing the fetus's right to life and advocates emphasizing the woman's right to choose.[7] This perceived conflict extended beyond abortion, impacting the rights of women in workplaces and medical care facilities.[8] Antiabortion activists in groups like Operation Rescue, Prisoners of Christ, and the Army of God adopted violent tactics that included bombing abortion clinics and assassinating abortion providers. Between 1977 and 1998, antiabortion activists were responsible for 269 bombings, arson attacks, or attempted bombings and attempted arson attacks on clinics; 790 bomb threats and death threats; 16 attempted murders, and 7 murders of doctors, clinic escorts, and clinic staff.[9] At the same time, groups like the National Right to Life Committee,

Americans United for Life, Concerned Women for America, and Focus on the Family were developing a less incendiary and more incrementalist antiabortion strategy that invoked a concern for women along with a concern for the unborn.[10] The mission statement of Americans United for Life (AUL) put it this way:

> The social experiment in abortion on demand, imposed by the judiciary in 1973, has disastrously failed by ending the lives of more than 30 million children while damaging the physical and emotional health of millions of women.... [A]bortion is a violent deception that results in two victims: the child whose life is destroyed, and the woman who suffers devastating physical and psychological harm.[11]

AUL's list of legislative objectives included one to "mandate standards for abortion clinics to protect the health and safety of women and correct often substandard conditions" and one to "inform women of the health risks of abortion including the link between abortion and breast cancer."[12] Similarly emphasizing abortion's impact on women, Focus on the Family's website quoted an anonymous woman's description of her experience after having undergone an abortion: "The following weeks and months brought a myriad of emotions. My relief quickly turned to grief.... Before long, I wanted to die.... My relationship ended.... I became promiscuous, drank, and experimented with lesbianism."[13] The National Right to Life Committee (NRLC) issued a pamphlet on "Abortion's Psycho-Social Consequences," warning that abortions may lead to psychological trauma, guilt, regret, divorce, promiscuity, child abuse, lesbianism, eating disorders, reckless behavior, substance abuse, and suicide.[14] Another NRLC pamphlet titled "Is Abortion Safe?" listed dangers including permanent infertility, hemorrhage, death, and breast cancer.[15] Concerned Women for America (CWA) similarly framed their opposition to abortion by emphasizing "the physical, emotional and spiritual harm to women, men and their families."[16] In a new iteration of arguments made during late nineteenth-century efforts to criminalize abortion, this approach intended to attract supporters in a "kinder gentler nation" who were turned off by the bombing of abortion clinics but might be drawn to a movement dedicated to protecting women while also protecting the fetus.[17] But then and now, these women-centered arguments against abortion obscure a much broader agenda than that single issue.

Just as antiabortion efforts at the turn of the twentieth century reflected a commitment to an ideology then called "separate spheres" so too do efforts at the turn of the twenty-first century reflect a commitment to an ideology of what its supporters call "family values." And just as the ideology of separate spheres encoded racial assumptions and class anxieties through prescribed traditional gender roles, so too does the ideology of family values.[18] For example, whereas nineteenth-century antiabortion activists like Horatio Storer worried about race suicide, today's antiabortion activists link the issue to immigration. In November 2006, the Missouri House of Representatives issued a report concluding that abortion was a factor in the rise of illegal immigration because it created a shortage of American-born workers. As its author Representative Edgar Emery (R) said, "If you kill 44 million of your potential workers, it's not too surprising we would be desperate for workers."[19] Dr. J. C. Willke—past president of the National Right to Life Committee, founder of the International Right to Life Federation, current president of Life Issues, and the originator of the "Why can't we love them both?" campaign, gave the following testimony in front of the South Dakota Taskforce to Study Abortion that was considering the Women's Health and Human Life Protection Act:

> Muslim countries forbid abortion. Furthermore they have large families....Germany's birth rate is 1.2....That is the Aryan Germans. What is happening? They're importing Turkish workers who do all of the more menial labor and right now there are over 1,500 mosques in Germany. The Muslim people in Germany have an average of four children. The Germans are having about one. So it's only a question of so many years and what do you think Germany is going to be? It's going to be a Muslim country.[20]

In conflating post-9/11 fears about Muslims with assertions about the relationship between legal abortion, economic imperatives, and immigration patterns in Germany, Wilke implicitly invites listeners to make those same connections in an American context. Phyllis Schlafly, president of the Eagle Forum and founder and chair of the Republican National Coalition for Life, has gone so far as to challenge the Fourteenth Amendment's guarantee of citizenship to anyone born in the United States, saying that "it's not the physical location of birth that defines citizenship, but whether your parents are citizens."[21] At the same time, though, the Republican National Coalition for Life endorses "legislation to make clear that the Fourteenth Amendment's protections apply to unborn children."[22] So, paradoxically, Schlafly and her organization argue against the Fourteenth Amendment's guarantee that "all persons born or naturalized in the United States and subject to the jurisdiction thereof, are citizens of the United States," while simultaneously arguing that the Fourteenth Amendment should apply to unborn children. It would appear that her suggestion is that the fetus should be considered a "person" with the attendant protections of due process and equal protection, but not a citizen, with the "privileges and immunities" associated with that status.

This contradiction troubles neither her nor Gary Bauer, past president of the Family Research Council and Republican presidential candidate in 2000, who worries that "hyphenated Americans put other countries and affiliations first, and they drive a wedge into the heart of 'one nation'" but also supports a human life bill that "defines unborn children as persons under the Fourteenth Amendment."[23] In *The Death of the West,* Patrick J. Buchanan clearly articulates the link between nativism and antiabortion arguments: "The West is dying. Its nations have ceased to reproduce, and their populations have stopped growing and begun to shrink. Not since the Black Death carried off a third of Europe in the fourteenth century has there been a graver threat to the survival of Western civilization."[24] At the same time that antiabortion and family values activists and organizations were focusing less on overturning *Roe* and more on trying to restrict abortion through partial-birth abortion bans, informed consent requirements, and waiting periods, and trying to protect the fetus through laws like the Unborn Victim of Violence Act, those same individuals and organizations began invoking arguments about fetal pain to link their "pro-life" politics to a larger worldview about the cultural fragility of a white Christian America.

The issue of fetal pain came to national attention on January 30, 1984 when, in a much-publicized address to the National Religious Broadcasters convention, President Ronald Reagan announced that "[m]edical science doctors confirm that when the lives of the unborn are snuffed out, they often feel pain, pain that is long and agonizing."[25] The contested nature of this claim was immediately exposed in the conflicting responses from physicians. The American College of Obstetricians and Gynecologists, representing the mainstream medical community's position, immediately issued the following statement:

> We know of no legitimate scientific information that supports the statement that a fetus experiences pain early in pregnancy. We do know that the cerebellum attains its final configuration in the seventh month and that mylenization of the spinal cord and the brain begins between the 20th and 40th weeks of pregnancy. These, as well as other neurological developments, would have to be in place for the fetus to receive pain. To feel pain, a fetus needs neurotransmitted hormones. In animals, these complex chemicals develop in the last third of gestation. We know of no evidence that humans are different.

At the same time, a group of twenty-six physicians rejected that statement in a public letter they wrote to Reagan, expressing their admiration for his success in "drawing the attention of people across the nation to the humanity and sensitivity of the human unborn."[26] For the antiabortion movement, resolving neurologists' debates about how to define, identify, and assess pain was ultimately less important than shifting the location of the fetal pain debate from peer-reviewed medical journals to emotionally charged public forums, changing the standard of proof from empirical evidence to visceral response, and transforming what had previously been a scientific and philosophical question about how to define and identify pain into an emotional and political one.[27]

Sympathetic physicians, lawyers, and philosophers bolstered this transformation. In his influential article "The Experience of Pain by the Unborn," Catholic philosopher and legal scholar John T. Noonan explained the strategic utility of the concept of fetal pain:

> We live in a society of highly developed humanitarian feeling, a society likely to respond to an appeal to empathy. There are those who either will not respond to an argument about killing because they regard the unborn as a kind of abstraction, or who will not look at actual death photographs of the aborted because they find the fact of death too strong to contemplate, but who nonetheless might respond to evidence of pain suffered in the process of abortion.[28]

Noonan's essay anticipated, albeit with a different political purpose, literary scholar Elaine Scarry's argument that pain is "something that cannot be denied and something that cannot be confirmed" and that the belief or disbelief in someone's pain serves as an "example of conviction, or alternatively, as an example of skepticism."[29] Historian Martin Pernick and journalist Annie Murphy Paul make the similar point that "pain has long played a special role in how society determines who is like us or not like us."[30] The differentiating power of pain is expressed in Shylock's question "If you prick us, do we not bleed?"; in the Grimm's fairy tale about a princess so sensitive that she could detect a pea buried beneath countless mattresses; and in nineteenth-century beliefs that blacks did not experience pain the same way that whites did.[31] Scarry's claim that "when some central idea or ideology or cultural construct has ceased to elicit a population's belief...the sheer material factualness of the human body will be borrowed to lend that cultural construct an aura of 'realness' and 'certainty,'" suggests why so much was at stake in arguments about fetal pain.[32] Explicitly adopting Noonan's antiabortion strategy and perhaps implicitly understanding Scarry's insights, Americans United for Life led the effort to invoke pain in its campaign to substantiate the fetal body.

AUL used their journal *Studies in Law and Medicine* as a platform from which antiabortion physicians could give their arguments the legitimacy of scientific authority, and could translate that realness and certainty, that material factualness, into political sway.[33] In "Fetal Pain and Abortion: The Medical Evidence," Dr. Vincent J. Collins, one of the physicians who had signed the letter supporting

Reagan, invoked the authority of data and evidence, but ultimately relied on making emotional claims to the heart:

> The prospect of fetal pain—pain that results from abortion—cuts through philosophical abstractions and scientific nomenclature, proceeding directly to the heart. A being that feels pain makes an urgent demand for recognition, a demand we know through the experience of our own bodies rather than because of any cool, deductive need in our minds for logical consistency.... The demand is based on empathetic or sympathetic impulses that have little to do with reason or notions of justice. Abortion is approved or tolerated largely because of feelings of sympathy with the pregnant woman...but an understanding of fetal pain...counterbalances the claim the woman makes on the emotions.[34]

Dr. Bernard Nathanson took this idea of inciting "empathetic or sympathetic impulses" on behalf of the fetus rather than on behalf of the woman outside of theory and put it into practice. One of the original founders of the National Association for the Repeal of Abortion Laws (NARAL), Nathanson had become a dedicated antiabortion activist in 1975.[35] After hearing Reagan's speech, Nathanson decided to make the argument for fetal pain visually, and he produced a twenty-eight-minute film of an abortion performed on a twelve-week-old fetus.[36] He introduced the purpose of the film: "Now, for the first time we have the technology to see abortion from the victim's vantage point. We are going to watch a child being torn apart, dismembered, disarticulated, crushed and destroyed by the unfeeling steel instruments of the abortionist." Throughout the film, Nathanson narrated ultrasound images, ascribing emotion, sensation, and intent to the twelve-week-old fetus, identified throughout as "the child": "The child will rear away from it [the suction cannula] and undergo much more violent, much more agitated movements. The child is now moving in a much more purposeful manner. The child is agitated and moves in a violent manner." Nathanson described the end of the procedure with the statement that would provide the title of the film: "We see the child's mouth open in a silent scream. This is the silent scream of a child threatened immediately with extinction."[37] Reverend Jerry Falwell, president of the Moral Majority, indicated his immediate understanding of the potential political power of this film, suggesting that it "may win the battle for us," and indeed, the NRLC distributed ten thousand prints of *The Silent Scream*, including copies to members of Congress and the justices of the Supreme Court.[38]

Leading neurologists and neuroembryologists challenged the basic assumptions of Nathanson's film, arguing that because a twelve-week fetus had not developed the nerve cell pathways in the cortex that would allow an electrical nerve impulse to travel from the brain to the muscle, it would be virtually impossible for a fetus at that developmental stage to experience pain. Dr. Robert Eiben, president of the National Child Neurology Society, said that it was a "desperately bad thing to imply" that fetuses felt pain.[39] Dr. Hart Peterson, acting chairman of pediatric neurology at New York Hospital at Cornell Medical Center in New York, said, "[T]he notion that a 12-week fetus screams in discomfort is erroneous."[40] Dr. Edwin C. Myer, chairman of the department of pediatric neurology at the Medical College of Virginia in Richmond, put it this way: "To make a statement that the fetus feels pain is a totally ridiculous statement. Pain implies cognition. There is no brain to receive the information."[41] Dr. Pasko Rakic, chairman of neuroanatomy at Yale University School of Medicine and one of the nation's leading experts in neuroembryology agreed, explaining that the absence of synapses in the cortex made it impossible to feel pain.

Planned Parenthood attacked the film for what it called "scientific, medical, and legal inaccuracies, misleading statements, and exaggerations," and convened a group of "internationally known and respected physicians" to identify the medical inaccuracies in the film.[42] Rejecting the claim that the twelve-week fetus experiences pain, these experts explained that "at this stage of pregnancy, the brain and nervous system are still in a very early stage of development.... Most brain cells are not developed. Without a cerebral cortex, pain impulses cannot be received or perceived."[43] The physicians also challenged Nathanson's description of the fetus moving in an "agitated" manner "in an attempt to avoid suction cannula."[44] Fetal movement, the physicians said, "is reflexive in nature, rather than purposeful, since the latter requires cognition, which is the ability to perceive and know."[45] The convened experts also concluded that the "videotape of the abortion was deliberately slowed down and subsequently speeded up to create an impression of hyperactivity."[46] Other criticisms included the fact that the "fetal model displayed during the abortion procedure is much larger than a fetus of a 12 weeks' gestation model visualized by ultrasonography."[47] Although including these criticisms in their reviews of and articles about the film, the press did not try to assess the science, but instead presented both arguments uncritically, implying that there were two equally legitimate interpretations of the status of fetal pain and leaving the reader or viewer to choose which explanation to believe.

Although the fetus was clearly the central victim in this film, central to its argument was also the claim that women frequently suffered severe and lasting psychological damage after having an abortion. The film ended with a montage of women Nathanson describes as "victims" who, because of the "conspiracy of silence with respect to the true nature of abortion," had had abortions with "no true knowledge" and were subsequently "full of extreme regret and sorrow."[48]

Nathanson's conclusion picked up on a phenomenon first identified by psycho-therapist Vincent Rue at a 1981 congressional hearing on "Abortion and Family Relations" as "post-abortion syndrome."[49] *The Silent Scream* reintroduced this idea, which became increasingly central to the antiabortion movement. The same year as the release of *The Silent Scream,* psychologist David Reardon surveyed members of a group called Women Exploited by Abortion (WEBA) and con-cluded that that there was a relationship between having an abortion and high rates of nervous breakdowns, substance abuse, violence, and suicide attempts.[50] Reardon founded the Eliot Institute, an organization dedicated to what he calls a "woman-centered" approach to opposing abortion, generates papers on post-abortion syndrome, and advocates for women he calls "abortion survivors."[51] Organizations like Rachel's Vineyard Ministries, which offers "a safe place to renew, rebuild, and redeem hearts broken by abortion," Safe Haven, which offers "a place for healing for the trauma of abortion," Victims of Choice, and Healing Hearts, among others, provide online counseling and online communities and message boards for women suffering from postabortion trauma.[52] Comparing postabortion stress to the posttraumatic stress disorder afflicting many Vietnam veterans, psychologist Anne Speckhard described women experiencing flash-backs and hallucinations, and reporting intense nightmares, such as images of discarded fetuses in garbage heaps or babies trying to locate their mother.[53]

The public may have first learned of postabortion trauma during the trial of Lorena Bobbitt, who, in 1994, cut off almost half of her husband John's penis. David Reardon provided the defense with the argument that Bobbitt's attack, which took place almost exactly three years after her husband coerced her into having an abortion, was a manifestation of postabortion trauma:

> Lorena Bobbitt's abortion was unwanted. It violated her moral beliefs and signified the destruction of her dream to have a family just like the one in which she had grown up. It was an attack on her self-identity and her maternal self. By understanding how her abortion traumatized Lorena, we can under-stand why she mutilated John in the way she did.... It takes no leap of imag-ination to see how a woman, such as Lorena who, on an unconscious level felt that she had been sexually mutilated by her abortion, would, in a moment of bitter passion, attempt to "castrate" her husband.[54]

Rue, founder and codirector of the Institute for Pregnancy Loss, concurred, saying that, "from the evidence accumulated in the course of her trial, it is very likely that Lorena Bobbitt's actions were a direct result of both her traumatic coerced abortion experience and her longstanding abusive relationship with her husband."[55] In linking abortion and domestic violence as related forms of abuse with similarly damaging consequences for women, Rue and Reardon provide a way for antiabortion activists to frame their argument in terms difficult for feminists to dispute.

Another strategy deployed by antiabortion activists wanting to position themselves as "women-centered" was their active promotion of the idea that there was a link between breast cancer and abortion. Joel Brind, a professor of endocrinology and biology at Baruch College, as well as an evangelical Christian and member of the NRLC, reviewed and analyzed a collection of epidemiological studies of that relationship, publishing his conclusions in the *Journal of American Physicians and Surgeons:*

> [I]nduced abortion is indeed a risk factor for breast cancer, despite the strong and pervasive bias in the recent literature in the direction of viewing abortion as safe for women.... It is deplorable that in an era in which women's rights appear so prominently on the political and public health landscape, women should be denied the right to know about the breast-cancer risk-increasing effect of such a common matter of choice as induced abortion.[56]

In journal articles, testimony in trials and in legislative debates, and in publications for antiabortion journals, Brind pushed this link through his advocacy for laws requiring clinics to warn women that one of the risks of an abortion was breast cancer. In 1999, he founded the Breast Cancer Prevention Institute, dedicated to publicizing what he called the abortion-breast cancer (ABC) link. In addition to a brochure titled "The Single Most Avoidable Risk for Breast Cancer Is Elective Abortion," the institute provides seven online fact sheets explaining the link.[57] Other organizations like the Coalition on Abortion/Breast Cancer spread similar ideas, selling magnets, bumper stickers, and T-shirts featuring their logo, a red ribbon outlined in pink, with pink text reading "Abortion Hurts Women" on one side and a pink breast cancer symbol on the reverse. Suggesting that the mainstream medical community is repressing information about this link, the coalition draws an analogy to the Tuskegee syphilis study, saying, "Just as the men in the Tuskegee study weren't told that their health was at risk, women who've had abortions haven't been told they're at greater risk for breast cancer. For this reason, they're less likely to seek early detection or to reduce their risk for the disease."[58] In addition to being scientifically suspect, these women-centered arguments mask a certain double message. Reardon's analysis of the Bobbitt case emphasized the impact on women of postabortion trauma, but it could easily be interpreted as a quite graphic object lesson about the dangers abortion poses to men. And Brind's explanation that "if a woman ignores the life of her unborn baby, maybe we can reach her through education concerning proven risks to herself," could be interpreted as an argument on behalf of women, but could also be read as a not-so-subtle suggestion that the purported link between breast cancer and abortion might be effective because a woman's self-interest is more powerful than her maternal instinct.[59]

Just as the mainstream medical profession had challenged the idea that the fetus could feel pain, it also challenged the concept of postabortion trauma and the myth of a link between breast cancer and abortion. A 1997 Danish study published in the *New England Journal of Medicine* was considered the authoritative study debunking Brind's argument. Despite that, in 2002, the National Cancer Institute responded to pressures from Brind, Representative Tom Coburn (R-OK), and the Bush administration to provide information about the ABC link on their website. Pro-choice organizations and NCI scientists succeeded in having that information removed, and in 2003, the NCI released a study that concluded, "[H]aving an abortion or miscarriage does not increase a woman's subsequent risk of developing breast cancer."[60] The American Psychological Association issued a report concluding that "the weight of the evidence" indicates that first-trimester abortion of an unwanted pregnancy "does not pose a psychological hazard for most women."[61] And in a comprehensive literature review published in the *Journal of the American Medical Association*, psychiatry professor Nada Stotland concluded that "there is no evidence of an abortion-trauma syndrome."[62]

But although postabortion trauma, fetal pain, and an ABC link did not have scientific backing, they did have strong emotional resonance and popular currency. And activists promoting all three phenomena were at least as interested in getting media attention as they were in gaining scientific legitimacy. Rather than publishing in refereed journals, activists were happy to have their research debated in the mass media, where the public could interpret the science through the familiar lens of politics instead of by the highly nuanced standards of epidemiology. Because scientific studies can rarely, if ever, prove a negative— they cannot, for example, prove that abortion does not cause breast cancer, that there is no such thing as postabortion syndrome, and that fetal pain does not exist—scientists who opposed the arguments of Reardon, Brind, and others were forced into making less conclusive arguments. This left the media to present the issue as a debate between two different but equally legitimate positions, leaving the public to decide which position they preferred.

For Nathanson and his supporters, the real success of his film would not be measured by its medical facts and scientific accuracy but by its emotional power and political efficacy. On those terms, the film was an unqualified hit. Following a screening of the film, Ronald Reagan said, "[I]f every member of Congress could see that film, they would move quickly to end the tragedy of abortion." David O'Steen, the executive director of the National Right to Life Committee, said he believed the film would do for the antiabortion movement what Harriet Beecher

Stowe's 1852 novel *Uncle Tom's Cabin* had done for the antislavery movement.[63] On May 21, 1985, the Senate Subcommittee on the Constitution of the Committee of the Judiciary, chaired by Senator Orrin G. Hatch (R-UT), held hearings on fetal pain.[64] Hatch's opening statement declared that fetal pain called upon "the humanitarian character of our Nation," indicating that in these hearings, emotion and anecdote would trump scientific evidence. The main witness in the hearings was Dr. Bernard Nathanson, who opened his testimony by showing clips from *The Silent Scream* and restating many of the film's interpretive claims.[65]

Although using fetal pain to make an argument against abortion was the ostensible purpose of these hearings, a less obvious, perhaps less conscious, phenomenon was that many of those who believed in the existence of fetal pain appropriated the language and undermined the politics of 1960s liberalism. Arguments putting fetal pain at the center of antiabortion rhetoric countered liberalism's monopoly on compassion with compassion for the fetus; appropriated liberalism's commitment to the tolerance of different views by insisting that anecdotal claims by politicians and laypeople be treated as seriously as scientific evidence from experts; and challenged liberalism's commitment to a woman's "right to choose" with an emphasis on a woman's "right to know."

The argument about fetal pain was, in part, an argument over the ownership of compassion. Joseph Sobran, senior editor at the *National Review*, argued in 1984 that "the fifteen million children killed in the womb since 1973 deserve to be called the victims of liberalism," and that liberals' refusal to accept the existence of fetal pain threatened to "explode their humanitarian pretensions."[66] Liberalism, Sobran suggested, "has organized itself historically around a series of 'suffering situations': slavery, child labor, racial discrimination, poverty. Liberalism's claim to power and authority was that it relieved pain. . . . Its entire claim to legitimacy was that it could make things stop hurting."[67] The consequences of this, for Sobran, are immense. "Private property, the work ethic, and of course the sanctity of life itself," he argued, "have all been forced to yield to the liberal imperative of relieving pain and misery of various kinds." But at the same time, he argues that liberalism is

> interested in those kinds of suffering that can be defined as "social problems" susceptible to collectible organized "solutions." . . . The liberal is interested in suffering only insofar as it can be exploited to force 'social change' and produce a secular order liberalism aspires to. . . . Permitting abortion is part of the scheme. Limiting abortion would disrupt the scheme. Therefore the pain of the aborted fetus is ineligible for the liberal's selective but purposeful "compassion."[68]

Sobran suggested that compassion was always just a tool used by liberals in their larger "purpose of subverting the morals and institutions of traditional America." Conversely, exposing liberals' "humanitarian pretensions" through the debate about fetal pain would, he contended, provide "a great service for the unborn" as well as for "the moral tradition to which America by right belongs."[69] Sobran's argument outlines the premise of "compassionate conservatism"—as articulated by Marvin Olasky in his 2000 book of that title and championed by George W. Bush in his 2000 presidential campaign—that would become central to the rhetoric of the Republican Party in the early twenty-first century.[70]

Recognizing that the issue of fetal pain could be leveraged into a wholesale attack on liberalism, some critics tried to expose the motives and politics behind the film. Psychologist James W. Prescott argued that the "motivation for 'The Silent Scream' was not fetal well-being.... The anti-abortion motivation behind the producers and supporters of 'The Silent Scream' resides in an authoritarian control and denial of the fundamental human right of self determination."[71] After analyzing the voting patterns of senators on a series of bills involving abortion, capital punishment, "no-knock" laws (laws that allowed police officers with warrants to enter homes without knocking), and gun control, Prescott identified a strong relationship between opposing abortion and supporting capital punishment; between opposing abortion and supporting no-knock laws; and between opposing abortion and opposing handgun control.[72]

Similarly, Catholics for a Free Choice developed what they called a "Pro-Child Life Score," by analyzing congressional support for child nutrition programs, Medicaid, Aid for Families with Dependent Children, Head Start, and food stamps—programs established as part of Lyndon B. Johnson's Great Society and War on Poverty in order to improve the health and well-being of children. Hoping to expand the discourse about what it meant to be pro-child beyond abortion, Catholics for a Free Choice compared the voting records of 100 congressional representatives who supported legalized abortion to the voting records of 100 representatives who opposed legalized abortion. The comparison revealed that the average Pro-Child Life Score of the representatives who support abortion rights was 92, and the average Pro-Child Life Score of the representatives who oppose legal abortion was 49.[73] It appeared that there was a clear relationship between one's position toward abortion and one's position toward the programs of 1960s liberalism, a relationship that suggests that abortion was about more, or less, than fetal life. And even on the specific issue of alleviating pain, an analysis of those same 200 representatives' votes on the Compassionate Pain Relief Act, which would permit the use of parenteral diacetylmorphine (heroin) for the relief of intractable pain when "pain could not be effectively treated with currently available analgesic medications" indicated that 72 percent of those who supported abortion rights supported the Human Pain Relief Act and 95 percent of those who opposed abortion rights opposed the Human Pain Relief Act.[74] What all of this suggests, according to Prescott, is that "the production of 'The Silent Scream' is another attempt by the anti-abortion movement to mislead the public and legislators into believing that the anti-abortion movement has a fundamental concern and compassion about human pain, suffering, and violence."[75] Whether the antiabortion movement intended to lead or mislead, it did succeed in shifting the terms of debate from competing political or legal perspectives to competing assumptions about knowledge and expertise.

Whereas the debate between Sobran and Prescott revolved around one of the tenets of liberalism, compassion, the debate between expert witnesses in the *Fetal Pain* hearings allowed antiabortion representatives to appropriate liberalism's commitment to multiple perspectives by challenging the authority of scientific expertise. Expert witnesses presenting scientifically complicated explanations for why the fetus does not feel pain were dismissive of the emotionally resonant arguments of Nathanson. Dr. Richard L. Berkowitz, acting chairman of the Department of Obstetrics and Gynecology at Mount Sinai Medical Center in New York, characterized those claims as "pseudoscientific" and "fanciful."[76] Dr. Jeremiah Mahoney, professor of human genetics, pediatrics, obstetrics, and gynecology at Yale University School of Medicine, addressed the issue this way: "Does the human fetus, early in its development within the womb, experience pain? Can the human fetus be aware of pain? Can the human fetus be in fear of pain? I believe that all scientifically derived evidence and observations available today which bring light to these questions say no."[77] Others repeatedly invoked the quantity and quality of scientific evidence mitigating against the existence of fetal pain.

Notwithstanding the impressive academic credentials of the witnesses testifying against fetal pain, the committee members focused their question-and-answer session not on the substance of the evidence, but on the politics of those witnesses. In a lengthy exchange, Representative Hyde kept pushing Berkowitz to "reveal" his political beliefs and Berkowitz refused, insisting that his politics were irrelevant as his testimony was based on his scientific knowledge, not his political positions. The emphasis on ascertaining whether those witnesses were pro-life or pro-choice suggests that the goal of the hearing was not to explicate the different interpretations of scientific evidence on pain, but to deploy the claim of fetal pain in service of one political argument, while at the same time undermining the conclusions of the medical experts as being politically motivated. The exchange between Hyde and Berkowitz demonstrates how arguments that knowledge was socially and politically constructed and that multiple truths could coexist—arguments generally associated with the academic and activist left—were now being appropriated and used to attack the credibility and legitimacy of experts who argued against the existence of fetal pain.

The third premise of liberalism challenged by arguments about fetal pain was the primacy of rights, which involved shifting the debate from a woman's "right to choose" to a woman's "right to know." Illustrating that shift was an exchange between Senator Gordon Humphrey (R-NH) and Dr. Kathryn Moseley, a pediatrician and neonatologist. Moseley testified that she found it "paradoxical" that when she was treating a sick child, she had to "go with a long paper of an informed consent for the parents," but that in the case of performing an abortion, "a woman, not really intent, in not knowing the full extent of what she is doing, gets no information whatsoever with regard to any pain it might experience upon the abortion of an unborn child."[78] Humphrey asked Moseley the following question:

> In your capacity as not only a physician, but also a physician who also happens to be a woman, you have a special perspective that our other witnesses do not have. Then as a woman who is a physician, or as a physician who is a woman... do you feel that knowledge of pain has been withheld from women, and do you feel that women should be more apprised of that possibility?[79]

Moseley responded, "I think knowledge not only of the possibility of pain perception of the fetus, but the uterine development of the fetus has been withheld."[80] Notwithstanding the weight of the evidence suggesting that the fetus does not feel pain, the issue had taken on a meaning of its own and had become entangled with the question of informed consent. Reverend James A. DeCamp put it this way: "Surely, at the least, those mothers who are aborting their unborn children should know the suffering they are putting their babies through. Shouldn't the woman's 'right to choose' carry with it a 'right to know' about this pain her child will feel?"[81] The woman's "right to know" would become crucial in efforts to restrict abortion through informed consent laws, efforts that had failed in the 1980 case of *Charles v. Carey*, the Seventh Circuit Court of Appeals had struck down several informed consent provisions in Illinois, including a restriction requiring physicians to provide all abortion patients with information regarding any "organic pain to the fetus."[82] Finding that that particular provision placed a direct and unwarranted burden on a woman's decision and created an unwarranted intrusion into the privacy of the physician-patient relationship, the court characterized the informed consent provisions as "medically meaningless, confusing, medically unjustified, and contradicted, causing cruel and harmful stress to... patients."[83] But in 1992, more than ten years after that decision, and almost twenty years after *Roe*, the

Supreme Court rendered a ruling in the *Planned Parenthood of Southeastern Pennsylvania v. Casey* decision that would enlarge the scope of informed consent and radically transform the landscape of abortion politics.

In 1988 and 1989, the Pennsylvania legislature amended its abortion law to require doctors to provide particular information about the health risks and possible complications of an abortion, establish a twenty-four-hour waiting period prior to the procedure, and require parental consent for minors and spousal notification for married women. Challenged by a group of abortion clinics and physicians, the laws were upheld first by a federal appeals court in 1991 and then by the Supreme Court in 1992. In a 5–4 ruling, *Planned Parenthood of Southeastern Pennsylvania v. Casey* reaffirmed *Roe* while also upholding all of the provisions except the spousal notification requirement.[84]

Three justices—Sandra Day O'Connor, David Souter, and Anthony Kennedy—wrote the plurality opinion, which established a new standard to determine whether laws restricting abortion were a violation of women's constitutional right to an abortion as determined by *Roe v. Wade*. The *Casey* decision held that states could regulate abortion in accordance with their "compelling interests" so long as those regulations did not have the purpose or effect of imposing an "undue burden," defined by the court as a "substantial obstacle in the path of a woman seeking an abortion."[85] Whereas the *Roe* decision had required states to completely rewrite their abortion statutes, most often dramatically liberalizing them, the *Casey* decision offered states the opportunity to revisit those statutes, and to construct new laws that did not constitute an "undue burden" but did restrict the availability of abortions.[86] Peter Samuelson, president of Americans United for Life, describes his organization's response to the *Casey* decision:

> After *Casey* it became very clear the Supreme Court is just not going to reverse *Roe*. But with *Casey* they said, "We'll open it up for state regulation. We understand there are other interests at stake, that the state has an interest in protecting the women and in the life of the unborn child." And so since then Americans United for Life and other groups have been working very incrementally trying to identify opportunities where we can protect the woman within what are the constitutional bounds today of her right to an abortion. . . . What we do with incremental laws is we invite people to think about it. We invite people to think about the negative impact of abortion on women. Abortion creates all sorts of psychological and health problems for women. It's a very difficult thing. It's not a good solution to the problem they're facing with the unwanted pregnancy.[87]

This new strategy, constructing women as the sympathetic victims of abortion, rather than as the selfish perpetrators of it, would be used to weave together the decade-old debate about fetal pain, the ABC link, and postabortion trauma with the new issue that was beginning to dominate abortion politics, the controversial late-term abortion procedure termed by the antiabortion movement "partial birth abortion."

Three months after the Supreme Court issued the *Casey* decision, at the National Abortion Federation Risk Management Seminar, a seminar for physicians, Cincinnati physician Dr. Martin Haskell presented a paper titled "Dilation and Extraction for Late Second Trimester Abortion," in which he described a new surgical procedure in which the physician would remove an intact fetus feet first until the head lodged against the cervix, and then depress its skull, and remove its intact body from the patient.[88] Haskell explained why this "intact dilation and extraction" (D&X) procedure was faster, cleaner, and safer than dismembering and then removing the fetus with the standard dilation and evacuation (D&E) method used in second-trimester abortions.[89] The NAF published Haskell's talk, along with detailed instructions on the procedure, in a volume on the proceedings of the seminar. When Jenny Westberg, an antiabortion activist on the NAF mailing list, received the proceedings, she decided to write about it, and include an illustration of the procedure, in *Life Advocate* (figure 5.1).[90]

When National Right to Life Committee lobbyist Douglas Johnson read the article and saw the illustrations, he decided to move the discussion of this procedure from a medical conference to the political stage.[91] In 1995, Johnson met with Representative Charles Canady (R-FL) and his legislative aide Keri Folmer, who before working for Canady had worked as a lawyer for the NRLC. It was at that meeting, according to Folmer, that the term "partial-birth abortion" was coined.[92] "We called it the most descriptive thing we could call it," Folmer explains. "We were throwing around terms. We didn't want it to be inflammatory. We wanted a name that rang true."[93] Whether intended to inflame or inform, the term partial-birth abortion did more of the former than the latter.

As the chair of the House Judiciary Subcommittee on the Constitution, Canady introduced the Partial-Birth Abortion Ban Act on June 14, 1995.[94] The bill defined partial-birth abortion as "an abortion in which the person performing the abortion partially vaginally delivers a living fetus before killing the fetus and completing the delivery" and held that physicians performing this procedure would be fined or imprisoned for up to two years.[95] Jenny Westberg's images were front and center of the debate about this bill. Objecting to the use of the illustrations as evidence, one physician wrote the following letter to Representative Canady:

There are many substantive inaccuracies in the drawings presented. For example, the clear implication of the drawings is that the fetus is alive until

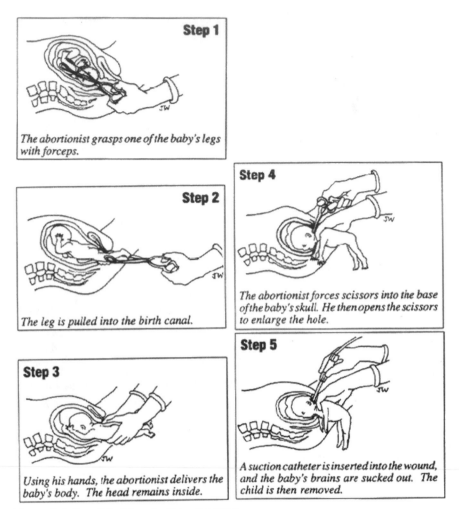

Step 1

The abortionist grasps one of the baby's legs with forceps.

Step 2

The leg is pulled into the birth canal.

Step 3

Using his hands, the abortionist delivers the baby's body. The head remains inside.

Step 4

The abortionist forces scissors into the base of the baby's skull. He then opens the scissors to enlarge the hole.

Step 5

A suction catheter is inserted into the wound, and the baby's brains are sucked out. The child is then removed.

Figure. 5.1 From *Life Advocate*, February 1993

the end of the procedure, which is untrue. The stylized illustrations further imply that the fetus is conscious and experiencing pain or sensation of some kind—which is also obviously untrue. Finally, the fetus depicted is shown as perfectly formed (indeed proportionally larger in relationship to the woman than it ought to be), when in fact a great number of such procedures are performed on fetuses with severe genetic or neurological defects. All of these factors, as well as the rudimentary, even crude, nature of the sketches added up to a picture that is, as I previously stated, highly imaginative and misleading.[96]

Despite this letter, and others like it, 332 members voted to allow the pictures to be submitted as exhibits in the House debate.[97] The schematic images and the graphic captions—one reads, "The abortionist jams scissors into the baby's skull"; another, "The child's brains are sucked out. The dead baby is then removed"—were a compelling background for the attacks on the procedure that either manipulated or appropriated elements of liberalism to make their point.

Representative Ed Bryant (R-TN), for example, compared the procedure to the death penalty:

If they brought Ted Bundy into the electric chair or were about to execute him after these years of appeal and all of this, and the power failed…and someone came and asked Mr. Bundy to put his head down and they hit him over the head with a screwdriver and knocked a hole in his head, and drained out his brain, sucked out his brain, does the gentleman from Florida think that would be any cause for civil libertarians in terms of cruel and inhuman punishment via this type of execution?[98]

This not-so-subtle maneuver implies that a civil libertarian would let Ted Bundy live while allowing an unborn baby to die in a gruesome manner. Others compared the procedure to historical wrongs like slavery, comparing the partial birth abortion ban to the movement to ban the slave trade, and identifying the bill's supporters with the abolitionist William Wilberforce. Others, like Representative Ernest Istook (R-OK), invoked more recent historical barbarities: "Some people may not want to recognize the practice that we seek to prohibit. Some people did not want to look when Hitler was slaughtering the Jews or Stalin was slaughtering his countrymen. If we do not look, if we do not understand what is being done…instead of barbarity they call it choice."[99] Here, the moral courage to support H.R. 1833 was compared to the same courage required to abolish slavery, defeat Hitler, and fight Communism.

Opponents of the bill countered these historically mythic comparisons with detailed stories from real women who had undergone this procedure. Vikki Stella described her decision this way:

I've been told that mothers like me are selfish and only want perfect babies; that we're having third trimester abortions because of cleft palates and missing fingers. Well, yes, my son had a cleft palate. I wish to God that was all that was wrong! He wasn't just imperfect—his condition was incompatible with life. The only thing keeping him alive was my body. He could never have survived outside my body. I took my son off life support.[100]

Tammy Watts told Congress a similar story:

We had wanted this baby so much. We named her Mackenzie.... I remember getting on the plane, and as soon as it took off we were crying because we were leaving our child behind. The really hard part started when I got home. I had to go through my milk coming in, everything you go through if you have a child. I don't know how to explain the heartache. There are no good words.... I never blamed God for this, I'm a good Christian woman.... I've still got my baby's room, and her memory cards from her memorial service, her foot and handprints.[101]

Testifying before Congress, Claudia Crown Ades described her experience this way:

We loved this baby. We wanted this baby desperately. This was our son. We were preparing our family and our world for him. And now, we had to prepare for a tragedy. Away went the baby name books. Away went the shower invitations. Away went the first birthday party, the baseball games, the bar mitzvah. Away went our dream.... Ironically, the final day of the procedure was Yom Kippur, the holiest day of the Jewish year. On Yom Kippur, we are asked to mourn those who have passed and pray to God to inscribe us into the Book of Life. I prayed more than one person can pray. I was praying for all of us.[102]

These women had been carefully selected to embody the characteristics most likely to elicit sympathy—they were married, they were mothers, they had wanted these pregnancies, they were white, they were middle class, they were religious, and they were heartbroken. Nonetheless, their experiences were easily dismissed by Representative Jim Bunning (R-KY):

As a father of 9 children and a grandfather of 28, I have had a lot of experience in the wonders of a new life being brought into this world. When a baby is born, it is the most innocent of creatures, its hands stretch and kick with energy, and its cry is filled with life. Compare this to what occurs during a partial-birth abortion. The baby exits the uterus, its hands extend to hold its mother, its legs kick wildly, in the air as the child attempts to breathe, but its first breath will never come.[103]

Bunning trumped the stories of women making devastating decisions to terminate their pregnancies and describing their genetically damaged fetuses with his personal story of fatherhood and his universalized narrative about a genetically perfect fetus. On November 1, 1995, the House of Representatives passed the Partial-Birth Abortion Ban Act by a vote of 288 to 139.[104]

The following week, when the bill went to the Senate, Gordon Smith (R-NH) further personalized the abstract fetus by reminding the senators that they had once been in that same position:

Think about it, my colleagues, because this is a very personal matter. Each and every one of us—each and every one of us—started out life as an unborn child. Just like the one depicted in the first illustration that I showed earlier today. When you were born as you came through the birth canal your little fingers moved, your little feet moved, you kicked your legs, you moved your arms.... We slept, we woke, we felt pain, we were happy, we were sad.... As I close, I am reminded of a great maxim. Do unto others as you have them do unto you.... You and I deserved to be protected by law from a partial-birth abortion when you and I lived in our mothers' womb.... We had value. We had worth. We had rights. We became U.S. Senators. And those little babies have the same rights that we have under the Constitution. As the Old Testament tells us, Almighty God knew us even then, and he loved us. Our fellow human beings, these youngest of Americans, deserve no less.[105]

Having asked each senator to imagine himself in place of the fetus, Smith looked to the nation's future, compromised and weakened by the practice of abortion:

As I look at that depiction of that little baby in the womb, hanging there limp, you know what I say to myself? How many U.S. Senators are there in that 700 [partial-birth abortions]? How many doctors, lawyers, Nobel Peace Prize winners, teachers? How many? I do not know. We will never know. We will never know. The first black president, is he or she in there? We will never know. First Hispanic president? We will never know. First woman president? We will never know. Cure for cancer? It may be one of those seven hundred...we will never know.[106]

Again, there is an appropriation and undermining of liberalism as Smith implied that the reason that no black, Hispanic, or woman had been elected president was not historical patterns of racism and sexism, as liberals might have it, but abortion. Smith went on to speak directly to President Clinton:

President Clinton, you were an unborn child once. The President's father died, you know, while his mother was pregnant. Is that not interesting? She faced a very tough decision. Do I raise a child alone without a father? Bill Clinton's mother chose life. Regardless of party, regardless of ideology, I think we could say we are thankful. He became a President of the United States. He could have been a victim. Bill Clinton could have been a partial-birth abortion.

Notwithstanding that plea, and the fact that the Senate had passed the bill by 55 to 44, President Clinton vetoed the bill.[107]

Hoping to override Clinton's veto, the Republican leadership scheduled a second set of hearings on the bill for March 21, 1996.[108] On the morning of the hearings, the House Judiciary Committee's Subcommittee on the Constitution focused on the question of whether or not the anesthesia used to reduce the woman's pain eliminated pain to the fetus. It turned into a sort of "he said/she said" contest between expert witnesses, and in the afternoon experts offered competing claims for sympathy.[109] The afternoon's first witness, Brenda P. Shafer, a registered nurse, described what she observed while assisting in an abortion by dilation and extraction:

> The baby's little fingers were clasping and unclasping, and his feet were kicking. Then the doctor stuck the scissors through the back of his head, and the baby's arms jerked out in a flinch, a startle reaction, like the baby does when you throw him up in the air and he thinks he might fall. The doctor opened up the scissors, stuck a high-powered suction tube into the opening, and sucked the baby's brains out. Now the baby went completely limp.[110]

To counter that graphic testimony, the opponents of the ban stuck to their strategy that women's stories would be the best argument for the procedure's necessity and called upon Mary-Dorothy Line and Coreen Costello to testify about their experiences.

In April 1995, Line and Costello confronted the most difficult decisions of their lives. Line, who describes herself as a "registered Republican and a practicing Catholic," had been married to her husband Bill for fourteen years when she became pregnant for the first time. Following her ob/gyn's recommendation, she had an alpha-fetoprotein (AFP) test to screen for neurological anomalies, including spina bifida. When the test indicated an abnormal AFP level, Line decided to have a follow-up amniocentesis, explaining that she and her husband "needed to know what we were dealing with."[111] The ultrasound given in preparation for the amniocentesis indicated that the fetus had a very advanced case of hydrocephalus, an abnormal accumulation of cerebrospinal fluid within ventricles in the brain. "We asked about *in utero* operations and drains to remove the fluid," Line said, "but Dr. Carlson said there was absolutely nothing we could do. The hydrocephaly was too advanced. Our precious little baby was destined to be taken from us. Dr. Carlson recommended that we terminate the pregnancy." Line underwent an intact dilation and evacuation, a three-day procedure she describes as "the worst days of our life. We had lost our son before we even had him."[112]

Costello was in her seventh month of pregnancy when she began experiencing contractions and rushed to the hospital for an ultrasound. She describes how "the physician became very silent. Soon more physicians came in.... My husband reassured me that we could deal with whatever was wrong. We had talked about raising a child with disabilities and there was never a question that we would take whatever God gave us."[113] Physicians said that "they did not expect our baby to live.... This poor precious child had a lethal neurological disorder...her vital organs were atrophying. Our darling little girl was going to die."[114]

A self-described "full-time, stay-at-home wife," Costello explains her political and religious beliefs: "I am a registered Republican, and very conservative. I don't believe in abortion. Because of my deeply held Christian beliefs, I knew I would never have an abortion."[115] Costello decided to try to maintain the pregnancy and deliver the baby, whom she and her husband had named Katherine Grace. Over the next two weeks, Katherine Grace's condition continued to deteriorate, and Costello describes realizing "that terrible truth...that if she were born, her passing would not be peaceful or painless.... We decided to baptize her *in utero,* while she was still alive." After being told by a doctor that it would be extremely risky to her life and health to deliver Katherine Grace, Costello decided to have an abortion by dilation and extraction.[116]

In contrast to the women whom Representative Bob Inglis (R-SC) described as "deceived and now realize that they wish they had not had an abortion," these women clearly understood the choices they were making. But tragic as their choices were, these women's stories could not compete with the unborn victims. At any rate, the hearings were more of a staged drama than a real effort to pass legislation, as it was clear from the outset that the bill would pass both houses of Congress but would not garner enough votes to override Clinton's veto. And indeed, when Congress passed the same bill the following year, Clinton vetoed it for a second time.

Because Congress did not have enough votes to override a presidential veto, the passage of a federal ban was extremely unlikely, and antiabortion activists refocused their efforts on passing legislation at the state level. By 2000, thirty-one states had passed partial-birth abortion bans, and the Supreme Court was considering the constitutionality of Nebraska's ban.[117] In June 2000, in the case of *Stenberg v. Carhart,* the Supreme Court ruled that because the Nebraska statute did not provide an exception for the health of the woman and did not accept that a significant body of medical authority viewed the procedure as the safest one in certain circumstances, it constituted an "undue burden."[118] The ruling invalidated similar laws in twenty-nine out of thirty-one states. Although a setback for antiabortion activists, the decision intensified their desire to pass a federal law rather than continue to work state by state, especially given that they were facing a more favorable political climate with a Republican Congress and Republican president.

Congress's third debate over the federal law pushed familiar emotional buttons. One representative asked, "[I]s there no limit, no amount of pain, is there no procedure that is so extreme that we can apply to this unborn child or this fetus that we are willing as a country to say that just goes too far?"[119] But proponents of the ban knew that they needed to do more than highlight the specifics of a gruesome procedure in order to pass a law that would withstand Supreme Court scrutiny after *Stenberg*. The *Stenberg* decision had offered a template for how to fix the law in order to make it compliant with the *Casey* standards, and when the House of Representatives and Senate passed a Partial-Birth Abortion Ban Act in 2003, it did include an exception for the life of a mother. The PBABA did not, though, include an exception for the woman's health, even though the *Stenberg* decision had explicitly identified that exception as necessary in order to make the ban constitutional. By including an extensive "findings" section that stated that "partial birth abortion is never medically necessary and that the procedure itself poses health risks to women," Congress was exploring how far they could push the assumption of judicial deference to legislative findings.[120] The Republican Congress was arguing that a health exception was unnecessary because the Supreme Court was required to "defer to congressional 'findings of fact' regarding the safety of D&X and the need for a health exception."[121] Senator Rick Santorum (R-PA) argued that Congress had the right to make findings that challenged the Supreme Court's decision because Congress had done "a heck of a lot more exhaustive study, in our deliberations with hearings and other testimony, than the Supreme Court can."[122] Representative James Sensenbrenner (R-WI) made a similar argument, saying that he hoped the Court would "give the same type of deference that it has done in the past civil rights and employment cases."[123] Representative John Conyers, Jr. (D-MI), strongly criticized this logic, arguing that "Gainsaying, no matter how presented, is not the same as fact-findings.... Congress cannot simply refute findings of fact made by the District Court by presenting its own 'findings.'"[124] This conflict was both a test of the Supreme Court's understanding of its relationship to Congress, as well as the natural result of the antiabortion activists efforts to challenge scientific expertise by creating their own experts.

The bill's supporters had explicitly and persuasively argued that the ban was as concerned with protecting women as it was with protecting the fetus. Senate Majority Leader Bill Frist (R-TN) claimed that partial-birth abortions "carry the danger of doing unnecessary harm to a mother, to an infant, and to our conscience as a nation that values the sanctity of human life."[125] When Bill Clinton vetoed the bill, he was surrounded by women whose pregnancies had been aborted with the D&X procedure. When George Bush signed the bill, he was surrounded by an all-male, all-white group of legislators. Although these women-centered antiabortion arguments focused rhetorically on a series of unfounded claims about the risks abortions posed to women, the consequences of those arguments are quite serious in presenting women with misinformation about the risks of abortions, and in limiting their physicians' ability to determine the best and safest procedure.

Two days after President Bush signed the PBABA into law on November 5, 2003, abortion providers in San Francisco, New York, and Nebraska obtained temporary restraining orders from federal district courts preventing the law from taking effect.[126] The decisions of these courts included harsh condemnations of Congress's fact-finding process. San Francisco Judge Phyllis Hamilton said that "the oral testimony before Congress was heavily weighted in favor of the Act.... [I]t is apparent to this court ... that the oral testimony before Congress was not only unbalanced, but intentionally polemic."[127] Nebraska Judge Richard G. Kopf found that the congressional findings were "unreasonable," that the "overwhelming weight of the trial evidence proves that the procedure is safe and medically necessary in order to preserve the health of women under certain circumstances," and that the ban was unconstitutional both in failing to provide a health exception and because it imposed an undue burden on women seeking abortions by banning some D&E procedures, in addition to all D&X procedures.[128] New York Judge Richard Conway Casey reached similar conclusions, arguing that "the evidentiary standard established by the Supreme Court does not permit the government to legislate in the face of medical uncertainty" and that "Congress did not hold extensive hearings, nor did it carefully consider the evidence before arriving at its findings.... This Court heard more evidence during its trial than Congress heard over the span of eight years.... Even the Government's own experts disagreed with almost all of Congress's factual findings."[129]

But although Judge Casey agreed with Judges Hamilton and Kopf that Congress had overstepped its bounds in claiming that the Supreme Court should defer to congressional findings over trial and appellate court testimony, he disagreed on a closely related issue of fetal pain. Judge Casey called the D&X procedure "gruesome, brutal, barbaric, and uncivilized," and agreed that the evidence supported the conclusion that the procedure "subject[s] fetuses to severe pain." In contrast, Judge Hamilton wrote that "much of the debate on this issue is based on speculation and inference" and that "the issue of whether fetuses feel pain is unsettled in the scientific community."[130]

For the most part, though, that issue had been settled. In August 2005, the *Journal of the American Medical Association* published a report concluding that "evidence regarding the capacity for fetal pain is limited but indicates that fetal perception of pain is unlikely before the third trimester."[131] The article makes a distinction between pain, which "requires cortical recognition," and "nociception," a system of physical reflexes driven by "peripheral sensory receptors," and concludes that the "capacity for conscious perception of pain can arise only after thalomocortical pathways begin to function, which may occur around 29 to 30 weeks' gestational age."[132] The *JAMA* article immediately intersected with a heated political debate about the existence and implications of fetal pain.[133] The authors' findings, based on a multidisciplinary review of several hundred scientific papers on fetal pain and fetal anesthesia and analgesia, led the authors—experts on anesthesia, neuroanatomy, obstetrics, and neonatal development—to conclude that "discussions of fetal pain for abortions performed before the end of the second trimester should be noncompulsory. Fetal anesthesia or analgesia should not be recommended or routinely offered for abortion because current experimental techniques provide unknown fetal benefit and may increase risks for the woman."[134] Antiabortion groups immediately attacked the article, with the NRLC issuing a statement that two of the article's authors were "pro-abortion activists" whose conclusions were "predetermined by their political agenda."[135]

Judge Casey's decision and this *JAMA* report reinvigorated the discussion of the pending Unborn Child Pain Awareness Act, sponsored in 2007 by Senator Sam Brownback (R-KS) and Representative Chris Smith (R-NJ). Pro-choice organizations struggled with how to respond to this issue. NARAL Pro-Choice America, perhaps the nation's leading abortion rights group, issued the following statement: "Pro-choice Americans have always believed that women deserve access to all the information relevant to their reproductive health decisions. For some women, that includes information related to fetal anesthesia options. NARAL Pro-Choice America does not intend to oppose this legislation."[136] But Planned Parenthood Federation of America, the National Abortion Federation, and the Center for Reproductive Rights all vigorously opposed the legislation. "It's really inflammatory antiabortion propaganda," said Janet Crepps, a lawyer with the Center for Reproductive Rights, headquartered in New York. "Right out of the box, I think it's an inappropriate exercise of congressional power. Congress is taking sides in a very controversial medical debate. It's a very fuzzy area."[137]

Opponents of so-called fetal pain legislation suggested that it manipulated scientific evidence and that "distribution of false and misleading information places an unconstitutional burden on a woman's right to choose," whereas proponents argued that it merely extended "existing state laws that mandate that patients receive information about abortion procedures before giving their consent."[138] The UCPAA was debated in the House and Senate in 2005, and remained in committee until December 6, 2006, when, in one of their last acts, the Republican-controlled House of Representatives of the 109th Congress called a vote on a revised version of that bill. Whereas Representative Lois Capps (D-CA) described the revised bill (H.R. 6099) as a "sham bill...laden with rhetoric but very little science... yet another partisan political ploy that misguidedly attempts to insert the government into private medical conversations between women and their doctors," Representative Phil Gingrey (R-GA) characterized it as "a compassionate piece of legislation to take informed consent to the level it should be at."[139] Although the vote was 250–162 in favor of the bill, it failed to get the two-thirds majority required to pass.[140] Nonetheless, as of October 2009, nine states had passed similar bills.[141]

At the same time that state legislatures and the U.S. Congress were debating fetal pain bills, the Supreme Court was hearing arguments from plaintiffs in the combined cases of *Gonzales v. Carhart* and *Gonzales v. Planned Parenthood Federation,* challenging the constitutionality of the Partial Birth Abortion Ban Act of 2003.[142] In oral arguments, Solicitor General Paul Clement argued that the law distinguished between the still-legal D&E (dilation and evacuation) procedure and the banned D&X (intact dilation and extraction) procedure, based on the fact that in the first case, "fetal demise takes place in utero," whereas in the second case, "the lethal act takes place when the fetus is more than halfway out of the mother."[143] Because the law did not differentiate between abortions performed pre- and postviability, Justice Ruth Bader Ginsburg pushed Clement on this question, asking why the law drew the line between a legal and illegal abortion not developmentally but geographically. Clement responded that the law recognized a "bright line" between abortion and infanticide, and that although that line was at times "temporal," it also had a "spatial dimension.... [T]hat line is basically in womb, outside of womb." He asked the justices to imagine a situation in which "there is a problem with the mother's health, there is a problem in her life so it's a lawful post-viability abortion. I don't think anybody thinks that the law is or should be indifferent as to whether in that case fetal demise takes place *in utero* or outside the mother's womb. The one is abortion, the other is murder."[144] Clement presented this scenario as one that everyone could agree upon. But Clement also agreed with Justice John Paul Stevens's statement that "[i]t [the ban] is not preventing the lethal act, it is requiring that the lethal act be performed prior to any part of the delivery, because there is no doubt that there will be a lethal act."[145]

These exchanges with the justices about why the "where" of the procedure mattered more than the "when" or "if" of the procedure echoed much of the testimony during the Edelin trial, revisiting the debate over how to distinguish between legal abortion and criminal infanticide that was as contested in 2006 as it had been in 1975. Also reminiscent of the Edelin trial, Clement and the justices used different terminology—Clement using *baby,* and Stevens, Bader Ginsburg, and Souter using *fetus*—throughout. At one point, Stevens said, "Some of these fetuses I understand in the procedure, are only four or five inches long. They are very different from fully formed babies." Somewhat surprisingly, Clement conceded the point, saying, "Justice Stevens, again, you're right," only to be interrupted by Justice Antonin Scalia's somewhat sarcastic comment that "when it's halfway out, I guess you can call it either a child or a fetus. It's sort of half and half, isn't it?"[146]

On April 18, 2007, the Court released their 5–4 decision in *Gonzalez v. Planned Parenthood* and *Gonzalez v. Carhart,* upholding the constitutionality of the Partial Birth Abortion Ban Act. The majority opinion, written by Justice Kennedy and joined by Chief Justice John Roberts, Justice Samuel Alito, Justice Antonin Scalia, and Justice Clarence Thomas, began by emphasizing their deference to the congressional findings that there was never a medical reason to perform this procedure other than to save the life of the mother, and then focused on the details of the procedure itself. Kennedy contrasted the description provided by Dr. Haskell, the physician who had presented the procedure at the National Abortion Federation Risk Management Seminar, to the description given by a nurse. He quotes Haskell's description:

> At this point, the right-handed surgeon slides the fingers of the left [hand] along the back of the fetus and "hooks" the shoulders of the fetus with the index and ring fingers (palm down). While maintaining this tension, lifting the cervix and applying traction to the shoulders with the fingers of the left hand, the surgeon takes a pair of blunt curved Metzenbaum scissors in the right hand. He carefully advances the tip, curved down, along the spine and under the middle finger until he feels it contact the base of the skull under the tip of his middle finger. The surgeon then forces the scissors into the base of the skull or into the forearm magnum. Having safely entered the skull, he spreads the scissors to enlarge the opening. The surgeon removes the scissors and introduces a suction catheter into this hold and evacuates the skull contents. With the catheter still in place, he applies traction to the fetus, removing it completely from the patient.[147]

He then quotes the description that nurse Brenda Shafer provided during the congressional debate over the act:

> Dr. Haskell went in with forceps and grabbed the baby's legs and pulled them down into the birth canal. Then he delivered the baby's body and the arms— everything but the head. The doctor kept the head right in the uterus....The baby's little fingers were clasping and unclasping, and his little feet were kicking. Then the doctor stuck the scissors in the back of his head, and the baby's arms jerked out, like a startle reaction, like a flinch, like a baby does when he thinks he's going to fall. The doctor opened up the scissors, stuck a high-powered

suction tube into the opening and sucked the baby's brains out. Now the baby went completely limp.... He cut the umbilical cord and delivered the placenta. He threw the baby in a pan, along with the placenta and the instruments he had just used.[148]

Kennedy turned to Shafer's description in explaining why he found persuasive the congressional findings that "implicitly approving such a brutal and inhumane procedure by choosing not to prohibit it will further coarsen society to the inhumanity of not only newborns, but all vulnerable and innocent life, making it increasingly difficult to protect such life," as well as the finding that the procedure "confuses the medical, legal, and ethical duties of physicians to preserve and promote life, as the physician acts directly against the physical life of a child, whom he or she had just delivered, all but the head, out of the womb, in order to deliver that life."[149] According to Kennedy, the *Casey* undue burden standard allows the "state to use its regulatory powers to bar certain procedures and substitute others, all in furtherance of its legitimate interests in regulating the medical profession in order to promote respect for life," and that Congress's concern with "draw[ing] a bright line that clearly distinguishes abortion and infanticide" clearly furthers the government's interests.[150] Kennedy goes on to conclude that not only does this ban not constitute an undue burden, but that it protects women from making uninformed and emotional decisions:

Respect for human life finds an ultimate expression in the bond of love the mother has for her child. The Act recognizes this reality as well. Whether to have an abortion requires a difficult and painful moral decision. While we find no reliable data to measure the phenomenon, it seems unexceptionable to conclude some women come to regret their choice to abort the infant life they once created and sustained. Severe depression and loss of esteem can follow. In a decision so fraught with emotional consequences some doctors may prefer not to disclose precise details of the means that will be used, confining themselves to the required statement of risks the procedure entails. From one standpoint this ought not to be surprising. Any number of patients facing imminent surgical procedures would prefer not to hear all details, lest the usual anxiety preceding invasive medical procedures become the more intense. This is likely the case with the abortion procedures here in issue. It is, however, precisely this lack of information concerning the way in which the fetus will be killed that is of legitimate concern to the State. The State has an interest in ensuring so grave a choice is well informed. It is self-evident that a mother who comes to regret her choice to abort must struggle with grief more anguished and sorrow more profound when she learns, only after the event, what she once did not know: that she allowed a doctor to pierce the skull and vacuum the fast-developing brain of her unborn child, a child assuming the human form.[151]

As an indication of her vehement opposition to what she called an "alarming" decision, Ruth Bader Ginsburg took the relatively unusual step of reading her dissent, which was joined by Justice John Paul Stevens, Justice David Souter, and Justice Stephen Breyer, out loud from the steps of the Supreme Court. She responded to Kennedy's decision point by point, beginning with a critique of his reading of the *Casey* decision. In determining whether or not a restriction constitutes an "undue burden," she argued that the court must consider the impact of the restriction not on "all women," "all pregnant women," nor even all women "seeking abortions." The restriction, Ginsburg explained, "must be judged by reference to those women for whom it is an actual rather than irrelevant restriction. Absence of health exception burdens all women for whom it is relevant—women who, in the judgement of their doctors, require an intact D&E because other procedures would place their health at risk."[152] And the standard for assessing whether a restriction is an undue burden must be measured not by the low bar of "rational basis," as Kennedy did, but by the higher bar of "heightened scrutiny."

She then condemned the majority's deference to congressional findings, suggesting that the findings did not reflect the tremendous weight of expertise on the argument that the procedure is at times the safest. Rather, she suggested, the findings reflected the antiabortion bias of Congress, and Kennedy's opinion indicated a similar hostility to *Roe* and *Casey*. She pointed out that throughout the opinion, Kennedy called the obstetrician-gynecologists who perform abortions "abortion doctors"; described the fetus as an "unborn child" and "baby"; described second-trimester previability abortions "late-term"; described medical judgments as "preferences" motivated by "mere convenience"; and referred to the "essential holding of *Roe*" not as "reaffirmed," which *Casey* did, but as "assumed for the moment."[153]

She concluded by rejecting entirely Kennedy's argument that the ban "protects" women from making bad decisions they may regret.[154] Ginsburg's strongest criticism came in her attack on the "antiabortion shibboleth" that "women who have abortions come to regret their choices, and consequently suffer from 'severe depression and loss of esteem.'"[155] Comparing this logic to the *Bradwell v. Illinois* decision, which in 1873 upheld an Illinois statute refusing to admit a woman to the bar because "the natural and proper timidity and delicacy which belongs to the female sex evidently unfits it for many of the occupations of civil life...the paramount destiny and mission of woman are to fulfill the noble and benign offices of wife and mother," and to the *Muller v. Oregon* decision, which in 1908 upheld limitations on women's hours of work because of women's "physical structure and a proper discharge of her maternal function," Ginsburg concluded that the *Gonzales* decision "reflects ancient notions about women's place in the family that have long since been discredited."[156]

Despite Ginsburg's powerful dissent, Kennedy's opinion illustrated the success of the women-centered arguments developed and deployed by the antiabortion movement over the previous two decades, while highlighting the fact that this case was at once about much more than and much less than the fetus. On the one hand, as Ginsburg made clear, not one more fetus will live as a result of the *Gonzales* decision, showing how opposition to partial-birth abortion was never about the saving of unborn life. The decision also suggested that those "ancient notions" that Ginsburg alluded to have not in fact been entirely discredited. Cheered by antiabortion activists and condemned by pro-choice activists as the biggest step taken toward banning abortion since the *Roe* decision, the *Gonzales* decision echoed nineteenth-century arguments for criminalizing abortion, arguments that emphasized a purported concern for women rather than the fetus. That similarity suggests that now, as then, the debate about abortion is less about the life and rights of the fetus than it is about women's role in society; and that now, as then, the court, and the country, remain conflicted about the relative authority of scientific authority and religious values, the connection between motherhood and citizenship, and the relationship of physical and physiological difference to the meaning of political and social equality.

EPILOGUE
FETAL MEANINGS

On January 20, 2009, hours before President-elect Barack Obama took the oath of office, the Provider Refusal Rule went into effect. Signed into law in the last days of President George W. Bush's administration, this "midnight rule" required the Department of Health and Human Services to cut off federal aid to health programs and institutions that discriminated against people who object to abortion on the basis of "religious beliefs or moral objections." The Provider Refusal Rule defined abortion to include "any of the various procedures—including the prescription, dispensing and administering any drug or the performance of any procedure or any other action—that results in the termination of the life of a human being in utero between conception and natural birth, whether before or after implantation."[1] This definition would include a variety of forms of birth control, including oral contraceptives and emergency contraception. Reflecting the belief that there is no meaningful difference between a fertilized egg and a third-trimester fetus, the HHS proposal exemplified the growing strategy of appropriating arguments from the liberal arsenal—in this case, arguments about religious tolerance—to achieve antiabortion ends. On March 2, 2009, President Obama directed the Department of Health and Human Services to rescind this law.

This was not the first time that Obama would directly overturn Bush administration policies limiting reproductive rights during his first months in office. Three days after his inauguration, he issued an executive order repealing rules that restricted federal money for international organizations that promote or provide abortions overseas.[2] On March 9, he lifted the Bush administration's strict limits on human embryonic stem cell research. And on March 23, the Food and Drug Administration changed their policy to make emergency contraception—also know as Plan B, or the "morning-after" pill—available without prescription to women seventeen years and older. These dramatic policy shifts reflect the enormous power of the state to construct and reconstruct fetal politics at a national level. But these shifts, enacted with a single signature, can obscure the ongoing struggles to define the meaning of the fetus.

In October 2009, Congress was debating whether or not the health-care reform plan would ban coverage of abortions under federally subsidized health insurance. Republicans opposed any federal subsidy going to pay for abortions, directly or indirectly; whereas Democrats were divided between their commitment to a public option, which could get lost over the abortion fight, and their commitment to reproductive rights. This debate reflected the ways that fetal discourses in the early twenty-first century are highly politicized struggles that take place in the arena of party politics.

At the state level, efforts to give personhood rights to the fetus continue. PersonhoodUSA is an organization that claims "each and every human being must be respected and protected from fertilization until natural death" and is dedicated to establishing the "pre-born, as legal persons with protection under the law."[3] PersonhoodUSA supports the Snowflake Embryo Donation and Adoption Awareness Program, which encourages people to adopt the more than five hundred thousand embryos currently in storage. They are also at the forefront of efforts to pass "personhood" laws that would establish the "pre-born as legal persons with protection under the law."[4] In February 2009, North Dakota's House of Representatives passed a personhood bill that requires state laws to apply to "any organism with the genome of *homo sapiens*," including a fertilized egg.[5] The state Senate voted down the bill in April of 2009 but passed a bill requiring abortion providers to inform a patient that "the abortion will terminate the life of a separate, unique, living human being."[6] Seventeen states are currently considering similar bills.[7] One of the most important rhetorical arguments made by PersonhoodUSA and represented in the so-called personhood bills is the shift in language from "unborn" to "preborn," a shift that suggests a natural continuum from preborn to born, as opposed to a discrete moment in time in which one changes from being unborn to born.

Contested fetal meanings, although not always as partisan as they have become since *Roe v. Wade,* have occupied an important place in the public sphere and collective imagination of the United States. And the stakes of these contests—for women in particular but for Americans in general—have always been high. The rhetoric and ideas of the antiabortion activists, the eugenicists, and the prenatal culturists of the Progressive Era echo throughout fetal discourses in the early twenty-first century. Debates about embryonic stem cell research, RU-486, and "partial-birth abortions" use the same "right to life" language as the early antiabortion movement. Arguments that declining birth rates among European-Americans, combined with escalating immigration rates from nonwhite countries auguring what conservative commentator Pat Buchanan called the "death of the West," echo Progressive Era fears of "race suicide." Concerns about the ethics of genetic testing and the quest for the perfect baby recall those about eugenics and stirpiculture. Books like *Super Baby: Boost Your Baby's Potential from Conception to Year One* and *While You're Expecting: Creating Your Own Prenatal Classroom,* products like the Em-bry-on-ics Learning System, which "provides developmentally appropriate stimulation to enhance the learning process in the womb," and organizations like the National Association for Prenatal Psychology and Education and the International Music Society for Prenatal Development could come straight out of Progressive Era theories of prenatal culture.[8] The image and idea of the fetus that motivated Horatio Storer in his campaign to criminalize abortion and that helped convict Kenneth Edelin remains a potent symbol for the pro-life movement. But although debates about the meaning and status of the fetus have taken place most explicitly in law and policy, they have also taken place in museums, cartoon strips, and in the cultural imagination.

In 2008, in celebration of their seventy-fifth anniversary, the Museum of Science and Industry in Chicago redesigned their "Prenatal Development" exhibit one more time.[9] As part of their planning process, the museum commissioned the Institute for Learning Innovation to conduct a study assessing visitors' responses to the current exhibit and to the one being planned. The report concluded that visitors rated the exhibit very highly—the average score was 8.4 out of 10—but it also identified a pattern of comments that reflected interest in and concern about the origins of the fetal specimens.

Many visitors identified the fetuses as their favorite part of the exhibit, praising their authenticity and "real-ness." Some praised the power of "seeing it right there, not in a book, seeing the actual human." One visitor said that she was "always thinking what happened to the babies.... I want to know what happened to each baby and mother." Other comments included the following: "It made me uncomfortable because they're babies on display"; "It's sad to think those babies died"; and "It's like being at a funeral, seeing an open casket.... It's a real person."[10] Other visitors asked whether the specimens were obtained during abortions, and one suggested that the exhibit was making a pro-life argument, asking, "How can you look at that and say it isn't a life?" Collectively, those surveyed praised the new plan for the future exhibit for being "respectful" to the fetuses. One visitor noted approvingly that it was "almost like a memorial."[11]

Given the cultural politics of the unborn in the contemporary United States, this wide range of responses is not surprising. Whether out of a practical need to attract visitors, a pragmatic desire to avoid becoming a target of protestors and activists, or a pedagogical inclination to let visitors interpret objects for themselves, the museum wanted an exhibit that would allow these competing interpretations to coexist. The consultants concluded their report with the recommendation that that "these potentially divisive issues should be monitored to ensure that the experience will be appealing and meaningful to the entire Museum visitorship," a recommendation that reflected the museum's commitment to an exhibit that allows for ambivalence and multiple meanings.[12]

In stark contrast to the museum's efforts to recognize multiple fetal meanings is the work of antiabortion cartoonist Gary Cangemi. The creator of the nationally syndicated comic strip featuring a "pro-life, prenatal cartoon baby" named Umbert, Cangemi is one of the most popular speakers at the Right to Life Committee's annual conventions.[13] In *Umbert the Unborn: A Womb with a View*, a book-length collection of these cartoons, Cangemi presents Umbert's nine months *in utero* chronologically, without differentiating visually the developmental process of gestation.[14] Umbert looks exactly the same in the cartoon labeled "First Trimester, Day 1," as he does in the cartoon labeled "Third Trimester, Day 270." Conflating nine fluid months of embryonic development into one static image of self-evident baby-ness, Cangemi gives narrative and illustrative form to his belief that "Umbert is a person from the moment of conception."[15] In addition to manipulating time, Cangemi's cartoons misrepresent space. Umbert's umbilical cord stops at the edge of a wavy line representing the placental barrier that encircles him, and the pregnant woman, Umbert's mother, is entirely left out.

Framing the fetus as an independent homunculus, as in Cangemi's cartoons, does more than make an argument against abortion.[16] Political scientist Rosalind Petchesky explains that because the fetus could not "possibly experience itself as dangling in space, without a woman's uterus and body and bloodstream to support it.... Every fetal image—including those projected on the display terminals of ultrasound machines—is an artificial construct, a fetish, representing the standpoint of neither an actual fetus nor a pregnant woman, but an outside observer."[17] In *Umbert the Unborn*, that outside observer is Gary Cangemi, from whose standpoint the fetus-as-fetish not only serves as an object lesson against abortion, but also makes arguments about gender roles, racial and ethnic identity, and American history.

Although described by Cangemi as a "pre-born infant of yet undetermined gender," Umbert is obviously a male, and his description of his mother and father suggests an uncritical acceptance of traditional gender roles. Umbert's mother is an exemplar of what journalist Gena Corea has called the "mother machine," meriting his attention only when she does something—plays classical music hoping to educate him but actually boring him, cries with excitement when she sees him in her first ultrasound, avoids alcohol for his benefit, eats nachos to his discomfort—that directly affects him.[18] In contrast, Umbert presents his father as someone who leads an interesting and busy life. Umbert eagerly anticipates the sound of a "really deep voice" at 6:00 P.M. signaling that "Dad's coming home from work," enjoys it when his father cheers on a football team, and worries when his father expresses concerns about the family finances.[19] And, after September 11, 2001, his father comforted his mother who was crying because "something terrible happened," and helped Umbert recognize his national identity: "Dad said they had to keep freedom alive for my sake. I'm proud to be conceived an American."[20]

One way that Cangemi connects Umbert to American history is by attributing to Umbert the identities of other famous Americans. One comic strip has three panels depicting Umbert as American presidents *in utero:* as George Washington, white wig on his head, he says, "I shall not tell a lie"; as Franklin D. Roosevelt, cigarette holder in his mouth, he says, "I will fear nothing but fear itself"; and as John F. Kennedy, big smile on his face, he says, "I will ask what I can do for my country."[21] And in another strip, his eighty-seventh day of gestation, he is depicted as Abraham Lincoln, with beard and hat, saying, "Four score and seven days ago, my parents brought forth a new life."[22] The subsequent panel shows Umbert-as-Umbert saying, "I wonder what kind of greatness I'm destined for."[23] Juxtaposed to Umbert's pride in being "conceived an American" is his argument that abortion might be depriving the nation of future greatness.

In Umbert's world, being "an American" implies embodying a particular gender, racial, and ethnic identity. Not only is Umbert male, but he is also presented as what Cangemi describes as a "warrior-hero." Cangemi wanted to give his creation a "heroic-sounding name . . . evoking the image of a warrior-hero, fighting for a noble cause—something that sounded like 'Richard the Lionhearted' or 'Peter the Great.'" Concerned that his first choice of a name "Umberto the Unborn" was too ethnic, Cangemi describes how he solved that problem: "I simply dropped the extra vowel," he explains, "and Umbert was "unborn."[24]

Despite his stated desire for Umbert to have no discernable ethnic identity beyond a normative whiteness, Cangemi draws one cartoon showing an African-American version of Umbert paraphrasing the spiritual with which Martin Luther King, Jr., famously concluded his speech at the 1963 March on Washington, saying, "Free at last, free at last, next month, I'll be free at last!"[25] The image of Umbert-as-King has dual meanings. Positioning Umbert, who is white, ethnicless, and male, as a member of a new oppressed minority group, the unborn, the antiabortion movement is presented as the logical descendant of the civil rights movement.[26] At the same time, having Umbert appropriate the language of the civil rights movement illustrates how pro-life ideology deploys the unborn as the metaphorical replacement for the white, ethnic-less, males whose rights have been oppressed by the civil rights movement and feminism.

In another example of Cangemi's desire to identify the antiabortion movement with historic efforts to resist oppression, and other historic struggles for rights and liberties, he shows Umbert invoking language from the Declaration of Independence and the American Revolution. In one cartoon, Umbert depicted as Umbert says: "I can't wait to celebrate my first Fourth of July. That's when they adopted the Declaration of Independence. I especially like the part about the right to life, liberty, and the pursuit of happiness. The Founding Fathers really looked after us unborn kids" (figure 6.1).[27] These references no doubt resonated with the many antiabortion activists who frequently linked their cause to the civil rights movement and the American Revolution. For example, the annual antiabortion "Oh Saratoga!" rally bills itself as a "turning point in the war against babies" just as the Battle of Saratoga was a turning point in the war against the British.[28] The website for that event features lyrics from the Civil Rights anthem "Eyes on the Prize" and a link to buy a "battlefield book" titled *A Manifesto for the Saving of the Unborn Child and the Restoration of the Republic.*[29] Sponsored by Operation Save America—the organization previously known as Operation Rescue—the "Oh Saratoga!" event highlights the rhetorical linkages between the antiabortion movement and a militant patriotism.[30]

A cartoon fetus articulating an antiabortion position, endorsing traditional gender roles, constructing a normative American identity as white and male, identifying as an oppressed minority, and drawing upon a particular interpretation of American history may not surprise readers living in contemporary America. *Ourselves Unborn* suggests that it would not have surprised readers at other times as well. There have been many different fetuses in twentieth-century America. From Armenouhie Lamson to Gary Cangemi, from Horatio Storer to Kenneth Edelin, from Franklin Mall to John Rock, from Oliver Wendell Holmes to Charles Condon, people have told stories about the fetus in prescriptive liter-

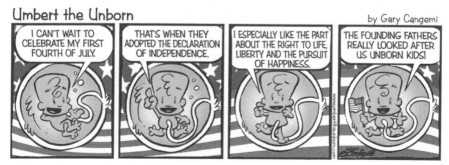

Figure. 6.1 Umbert the Unborn

ature and cartoons, in churches and courtrooms, in political parties and congressional debates, in museums and laboratories, in private homes and doctors' offices.

From the late nineteenth century through the early twenty-first century, the fetus has been a vehicle through which people have wrestled with assumptions about science and religion, anxieties about demography and democracy, beliefs about feminism and motherhood, and ideas about conservatism and liberalism. Recent efforts to protect "fetal rights" and fetal citizenship echoed but did not replicate late nineteenth-century efforts to protect the "right to be well-born" and the fears of race suicide. Appreciating the rhetorical continuities that link these claims together, as well as the historical specificities that differentiate them from one another, underscores the significance of fetal meanings in the history of modern America as well as the significance of modern America in the history of fetal meanings.

NOTES

Introduction

1. Rick Weiss, "New Status for Embryos in Research," A01.

2. State Children's Health Insurance Program; Eligibility for Prenatal Care and Other Health Services for Unborn Children; Final Rule, 67 Fed. Reg. 61955–61974 (2002) (to be codified at 42 C.F.R. pt. 457).

3. "U.S. District Judge Blocks Pregnant Woman's Deportation, Says Fetus Is U.S. Citizen."

4. Casper and Morgan, "Constructing Fetal Citizens."

5. *Roe v. Wade,* 410 U.S. 113 (1973).

6. NARAL Pro-Choice America Foundation, "Anti-Choice Violence and Intimidation," 2006.

7. National Abortion Foundation, "NAF Violence and Disruption Statistics," available at http://www.prochoice.org/about_abortion/violence/; (accessed July 19, 2008); Ginsburg, "Rescuing the Nation: Operation Rescue and the Rise of Anti-Abortion Militance," in *Abortion Wars,* ed. Solinger, 227–250.

8. Han, "Seeing Like a Family," in *Imagining the Fetus,* eds. Sasson and Law.

9. Needham, *A History of Embryology;* Speert, *Illustrated History of Gynecology and Obstetrics;* William Ray Arney, *Power and the Profession of Obstetrics;* and Ann Oakley, *The Captured Womb.*

10. Harrison, "Unborn: Historical Perspective of the Fetus as a Patient"; Kolata, *The Baby Doctors;* Harrison, Golbus, and Filly, eds., *The Unborn Patient;* and Casper, *The Making of the Unborn Patient.*

11. Blank, *Mother and Fetus;* Steinbock, *Life before Birth;* Roth, *Making Women Pay;* and Schroedel, *Is the Fetus a Person?.*

12. Dorland, *X-Ray in Embryology and Obstetrics;* Kevles, *Naked to the Bone;* Terry, "The Body Invaded"; and Cartwright, *Screening the Body.*

13. For work showing how the fetus is interpreted in other cultures, see Dettwyler, *Dancing Skeletons;* von Raffler-Engel, *The Perception of the Unborn Across the Cultures of the World;* LaFleur, *Liquid Life;* Oaks, "Fetal Spirithood and Fetal Personhood"; Conklin and Morgan, "Babies, Bodies, and the Production of Personhood in North America and a Native Amazonian Society"; Morgan, "Imagining the Unborn in the Ecuadoran Andes"; Ortiz, "'Bare-Handed' Medicine and Its Elusive Patients"; Hardacre, *Marketing the Menace Fetus in Japan;* Oaks, "Irish Trans/national Politics and Locating Fetuses," in *Fetal Subjects, Feminist Positions;* Moskowitz, *The Haunting Fetus.*

14. Becker, "From *Muller v. Oregon* to Fetal Vulnerability Policies"; Berrian, "Pregnancy and Drug Use"; Blank, *Fetal Protection in the Workplace;*, Cohen and Taub, eds., *New Reproductive Laws for the 1990s;* Daniels, *At Women's Expense;* Fineman and Karpin, eds., *Mothers in Law;* Roth, *Making Women Pay;* Samuels, *Fetal Rights, Women's Rights;* Williams, "Firing Women to Protect the Fetus."

15. *In re A.C.* 533 A.2d 611 (1987); *United Auto Workers v. Johnson Controls, Inc.,* 111 S. Ct. 1196 (1991; *Ferguson v. City of Charleston,* 183 F. 3d 469 (2001).

16. Cobb, *Generation;* Pinto-Correia, *The Ovary of Eve.*

17. Morgan, *Icons of Life;* Marsh and Ronner, *The Fertility Doctor;* McLaughlin, *The Pill, John Rock, and the Church;* Morgan, "Trafficking in Fetal Remains."

18. Casper, *The Making of the Unborn Patient.*

19. Brodie, *Contraception and Abortion in Nineteenth-Century America;* Mohr; *Abortion in America;* Reagan; *When Abortion Was a Crime;* Solinger, *Abortion Wars;* Petchesky, *Abortion and Woman's Choice.*

20. Zwerin and Shapiro, "Abortion: Perspectives from Jewish Traditions."

21. Mohammed, "Islamic Tradition and Reproductive Choice."

22. Schroedel, "Law, Religion, and Fetal Personhood."

23. Ibid.

24. Sasson and Law, eds., *Imagining the Fetus: The Unborn in Myth, Religion, and Culture.*

25. Noonan, ed., *The Morality of Abortion: Legal and Historical Perspectives;* William Saletan, *Bearing Right.*

26. Stabile, "Shooting the Mother"; Hartouni, "Fetal Exposures"; Rothman, *The Tentative Pregnancy.* Also see Petchesky, "Fetal Images"; Franklin, "Fetal Fascinations"; Bordo, "Are Mothers Person?"; Berlant, "America, 'Fat,' the Fetus," in *The Queen of America Goes to Washington City;* Hartouni, *Cultural Conceptions;* Mitchell and Georges, "Baby's First Picture"; and Taylor, "Images of Contradiction."

27. Martin, "The Fetus as Intruder: Mother's Bodies and Medical Metaphors"; Martin, *The Woman in the Body;* Casper, *The Making of the Unborn Patient;* Rothman, *The Tentative Pregnancy;* and Rapp, *Testing Women, Testing the Fetus.* Also see Cartwright, "The Logic of Heartbeats"; and Kahn, *Bearing Meaning.* For more general discussions of the ways in which gender ideologies are at work in the production of scientific knowledge, see Harding, *The Science Question in Feminism;* Hubbard, *The Politics of Women's Biology;* Laqueur, *Making Sex;* Longino, *Science as Social Knowledge;* Harding, *Whose Science? Whose Knowledge?;* Haraway, *Simians, Cyborgs, and Women: The Reinvention of Nature.*

28. Morgan, "Materializing the Fetal Body"; Hopwood, "'Giving Body' to Embryos"; and Hopwood, *Embryos in Wax.*

29. *The Silent Scream,* a 28-min. film produced by Donald S. Smith (American Portrait Films, 1984), script and visuals at http://www.silentscream.org (accessed July 14, 2008); *Gonzalez v. Carhart* 550 U.S. 124 (2007).

Chapter 1

1. Lamson, *My Birth.*

2. For reviews, see F.H.P., "My Birth," *Education* 37, no. 7 (March 1917): 468 and the *New York Times,* March 27, 1927.

3. Walsh, "*Doctors Wanted: No Women Need Apply*"; Morantz-Sanchez, *Sympathy and Science;* Abram, *Send Us a Lady Physician;* Drachman, "The Limits of Progress: The Professional Lives of Women Doctors."

4. Biographical information on Lamson comes from *Who Was Who Among North American Authors,* 1921–1929, vol. 2 (Gale Research Co, 1976) and "Armene Lamson: Social, Civic, UNICEF Leader," Obituary, *Seattle Post-Intelligencer,* September 23, 1970.

For references to Lamson's role in the suffrage movement, see Haarsager, *Bertha Knight Landes of Seattle;* Jaconi, "Inez Milholland: A Thanatography of the Suffrage Martyr."

5. Commager, *The American Mind;* Hayes, *The Response to Industrialism;* Wiebe, *The Search for Order;* Boyer, *Urban Masses;* Bruce, *The Launching of Modern American Science;* Rodgers, *Atlantic Crossings;* Livingston, *Pragmatism, Feminism, and Democracy;* Menand, *The Metaphysical Club.*

6. Upton Sinclair coined the term "white collar workers" in *The Brass Check;* "teener" was coined in 1894 and "teenage" originated in 1921, see "Etymology Online," available at http://www.etymonline.com/index.php?term=teenage; Ouida and Sarah Grand coined the term "New Woman," in their 1894 essay in the *North American Review,* see "New Woman," *The Cambridge Guide to Women's Writing in English,* Lorna Sage, Germaine Greer, and Elaine Showalter, eds. (Cambridge: Cambridge University Press, 1999), 465; Alain Locke, coined "New Negro" in his essay, "Enter the New Negro," *The Survey Graphic Harlem Number* 6, no. 6 (March 1925): 631–634.

7. Ballantyne, *Manual of Antenatal Pathology and Hygiene,* 3.

8. Lamson, *My Birth.*

9. Ibid., 148.

10. Hopwood, "Producing Development."

11. Wiebe, *The Search for Order;* Lippmann, *Drift and Mastery.*

12. Lippmann, *Drift and Mastery,* 148.

13. Gilbert, *A Conceptual History of Modern Embryology;* Clarke, *Disciplining Reproduction.*

14. Cobb, *Generation,* 2006, 11.

15. Aristotle, *The History of Animals* 7.3.583 and Aristotle, *On the Generation of Animals* 2.5.714, quoted in Grossinger, *Embryogenesis,* 122. Also see Noonan, "An Almost Absolute Value in History," in *The Morality of Abortion: Legal and Historical Perspectives,* 1–60.

16. Feen, "Abortion and Exposure in Ancient Greece."

17. Needham, *A History of Embryology;* Ford, *When Did I Begin?;* Dunstan, *The Human Embryo;* Tuana, "The History of Embryology"; and Horowitz, "The 'Science' of Embryology before the Discovery of the Ovum," 105–112.

18. Horowitz, "The 'Science' of Embryology," 109.

19. Pinto-Correia, *The Ovary of Eve,* 3.

20. Porter, *The Greatest Benefit to Mankind,* 201–226.

21. Pinto-Correia, *The Ovary of Eve,* 25; Porter, *The Greatest Benefit to Mankind,* 219–223.

22. Grossinger, *Embryogenesis,* 121.

23. Irwin, "Embryology and the Incarnation"; Roe, *Matter, Life, and Generation.*

24. Pinto-Correia, *The Ovary of Eve,* 4.

25. Cobb, *Generation,* 246.

26. Meyer, *The Rise of Embryology,* 198; Hertwig, *The Biological Problem of Today.*

27. Hertwig, *The Biological Problem of Today,* 248.

28. Buettner, "Franklin Paine Mall," *Embryo Project Encyclopedia* (Embryo Project Research Network of Arizona State University, 2007), available at http://embryo.asu.edu/view/embryo:124433? (accessed July 16, 2008; Mall, "A Human Embryo, Twenty-Six

Days Old"; Mall, "A Contribution to the Study of the Pathology of Human Embryos"; Mall, "A Plea for an Institute of Human Embryology." Formally, the term *embryo* refers to the developing human during the first eight weeks of gestation, but in the nineteenth and early twentieth centuries, the word *embryo* was used—colloquially and professionally—to refer to the developing human through all stages of development. For a discussion on terminology, see Lynn Morgan, "Embryo Tales," in Icons of Life, 264.

29. Hopwood, "Producing Development," 45.

30. Hopwood, "Pictures of Evolution and Charges of Fraud," 261.

31. Hopwood, *Embryos in Wax,* 69.

32. Morgan, "The Embryography of Alice B. Toklas," 309.

33. Morgan, "Embryo Tales," in *Icons of Life,* 265; Mall, "Report upon the Collection of Human Embryos at the Johns Hopkins University." Also see Mall, "Methods of Preserving Human Embryos"; Mall, "A List of Normal Human Embryos Which Have Been Cut into Serial Sections."

34. Morgan, "Trafficking in Fetal Remains." For a discussion of the use and display of fetuses in late-nineteenth-century France, see Menon, "Anatomy of a Motif"; Thelberg, "Instruction of College Students in Regard to Reproduction and Maternity"; Morgan, "The Rise and Demise of a Collection of Human Fetuses at Mount Holyoke College"; McLaren, "Why Study Early Human Development"; Clarke, "Research Materials and Reproductive Science in the United States"; Clarke, "Money, Sex, and Legitimacy at Chicago, circa 1892–1940"; and Morgan, "Materializing the Fetal Body."

35. Morgan, "'Properly Disposed Of,'" 248; Greg, "The Carnegie Human Embryo Collection: A Brief History." On the history of the Carnegie Institute of Embryology, see Sabin, *Franklin Paine Mall;* Corner, *The Seven Ages of a Medical Scientist;* McLaughlin, *The Pill, John Rock, and the Church,* 58–71; Brown, "The Department of Embryology of the Carnegie Institution of Washington," 92–96.

36. Morgan, "Properly Disposed of," 255.

37. Ibid., 255.

38. Ibid., 262.

39. Corner, *Ourselves Unborn,* 28.

40. The first of these statutes was in Connecticut. *Public Statute Laws of the State of Connecticut,* 1821 (Hartford, 1821), 153–53, reprinted in Tone, *Controlling Reproduction,* 138.

41. Mohr, *Abortion in America,* 149. In "Taking the Trade," Dayton makes a similar argument for the eighteenth century, arguing that abortion became problematic only when it exposed a failed courtship or illegitimacy, in which case it was attacked as dangerous for women, not as "the destruction of the fetus."

42. Brodie, *Contraception and Abortion,* 268–271; Dyer, *Champion of Women and the Unborn.*

43. Brodie, *Contraception and Abortion,* 270.

44. Storer, *Why Not? A Book Intended for Every Woman.* Also see Dyer, *Champion of Women and the Unborn.*

45. Brodie, *Contraception and Abortion,* 270; Beisel, *Imperiled Innocents.*

46. Storer, *On Criminal Abortion,* 13.

47. Storer, *On Criminal Abortion,* 11.

48. Hodge, *Foeticide, or Criminal Abortion,* 22.

49. Storer, *On Criminal Abortion,* 14.

50. Hodge, *An Introductory Lecture to a Course on Obstetrics,* quoted in Brodie, *Contraception and Abortion,* 266.

51. Hodge, *Foeticide, or Criminal Abortion,* 3.

52. *Boston Medical and Surgical Journal* 53, no. 20 (December 13, 1855): 409–411; Storer, *On Criminal Abortion,* 58; Sauer, "Attitudes to Abortion in America"; Nebinger, *Criminal Abortion: Its Extent and Prevention,* 21.

53. *New York Times,* August 27, 1871, 6.

54. Dorland, *A Manual of Obstetrics,* 96.

55. Hodge, *Foeticide, or Criminal Abortion,* 33.

56. Hodge, *Foeticide, or Criminal Abortion,* 29 and 37.

57. Ibid., 29.

58. "Procuring Abortions."

59. Degler, *At Odds,* 239. Although many Christian leaders condemned abortion, the Apostolic Constitutions (circa 380 CE) allowed abortions early in pregnancy but prohibited it if the fetus was of human shape and contained a soul: "Thou shalt not slay the child by causing abortion, nor kill that which is begotten. For everything that is shaped, and has received a soul from God, if slain, it shall be avenged, as being unjustly destroyed." (7:3). St. Augustine (354–430 CE) embraced the Aristotelian concept of "delayed ensoulment," arguing that because a human soul cannot live in an unformed body, an abortion early in pregnancy is not murder because no soul is destroyed. In the seventeenth century, the concept of *simultaneous animation,* the belief that an embryo acquires a soul at the time of conception, gained acceptance within the medical and church communities.

60. Quoted in Noonan, "An Almost Absolute Value in History," in *The Morality of Abortion,* 13. On the other hand, Tertullian also rejected contraception and abortion, saying that, "murder being once for all forbidden, we may not destroy even the foetus in the womb.... To hinder a birth is merely a speedier murder; nor does it matter whether you take away a life that is born or destroy one that is coming to the birth. That is a man which is going to be one; you have the fruit already in hand."

61. *The Decreten* ("determined to be the case") collected statements from religious and secular authorities and was the basic canon law textbook in Europe and the Catholic Church until 1917. Gilbert, Tyler, and Zackin, *Bioethics and the New Embryology,* 37.

62. Ryan, "Wrestling with the Angel"; McLaren, "Policing Pregnancies: Changes in Nineteenth-Century Criminal and Canon Law," in Dunstan, ed., *The Human Embryo,* 187–207.

63. Quoted in Stormer, *Articulating Life's Memory,* 71.

64. Kelly, "The Ethics of Abortion as a Method of Treatment in Legitimate Practice."

65. Mitchell, "Infanticide: Its Moral and Legal Aspects."

66. Stormer, *Articulating Life's Memory,* 23.

67. For a cogent analysis of the declining birthrate and increasing abortion rate, see Mohr, *Abortion in America,* 50–93.

68. Lears, *No Place of Grace*; Smith-Rosenberg, *Disorderly Conduct*; Cott, *The Grounding of Modern Feminism*; Mark Carnes, *Meanings for Manhood*; and Bederman, *Manliness and Civilization*.

69. Quoted in Guinn, "Figuring the Fetus," 24.

70. Storer, *Why Not?* Also see Dyer, *Champion of Women and the Unborn*.

71. Storer, *Why Not?* 85.

72. Stormer, *Articulating Life's Memory*, 23.

73. Theodore Roosevelt, "A Letter from President Roosevelt on Race Suicide"; physician quoted in Mohr, *Abortion in America*, 297.

74. Sinclair, *The Crowning Sin of the Age*, 19.

75. Stormer, *Articulating Life's Memory*, 8.

76. Jelliffe, *The Medical News*, 192.

77. Quoted in Reagan, *When Abortion Was a Crime*, 89; Holmes, "The Methods of the Professional Abortionist."

78. Sinclair, *The Crowning Sin of the Age*, 16.

79. Quoted in Reagan, *When Abortion Was a Crime*, 83; Reed, "Therapeutic and Criminal Abortion," 27.

80. Findlay, "The Slaughter of the Innocents," 35.

81. Quoted in Holmes, "The Methods of the Professional Abortionist," 542.

82. Quoted in Reagan, *When Abortion Was a Crime*, 83.

83. Quoted in ibid., 85; Taussig, *The Prevention and Treatment of Abortion*, 79.

84. Nix, *The Unborn*.

85. *Dietrich v. Inhabitants of Northampton*, 14.

86. Ibid., 15.

87. *Allaire v. St. Luke's Hospital*, 640.

88. Ibid., 640.

89. Ibid., 642. Also see *Walker v. Gt. Northern Railway Co.* and *Gorman v. Budlong*. See "The Rights of Unborn Children"; "Injuries to Infants *en ventre sa mere*"; and "Legal Protection to Unborn Children" for discussions of this trend.

90. *Allaire v. St. Luke's Hospital*, 640.

91. Herzog quoted in Marcy, "Education as a Factor in the Prevention of Criminal Abortion and Illegitimacy."

92. Robinson, *Fewer and Better Babies, or the Limitation of Offspring*, 121.

93. Smith, *A Plea for the Unborn*; Treub, *The Right to Life of the Unborn Child*; Smith, *The Color Line*; Rentoul, *Race Culture; or, Race Suicide?*; Dietrich, *The Melting Pot*; Dawson, *The Right of the Child to Be Well Born*; "The Rights of Unborn Children"; "The Rights of the Unborn"; Pollard, *The Rights of the Unborn Race*; and Guyer, *Being Well-Born*.

94. Rodgers, "In Search of Progressivism"; Kloppenberg, *Uncertain Victory*.

95. Bolotin and Laing, *The Chicago World's Fair of 1893*; Johnson, *A History of the World's Columbian Exposition Held in Chicago in 1893*.

96. Hopwood, *Embryos in Wax*, 1. *World's Columbian Exposition: Chicago, Official Catalogue Exhibition of the German Empire*, 279.

97. Bancroft, *The Book of the Fair*.

98. Hanson, *The World's Congress of Religions*.

99. Ibid., 25.

100. Wilcox, "Splendid Amazons and Pygmy Men," 36.

101. Moore and Moore, *In Search of White Crows;* Washington, *Madame Blavatsky's Baboon;* Satter, *Each Mind a Kingdom;* Braude, *Radical Spirits.*

102. Tingley, *The Gods Await.*

103. Dresser, *A History of the New Thought Movement,* 33.

104. Clymer, *By Means of the Art or Science Known as Stirpiculture,* 13.

105. Ibid., 19.

106. Bayer, *Maternal Impressions,* 4.

107. Ibid., 160.

108. Ibid., 81.

109. Wilcox, *The Heart of the New Thought.*

110. Smith, "Prenatal Education," 152.

111. Ibid., 154.

112. Champness, "Heredity versus the Power of Thought," 63.

113. Harman, *The Right to Be Born Well,* 13.

114. Ibid., 63.

115. Quoted in Miller, "The White City," 84. For more on the racial ideology of the fair, see Baker, *From Savage to Negro.*

116. *Harper's Magazine* 173 (September 1, 1893).

117. Jastrow, "The Section of Psychology," 50; Varigny, "The Experimental Psychology Laboratory of the University of Madison."

118. Bancroft, *The Book of the Fair.*

119. Quote from Ambert, "The Graphic Sphere," 15. For a more thorough examination of eugenics, see Selden, *Inheriting Shame;* Degler, *In Search of Human Nature;* Richards, *Darwin and the Emergence of Evolutionary Theories of Mind and Behavior;* and Hofstadter, *Social Darwinism in American Thought.*

120. Larson, "Tailored Genes," 1.

121. Noyes, "Essay on Scientific Propagation," 5.

122. Kern, *An Ordered Love;* Karp, "Past Perfect: John Humphrey Noyes, Stirpiculture, and the Oneida Community"; and Foster, *Women, Family, and Utopia.*

123. Haller, *Eugenics: Hereditarian Attitudes in American Thought;* Ludmerer, *Genetics and American Society: A Historical Approach;* Rosenberg, "The Bitter Fruit"; Duster, *Backdoor to Eugenics;* Degler, *In Search of Human Nature;* Rushton, *Genetics and Medicine in the United States;* Kevles, *In the Name of Eugenics;* Hasian, *The Rhetoric of Eugenics in Anglo-American T*hought; Paul, *Controlling Human Heredity, 1865 to the Present;* Selden, *Inheriting Shame;* Carlson, *The Unfit;* and Kline, *Building a Better Race.*

124. Rosenberg, *No Other Gods,* 89.

125. Galton, *Eugenics: Its Definition, Scope and Aims,* 45.

126. Gillham, *A Life of Sir Francis Galton,* 2001; Paul, *Controlling Human Heredity,* 5.

127. Laughlin, "The Scope of the Committee's Work," 7.

128. Selden, *Inheriting Shame,* 7.

129. In 1907, the first involuntary sterilization law was passed in Indiana; in 1927 the Supreme Court ruling in *Buck v. Bell* upheld the compulsory sterilization of "socially

inadequate person[s]"; and by 1932, twenty-six states had passed laws legalizing "forced sterilization of individuals considered feebleminded, retarded, delinquent, or otherwise unfit." Between 1907 and 1973, it is estimated that more than sixty thousand people were eugenically sterilized in the United States.

130. First quote from Paul, *Controlling Human Heredity*, 1; second quote from Pernick, *The Black Stork*, 1996, 43.

131. Lippincott, "'Something in Motion and Something to Eat Attract the Crowd.'"

132. Richards, *Euthenics*, 3. For more on Ellen Swallow Richards, see Hunt, *The Life of Ellen H. Richards;* Clarke, *Ellen Swallow;* Stage, "Ellen Richards and the Social Significance of the Home Economics Movement"; Yudkin, "Earth, Air, Water, Hearth: The Woman Who Founded Ecology"; Athey, "Eugenic Feminisms in Late Nineteenth-Century America: Reading Race in Victoria Woodhull, Frances Willard, Anna Julia Cooper, and Ida B. Wells"; Cooke, "Non-Sense and Anti-Sentimentality: Home Economics, Euthenics, and the 'Threat' to Race Betterment Efforts in America."

133. Richards, *Euthenics*, viii.

134. Turner, "The Significance of the Frontier in American History."

135. Ibid.

136. Holbo, "The Home-Making of Americans."

137. Lamson, *My Birth*, 61.

138. Ibid., x.

139. Ibid., 4.

140. Ibid., 4.

141. Ibid., 5.

142. Ibid., 7.

143. Ibid., 19.

144. The narrator begins as an egg, but because he will ultimately be born a boy, and identifies himself as male throughout the book, even when he was an egg, I will refer to the narrator as "he."

145. Lamson, *My Birth*, 33. For a critique of the narrative strategies that govern the telling of the story of conception, see Martin, "The Egg and the Sperm," 485–501.

146. Lamson, *My Birth*, 34.

147. Ibid., 37.

148. Ibid., 32.

149. Ibid., 69.

150. Ibid., 48.

151. Ibid., 53.

152. Ibid., 53.

153. Ibid., 134. Emphasis mine.

154. Ibid., 148.

155. Ibid., xxi.

156. Cooke, *The Baby Before and After Arrival;* Galland, *Maternity and Child Care;* Long, *Motherhood;* and Van Blarcom, *Getting Ready to Be a Mother.*

157. Ladd-Taylor, *Mother-Work.*

158. In 1870 the American Woman Suffrage Association founded its own magazine, *The Women's Journal*. Edited by Lucy Stone, *The Women's Journal* was published for forty-seven years before being replaced by *The Woman Citizen* in 1917.

159. Alsop, "The Right to Be Well Born," 30.

160. Ibid., 30.

161. Rydell, *All the World's a Fair*, 44.

162. Ibid., 47.

163. Selden, *Inheriting Shame*, 19.

164. *Buck v. Bell* 274 U.S. 200 (1927).

Chapter 2

1. Wax models of embryos had been displayed at the 1893 World's Fair Columbian Exposition and at the 1904 World's Fair in St. Louis, but these 1933 exhibits were the first to display organic specimens.

2. Liebling, "Masters of the Midway," 25.

3. Ibid., 25.

4. Liebling, *Telephone Booth Indian*, 8.

5. Carey, *Medical Science Exhibits*, 32.

6. Ibid., 34.

7. Liebling, "Masters of the Midway," 26.

8. Aprison, "The Prenatal Exhibit at the Museum of Science and Industry," 25.

9. Cole, "Sex and Death on Display," 48.

10. Liebling, "Masters of the Midway," 26.

11. Carey, *Medical Science Exhibits*, 33.

12. Ibid., 34; Carey, "Health Education at the Exposition."

13. Quoted in Taylor, "Ward Hall: King of the Sideshows."

14. Cole, "Sex and Death on Display," 48.

15. Butler, *Bodies That Matter*, 9–10; Grosz, *Volatile Bodies*; Csordas, "Introduction: The Body as Representation and Being-in-the-World," in *Embodiment and Experience*, 1–24; Conboy, Media, and Stenburg, *Writing on the Body*; Williams, "Modern Medicine and the 'Uncertain Body'"; Bermudez, Marcel, and Eilan, *The Body and the Self*; Weiss and Haber, *Perspectives on Embodiment*; Welton, *Body & Flesh*, 1041–1049; Price and Shildrich, *Feminist Theory and the Body*; and Weiss, *Body Images*.

16. Gilbert, *A Conceptual History of Modern Embryology*; Clarke, *Disciplining Reproduction*.

17. Corner, *Ourselves Unborn*, 28.

18. Thelberg, "Instruction of College Students in Regard to Reproduction and Maternity"; Morgan, "Zoology at Mount Holyoke"; McLaren, "Why Study Early Human Development"; Clarke, "Research Materials and Reproductive Science in the United States"; Clarke, "Money, Sex, and Legitimacy at Chicago"; and Morgan, "Materializing the Fetal Body," in *Fetal Subjects, Feminist Positions*.

19. "Conception in a Watch Glass"; Perone, "In Vitro Fertilization and Embryo Transfer," 698; Rock and Menkin, "In Vitro Fertilization and Cleavage of Human Ovarian Eggs."

20. Morgan, "Materializing the Fetal Body," in *Fetal Subjects, Feminist Positions,* 50–53.

21. Corner, *The Seven Ages of a Medical Scientist,* 289.

22. Rosof, "Embryo Use or Abuse Taints Groundbreaking Study."

23. Corner, *The Seven Ages of a Medical Scientist,* 289.

24. "New Test for Pregnancy."

25. "60-Minute Pregnancy Test," 51.

26. "Laboratory Conception," 74.

27. "Frozen Sperm Pregnancies," 292.

28. Cole, "Sex and Death on Display," 48.

29. May, *Homeward Bound.*

30. May, *Barren in the Promised Land,* 129.

31. Hildebrand, "How to Tell the Story of Birth," 32.

32. Sungard, *The Miracle of Growth,* 1.

33. Ibid.

34. Kogan, *A Continuing Marvel,* 121.

35. Hildebrand, "How to Tell the Story of Birth," 29.

36. "First Breath of Life," 56.

37. "In the Sixth Week of Life," 83.

38. "The Human Embryo," 79. Also see "Babies before Birth," 19; and Nilsson, "Drama of Life before Birth," 62.

39. "Embryo's Face," 115.

40. "German Measles Menace," 31.

41. Stratton, "X-Rays and Pregnancy," 37.

42. U.S. Department of Health, Education, and Welfare, "Protecting the Unborn Baby."

43. Sontag, *Annual Report.* The project is still operating and over the past seventy years has tracked several thousand people from conception to adulthood. In 1929, Dr. Arthur E. Morgan, the president of Antioch College in Ohio, approached his childhood friend Samuel Fels, a Philadelphia soap manufacturer and philanthropist, with the idea of developing an institute that would study human development from birth to adulthood. Fels agreed to fund the program but insisted that the institute should include the nine months between conception and birth. Agreeing to expand the mission of the project, Morgan named Dr. Lester W. Sontag, Antioch College's physician, the first director of the Samuel S. Fels Research Institute for the Study of Prenatal and Postnatal Environment.

44. Samuel S. Fels Fund website, http://www.samfels.org/index.html (accessed July 18, 2008).

45. Dewey, *Behavior Development in Infants,* 8. Also see Murchison, "Origin and Prenatal Growth of Behavior," 31–159; and Hooker, *A Preliminary Atlas of Early Human Fetal Activity.*

46. Carlisle and Carlisle, "Secrets of Life before Birth."

47. "Cornell Education Heads New Yale Child Center," 30; Gesell, *The Embryology of Behavior.*

48. "Expert Worrying."

49. Ibid.

50. Fodor, *The Search for the Beloved,* 1.

51. Montagu and Shalit, "New Light on Life Before Birth," 63.

52. Fasten, "The Myth of Prenatal Influences?" 27.

53. "Baby May Be Neurotic if Mother Is Disturbed," 376.

54. "Expectant Mothers' Emotions May Have Bearing on Child," 31; "Fears and Babies," 49.

55. May, *Barren in the Promised Land,* 170.

56. Philip Wylie, *Generation of Vipers;* Levy, *Maternal Overprotection;* Strecker, *Their Mother's Sons;* and Lundberg and Farnham, *Modern Woman: The Lost Sex.*

57. Articles are from the following journals, listed in chronological order: *Scientific Digest,* December 1943; *Ladies Home Journal,* November 1945; *Saturday Evening Post,* October 26, 1946; *Today's Health,* September 1949; *Ladies Home Journal,* March 1950; *Women's Home Companion,* July 1950; Philip Wylie, *Generation of Vipers.*

58. Strecker, *Their Mother's Sons,* 30.

59. Ibid.

60. Rapson, *Individualism and Conformity in the American Character;* Leinberger and Tucker, eds., *The New Individualists;* McClay, *The Masterless;* Shain, *The Myth of American Individualism;* and Cushman, *Constructing the Self.* For a different set of texts that embody this cultural anxiety, or obsession, with individuality, see Whyte, *The Organization Man;* and Wilson, *The Man in the Gray Flannel Suit.* These books express concern at the loss of masculine individuality through the conformity of suburban life. Although clearly not engaged in the same anxieties about individuality that are expressed in fetal discourses, the coexistence of this version of anxiety about the individual suggests that the problem of individuality took many forms in postwar culture.

61. Gilbert, *Biography of the Unborn;* Corner, *Ourselves Unborn,* ix.

62. Corner, *Ourselves Unborn,* 70.

63. Ibid., 36.

64. Ibid., 2.

65. Sungard, *The Miracle of Growth,* 30.

66. Berrill, *The Person in the Womb,* 3.

67. Strecker, *Their Mother's Sons,* 30.

68. Gruenberg, *The Wonderful Story of How You Were Born,* 5. For other examples from this growing genre of books for children about human reproduction, see Whiting, *The Story of Life;* Rostand, *Adventures before Birth;* Strain, *Being Born;* Meyr, *Your Own True Story;* Faegre, *Your Own Story;* Bibby, *How Life Is Handed On;* Buck, *Johnny Jack and His Beginnings;* Cockefair and Cockefair, *The Story of You;* Lerrigo and Southard, *A Story about You;* Appleman, *When Two Become Three.*

69. Parsons, "The Science Legislation and the Role of the Social Sciences"; "University Presses and the Popularization of Science"; "Science and the Public"; "Science and the Citizen"; "Scientific Thought in the Coming Decades"; "Rise of Scientific Understanding"; "Scientists: A Moral Obligation to be Intelligible"; "Does the Greater Understanding of Man and Nature Increase the Scientist's Social Responsibility?"; "Influence of Scientists"; "Place of Science in Society Today"; "Science and Human Values"; "Science and the Citizen"; "Scientists Succumb to Public Role"; "Obstetric and Gynecological Milestones."

70. Boyer, *By the Bomb's Early Light*; May, *Homeward Bound*; Gilbert, *Redeeming Culture*; Herman, *The Romance of American Psychology*; Henriksen, *Dr. Strangelove's America*. Boyer cites a 1946 Social Science Resource Commission survey that found a "generalized belief in the inexhaustibility of scientific invention," 23. May writes that "postwar America was the era of the expert … science and technology seemed to invade virtually every aspect of life, from the most public to the most private.…One study found that reliance on expertise was one of the most striking developments of the postwar years…despite the public's perception of scientific mastery and objectivity, professionals groped for appropriate ways to conceptualize and resolve the uncertainties of the time," 26.

71. "Man Tells Us What We Must Do," 173; Arendt, *Human Condition*, xxi.

72. Church, "Parents: Architects of Peace," 18–19.

73. Kogan, *A Continuing Marvel*, 122.

74. Schweitzer, *The Rights of the Unborn & the Peril Today*.

75. *Renslow v. Mennonite Hospital*.

76. *Bonbrest v. Kotz*. This case was unusual in that it dealt with a tort inflicted during delivery, rather than one inflicted earlier in pregnancy. The plaintiff chose to argue this case as one of prenatal harm, defining the victim as an infant *en ventre sa mere*, rather than as a born child. The briefs for this case no longer exist, so I do not know why they made this strategic decision, which seems usual given the strength of precedent against it.

77. *Dietrich v. Inhabitants of Northampton*.

78. Ibid., 15.

79. Mohr, *Doctors and the Law*; Horowitz, *The Transformation of American Law, 1870–1960*; Jasanoff, *Science at the Bar*; Faigman, *Laboratory of Justice*.

80. *Smith v. Luckhardt*.

81. "Fetal Rights," 47.

82. *Stemmer v. Kline*, 455.

83. Ibid., 455.

84. Ibid, 467.

85. *Bonbrest v. Kotz*, 469.

86. *Stemmer v. Kline*, 469.

87. Bonbrest v. Kotz, n. 13.

88. Jackson, "Infants: Actions."

89. Munsterman, "Torts: Right of a Viable Child to Maintain a Tort Action for Negligent Prenatal Injury," 431–436.

90. Seld, "Torts: Prenatal Injuries: Right of an Infant to Sue."

91. Kalman, *The Strange Career of Legal Liberalism*.

92. Wong and Nicotera, "Brown v. Board of Education and the Coleman Report."

93. *Verkennes v. Corniea*. This case dealt with the claim of a pregnant woman against her obstetrician. Beatrice Verkennes's uterus ruptured during labor, and her unborn child Baby Girl Rita Verkennes died *in utero*. Beatrice Verkennes claimed that the defendants' failure to care for her appropriately was the cause of her child's death.

94. *Williams v. Marion Rapid Transit Inc.*, 334.

95. Ibid., 335.

96. Alton, "Torts: Action by Child for Prenatal Injuries," 411. For similar statements of praise, see R.M.L., "Torts: Prenatal Injuries: Right of Infant to Sue"; Jordan, "Constitutional Law: 'Person' Within the Meaning of Section 16, Article I of the Constitution"; and Turner, "Torts: Recovery for Prenatal Injuries."

97. Fleishman, "Torts: Right of a Viable Infant to Maintain An Action for Negligent Prenatal Injuries."

98. *Williams v. Marion Rapid Transit Inc.*, 340.

99. Ibid., 334. *Woods v. Lancet,* This case was an action by Robert C. Woods, infant, and Estelle Woods, guardian, for injuries sustained while plaintiff was *en ventre sa mere* in the ninth month of pregnancy. The decision does not describe the events of the accident other than to find that the "negligence of the defendant" caused the infant to "come into this world permanently maimed and disabled," 693. *Mitchell v. Couch.* This case is an action by the administrator of the estate of a child born dead after a car accident. At issue was the viability of the child at the time of the accident.

100. Needham, *A History of Embryology.*

101. Williams, *Obstetrics;* Stander, *Williams Obstetrics.*

102. Horowitz, *The Transformation of American Law,* 1870–1960; Mohr, *Doctors and the Law;* Toumey, *Conjuring Science;* Jasanoff, *Science at the Bar;* Angell, *Science on Trial.*

103. In the late 1940s, law reviews and medical journals published an increasing number of articles delineating the increasingly imbricated relationship between law and medicine. In the 1940s, references to articles about medical jurisprudence take up several pages in the indexes to legal and medical periodicals, as opposed to the few lines that they had occupied merely ten years earlier.

104. *Williams v. Marion Rapid Transit Inc.*, 334.

105. Ibid., 335.

106. Dudziak, *Cold War Civil Rights;* and Borstelmann, *The Cold War and the Color Line.*

107. Spock, *Pocket Book of Baby and Child Care;* Kanner, *In Defense of Mothers.* Also see Weiss, "Mother: The Invention of Necessity."

108. Kanner, *In Defense of Mothers,* 34.

109. Ibid., 34.

110. *Hornbuckle v. Plantation Pipe Line, Co.*

111. "A New Theory in Prenatal Injuries: The Biological Approach."

112. Marcus, "Torts: Prenatal Injury: Right of Injury in Non-Viable Fetus."

113. For a discussion of the centrality of meiosis in determining life, see Schrödinger, *What Is Life?* For a discussion of the discovery of DNA, see Lewontin, *Biology as Ideology.*

114. Stason, Estep, and Pierce, *Atoms and the Law,* 202. For a contemporary analysis of preconception torts, see Greenberg, "Reconceptualizing Preconception Torts."

115. Eastman, *Williams Obstetrics,* 1945 and 1956.

116. "Torts: Child's Right of Action for Prenatal Injuries."

117. *Allaire v. St. Luke's Hospital,* 640.

118. *Application of Donald L. Clarke.* The extension of this statute to include the unborn child was added by constitutional amendment in 1925.

119. *Application of Donald L. Clarke,* 142.

120. Ibid., 142.

121. "HEW's Power to Grant AFDC Benefits to Technically Ineligible Individuals."

122. Melnick, *Between the Lines,* 102.

123. "Aid to the Unborn."

124. "Aid to Families with Unborn Dependent Children: May the State Withhold Benefits?"

125. Social Security Amendments of 1972, *Report of the Committee on Finance,* U.S. Senate, to accompany H.R. 1, To Amend the Social Security Act, and for Other Purposes, September 26, 1972 (U.S. Government Printing Office), 467; House Ways and Means Committee, *Report No.* 92–231, to accompany H.R. 1, printed in U.S. Code: Congressional and Administrative News, 92nd Cong., 2nd sess., 1972 (West), vol. 3, 4989.

126. Report on the Committee of Ways and Means, "Social Security Amendments of 1971."

127. Ibid.

128. *Burns v. Alcala.*

129. For excellent treatments of the struggles to overthrow and circumvent laws criminalizing abortion in the twentieth century, see the following works: Joffe, *Doctors of Conscience;* Solinger, *Wake Up Little Susie;* Garrow, *Liberty and Sexuality;* Reagan, *When Abortion Was a Crime;* Kaplan, *The Story of Jane;* Fried, *From Abortion to Reproductive Freedom;* Ginsburg and Rapp, *Conceiving the New World Order.*

130. Kinsey, *Sexual Behavior in the Human Female;* Calderone, *Abortion in the United States,* 84.

131. Luker, *Abortion and the Politics of Motherhood,* 62–65.

132. "Law on Abortion Called Too Strict"; the American Law Institute's Model Penal Code (1962) provided an important catalyst. The "tentative draft" of the code's section on abortion (§ 230.3), which was published in 195, proposed that abortion should be a felony, with the level of punishment to depend on whether the abortion took place up to or after the twenty-sixth week of pregnancy. It added, however, that "[a] licensed physician is justified in terminating a pregnancy if he believes there is a substantial risk to the physical or mental health of the mother, that the child would be born with serious physical or mental defects, or that the pregnancy resulted from rape or incest."

133. Luker, *Abortion and the Politics of Motherhood,* 63.

134. In 1960, Merrell, a pharmaceutical company, had applied to the FDA for approval, but, concerned by the data coming out of Germany about the teratogenic potential of thalidomide, Frances Kelsey had blocked its application. For an overview of the thalidomide controversy, see *New York Times,* August 2, 1962, 1. Also see Fine, *The Great Drug Deception;* and Sjostrom and Nilsson, *Thalidomide and the Power of the Drug Companies.*

135. For estimates regarding the decline in the abortion rate after the institution of hospital abortion boards, see Niswander, "Medical Abortion Practices in the United States." For general discussions of the problem, see Rosen, *Therapeutic Abortion;* Packer and Gambell, "Therapeutic Abortion: A Problem in Law and Medicine"; Russell, "Changing Indications for Therapeutic Abortions"; Loth and Hesseltine, "Therapeutic Abortion at the Chicago Lying-In Hospital"; Pearse and Ott, "Hospital Control of

Sterilization and Therapeutic Abortion"; Rosen, "The Psychiatric Implications of Abortion: A Case Study in Hypocrisy," 105; and Bolter, "The Psychiatrist's Role in Therapeutic Abortion: The Unwitting Accomplice."

136. Luker, *Abortion and the Politics of Motherhood*, 62–65.

137. *Journal of the American Medical Association* published a series of pro-reform editorials and *Modern Medicine* reported that 87 percent of American physicians favored less restrictive abortion laws.

138. Garrow, *Liberty and Sexuality*, 323, 329, 331; "Abortion History Timeline," National Right to Life website, *http://www.nrlc.org/abortion/facts/abortiontimeline. html* (accessed June 13, 2008). Also see "Chronology of Abortion Politics," in Solinger, *Abortion Wars*, xii.

139. Solinger, *Abortion Wars*, xii. Also see Nelson, "From Abortion Rights to Reproductive Freedom."

140. "Abortion Reform Bill Passes," 2.

141. See Garrow, *Liberty and Sexuality*; Faux, *Roe v. Wade*; Tribe, *Abortion*; Petchesky, *Abortion and Women's Choice*; and Weddington, *A Question of Choice*.

142. *Roe v. Wade*.

143. Ibid.

Chapter 3

1. The Massachusetts Grave-Robbing Statute of 1814, Massachusetts General Laws, c. 265 § 13. "Whoever, not being lawfully authorized by the proper authorities, willfully digs up, disinters, removes or conveys a human body or the remains thereof...shall be punished in the state prison for not more than three years or in jail for not more that two and one half years or by a fine of not more than two thousand dollars."

2. For general histories of grave robbing, see Richardson, *Death, Dissection, and the Destitute*; Schultz, *Body Snatching*; Michael Sappol, *A Traffic of Dead Bodies*.

3. Culliton, "Grave-Robbing."

4. Assistant District Attorney and Foreman of the Grand Jury, "A True Bill for the Indictment of Kenneth Edelin," Commonwealth of Massachusetts, April 11, 1975.

5. Paige, *The Right- to-Lifers*, 27. Paige explains that in 1978, the newly elected district attorney Newman Flanagan "dismissed charges against the 'grave-robbers' for reasons neither he nor their defense counsel will disclose." John A. Nucci, Court Clerk for the Massachusetts Superior Court of Suffolk County explains that all court records pertaining to that case have been sealed at the mutual request of the district attorney's office and the accused doctors. Author's phone call with Nucci, July 5, 2001.

6. In 1928, researchers in Italy transplanted fetal pancreatic tissue into a patient, and in 1939, researchers in the United States did the same. Vawter et al., "Chronology of Events in the Transplantation of Human Fetal Tissue," in *The Use of Human Fetal Tissue: Scientific, Ethical, and Policy Concerns*, 189–196. On the history of fetal research, see "An Assessment of the Role of Research Involving Living Human Fetuses in Advances in Medical Science and Technology," a report by the Battelle-Columbus Laboratories, commissioned by the National Commission for the Protection of Human Subjects of Biomedical and Behavioral Research, published in *Research on the Fetus: Appendix* (Washington, D.C.: U.S. Department of Health Education and Welfare,

DHEW Publication No. OS 76–128); Maynard-Moody, *The Dilemma of the Fetus;* Casper, *The Making of the Unborn Patient;* Hanna, *Biomedical Politics;* and Hellegers, "Fetal Research."

7. Roberts, "Potential Cure, Ethical Questions."

8. Enders, Weller, and Robbins, "Cultivation of the Lansing Strain of Poliomyelitis Virus in Cultures of Various Human Embryonic Tissues." Enders, Weller, and Robbins were awarded the Nobel Prize in Physiology and Medicine in 1954 for this achievement. Also see Salk, "Studies in Human Subjects on Active Immunization against Poliomyelitis"; Sabin, "Oral Poliovirus Vaccine"; Paul, *A History of Poliomyelitis.*

9. Vawter et al., "Chronology of Events," *The Use of Human Fetal Tissue.*

10. Ibid.

11. Zimmerman, *Rh: The Intimate History of a Disease and Its Conquest;* Rapp, *Testing Women, Testing the Fetus.*

12. Culliton, "Grave-Robbing," 421.

13. Paul, *A History of Poliomyelitis.*

14. Biographical information on doctors comes from Sheehan, "BCH Fetus Case: Research at Stake."

15. Philipson et al., "Transplacental Passage of Erythromycin and Clyndamycin."

16. Medical journals had been publishing the results of studies using fetal tissue since the early 1940s, but with the exception of the polio vaccine, none of these studies were covered in the mainstream press. See Mahoney, "The Nature and Extent of Research Involving Living Human Fetuses," Reference List, pp. 1.40–1.48, in *Research on the Fetus: Appendix,* for a discussion of fetal research throughout the twentieth century and for citations to articles on that topic published between 1890 and 1970 in *Journal of the American Medical Association.*

17. Holland, *The Human Embryonic Stem Cell Debate;* Maienschein, *Whose View of Life?;* Jones, *The Soul of the Embryo;* Herald, *Stem Cell Wars.* For an examination of the debate in the United Kingdom that highlights the intersection between cultural and scientific controversies, see Julkay, *The Embryo Research Debate: Science and the Politics of Reproduction.*

18. Knox, "Citizens Groups to Push BCH to Resume Abortion Services," 3.

19. Paige, *The Right to Lifers,* 11.

20. Bruzelius, "Edelin: A Dedicated Doctor," 2.

21. Sheehan, "BCH Fetus Case," 1.

22. Ibid. Estimates of MCL membership come from Joseph Reilly, director of MCL in 1983, quoted in Paige, *The Right to Lifers,* 14.

23. After serving one term in the statehouse, Delahunt was elected district attorney of Quincy in 1976, a position he held until 1996, when he was elected to represent the 10th Congressional District of Massachusetts. A pro-choice Democrat, Delahunt supports stem cell research.

24. Culliton, "Fetal Research: The Case History of a Massachusetts Law," 237.

25. Ibid.

26. Ibid.

27. Ibid.

28. See *Science* 178 (November 10, 1972) for a report on Nathan's work. Beta-thalassemia is an inherited disease that occurs in people of Mediterranean ancestry.

29. Ibid.

30. Culliton, "Fetal Research," 237.

31. Ibid.

32. Ibid.

33. Raymond L. Flynn represented South Boston and Dorchester in the Massachusetts Legislature for two terms, from 1971 to 1978, years when he vehemently opposed busing. He then served three terms on the Boston City Council from 1978 to 1983 and three terms as the mayor of Boston, from 1984 until 1993. In 1993, President Clinton appointed him U.S. ambassador to the Vatican. In 2001, Flynn was the host of a radio talk show in Boston.

34. Sheehan, "BCH Fetus Case," 1.

35. Ibid.

36. Massachusetts Racial Imbalance Act, St. 1965, c. 641, §§ 1 et seq., codified at GL c. 71, §§ 37C, 37D & c. 15 §§ 1I.

37. See Lukas, *Common Ground,* 137, for a discussion of Flynn's and O'Neil's role in the busing controversy and pp. 115–139 for a discussion of the formation of ROAR. See Paige, *The Right-to-Lifers,* 16, for a discussion of O'Neil's role in the grave-robbing/manslaughter hearings. For a documentary about the intersections between racism and abortion in Boston, see *Voices of a Divided City: Crisis to Crisis,* videocassette, series, CEBA Award Collection for the World Institute of Black Communications, pro-duced/directed by Romas V. Slezas, Henry E. Hampton, and Alvin H. Goldstein (United States: Corp. for Public Broadcasting, 1982).

38. Sheehan, "BCH Fetus Case," 1.

39. Ibid.

40. For discussions of the power of antielitism to bring together groups previously unaligned, particularly urban Catholics and southern Protestants, shake up party iden-tities, and create new grassroots activists, see Schulman, *The Seventies; Critchlow, Phyllis Schlafly and Grassroots Conservatism;* Rymph, *Republican Women;* Perlstein, *Nixonland;* and Schulman and Zelizer, *Rightward Bound.*

41. Paige, *The Right-to-Lifers,* 116.

42. Ibid.

43. Lukas, *Common Ground.*

44. Wilde, *Vatican II.*

45. Swerdlow, *Women Strike for Peace;* Kaplan, *Crazy for Democracy;* Jetter, Orleck, and Taylor, *The Politics of Motherhood;* Blee, *No Middle Ground;* McGirr, *Suburban Warriors.*

46. Paige, *The Right-to-Lifers,* 17.

47. Ibid.

48. Edelin, *Broken Justice,* 73.

49. Sheehan, "BCH Fetus Case," 1.

50. Ibid.

51. Ibid.

52. Ibid. Flanagan was also a member of the Knights of Columbus, a Catholic organization involved with antiabortion activism, and two of his brothers were priests.

53. Paige, *The Right-to-Lifers*, 19. *Boston Globe* court reporter Alan Sheehan reported that following the *Roe* decision, Flanagan asked a clerk to research all state and federal law regarding abortion, particularly regarding the legal definitions of life, birth, and viability. The clerk pointed out that the Supreme Court decision in *Roe* had not addressed the doctors' responsibility to a fetus born alive in the course of abortion. This "loophole" would become a key factor in the Edelin case.

54. "New Attack on Abortion," 84.

55. Knox, "BCH Trustees Reinstate 3 Indicted Doctors," 3.

56. Reinhold, "Boston Indicts Doctors in Fetus Case," 1.

57. Sheehan, "Manslaughter Is Charged in BCH Abortion," 1.

58. Ibid.

59. Knox, "Citizens' Groups Push BCH to Resume Abortion Services," 3.

60. Ibid.

61. "New Attack on Abortion," 84.

62. Bruzelius, "BCH to Resume Abortion When Way Is Clear," 4.

63. Culliton, "Grave-Robbing," 420.

64. Ibid.

65. Robert Reinhold, "Boston vs. the Doctors: Strange Case," 21.

66. DiGeorge syndrome is a genetic disorder that causes abnormal glandular growth in one in ten thousand newborns. Walters, "Ethical Issues in Fetal Research: A Look Back and a Look Forward"; Greeley et al., "The Ethical Use of Human Fetal Tissue in Medicine"; Nolan, "The Use of the Embryo or Fetus in Transplantation"; American Medical Association, "Medical Applications of Fetal Tissue Transplantation"; and Coutts, "Fetal Tissue Research."

67. Senate Subcommittee on Government Research of the Committee on Government Operations, *Hearings on S.J. Resolution 145*, 90th Cong., 2nd sess., March, 8–9, 21–22, and 27–28, and April 2, 1968. See also Curran, "The Law and Human Experimentation"; and Curran, "The Approach of Two Federal Agencies."

68. Senate Subcommittee on Health of the Committee on Labor and Public Welfare, *Joint Hearing of the National Advisory Commission on Health Science and Society*, 92nd Cong., 1st sess., November 9, 1971.

69. Barber et al., *Research on Human Subjects*; Lederer, *Subjected to Science*; Welsome, *The Plutonium Files*. On the Tuskegee scandal, see Rothman, "Human Experimentation and the Origins of Bioethics in the United States," 185–200; Jones, *Bad Blood*; and Reverby, *Tuskegee's Truth*. On the contraceptive studies, see Roberts, *Killing the Black Body*; Jessie Rodrique, "The Black Community and the Birth Control Movement," and Mason, "Minority Unborn." On the Willowbrook studies, see Rothman and Rothman, *The Willowbrook Wars*.

70. Harris Poll cited in Carroll, *It Seemed Like Nothing Happened*, 235.

71. On the disability right-to-life movement, see James Gustafson, "Mongolism, Parental Desires, and the Right to Life"; "Film Ponders the Right to Life of a Mentally Retarded Infant," 31; and "Medical Ethics: The Right to Survival, 1974," Hearings before

the Senate Subcommittee on Health of the Committee on Labor and Public Welfare, 93rd Cong., 2nd sess., June 11, 1974. For feminist perspectives on this issue, see Blumberg, "The Politics of Prenatal Testing and Selective Abortion"; and Saxton, "Prenatal Screening and Discriminatory Attitudes about Disability."

72. See Rothman, *Strangers at the Bedside;* Jonsen, *The Birth of Bioethics;* and Stevens, *Bioethics in America,* for different interpretations of how that concern generated the growth, professionalization, and institutionalization of the discipline and practice of bioethics.

73. Ramsey, *Ethics at the Edges of Life.*

74. Jonsen, "The Ethics of Research with Human Subjects: A Short History," *Source Book in Bioethics,* 7.

75. The Hastings Center was founded in 1969, with the mission of focusing on the conjunction of ethics and public policy, and the Kennedy Institute of Ethics (originally named the Kennedy Center for the Study of Human Reproduction and Development) opened at Georgetown University in 1971, with the mission to study ethical issues involved in reproductive research within the context of a liberal Catholicism.

76. Sarkos, "The Fetal Tissue Transplant Debate in the United States: Where Is King Solomon When You Need Him," 411.

77. Victor Cohen, "Live Fetal Research Debated."

78. Ibid.

79. Ibid.

80. Cohen, "NIH Vows Not to Fund Fetus Work," 1; and "NIH Bans Research on Live Fetuses," 253.

81. Department of Health, Education, and Welfare, National Institutes of Health, "Protection of Human Subjects: Policies and Procedures," 38 Fed. Reg. No. 221, Part II, November 16, 1973, 738–748.

82. *Congressional Quarterly Almanac* 29, no. 11 (September 1973): 512.

83. Senate Committee on Labor and Public Welfare, *Hearings on the National Research Act,* 92nd Cong., 1st sess., May 1973, 1326.

84. Rothman, *Strangers at the Bedside,* 184.

85. Kenneth John Ryan, M.D., Chief of Staff at Boston Hospital for Women was the chair of the commission. Other National Commission members were: Robert E. Cooke, M.D., Vice Chancellor for Health Sciences at the University of Wisconsin; Donald W. Seldin, M.D., Professor and Chairman, Dept. of Internal Medicine, University of Texas at Dallas; Joseph V. Brady, Ph.D., Professor of Behavioral Biology at Johns Hopkins University; Eliot Stellar, Ph.D., Provost of the University and Professor of Physiological Psychology, University of Pennsylvania; Albert R. Jonsen, Ph.D., Adjunct Associate Professor of Bioethics, University of California at San Francisco; Karen Lebacqz, Ph.D., Assistant Professor of Christian Ethics, Pacific School of Religion; Patricia King, J.D., Associate Professor of Law, Georgetown University Law Center; David W. Louisell, J.D., Professor of Law, University of California at Berkeley; Robert H. Turtle, LL.B., Attorney, VomBaur, Coburn, Simmons & Turtle, Washington, D.C.; and Dorothy I. Height, President, National Council of Negro Women, Inc. between 1975 and 1979, these twelve people produced the following eight reports: *Research on the Fetus, Research Involving Prisoners, Research Involving Children, Psychosurgery,*

Disclosure of Research Information, Research Involving Those Institutionalized as Mentally Infirm, Special Study, and *The Belmont Report.*

86. All codes and regulations, as well as all reports and papers submitted to the committee, were published separately as *Research on the Fetus: Appendix.* Reports and papers include: Maurice J. Mahoney, "The Nature and Extent of Research Involving Living Human Fetuses"; Sissela Bok, "Fetal Research and the Value of Life"; Joseph F. Fletcher, "Fetal Research: An Ethical Appraisal"; Marc Lappe, "Balancing Obligations to the Living Human Fetus with the Needs for Experimentation"; Richard A. McCormick, "Experimentation on the Fetus: Policy Proposals"; Paul Ramsey, "Moral Issues in Fetal Research"; Seymour Siegal, "Experimentation on Fetuses Which Are Judged to Be Nonviable"; LeRoy Walters, "Ethical and Public Policy Issues in Fetal Research"; Richard Wasserstrom, "Ethical Issues Involved in Experimentation on the Nonviable Human Fetus"; Stephen Toulmin, "Fetal Experimentation: Moral Issues and Institutional Controls"; Leon Kass, "Determining Death and Viability in Fetuses and Abortuses"; Richard E. Behrman, "Report on Viability and Nonviability of the Fetus"; A. M. Capron, "The Law Relating to Experimentation with the Fetus"; John P. Wilson, "A Report on Legal Issues Involved with Research on the Fetus"; Battelle-Columbus Laboratories, "An Assessment of the Role of Research Involving Living Human Fetuses in Advances in Medical Science and Technology"; and Michael Bracken, "The Stability of the Decision to Seek Induced Abortion."

87. *Research on the Fetus: Appendix,* 92.

88. The Department of Health and Human Services (DHHS), Title 45, part 46, of the Code of Federal Regulations. Subpart B of 45 CFR part 46, promulgated on August 8, 1975, pertains to research involving fetuses, pregnant women, and human in vitro fertilization. The 1975 regulations were jointly published in the *Federal Register* with the report and recommendations of the National Commission for the Protection of Human Subjects of Biomedical and Behavioral Research, *Research on the Fetus* (40 Fed. Reg. 33526). Subsequent changes were incorporated January 11, 1978 (43 Fed. Reg. 1758); November 3, 1978 (43 Fed. Reg. 51559); and June 1, 1994 (59 Fed. Reg. 28276).

89. Nolen, *The Baby in the Bottle,* 71.

90. Ibid., 73.

91. Ibid., 88.

92. Ibid., 71.

93. Edelin, *Broken Justice,* 1.

94. Biographical information on Edelin comes from his memoir, *Broken Justice,* and also from Bruzelius, "Edelin: A Dedicated Doctor," 2; and Paige, *The-Right-to-Lifers.* Edelin quote comes from interview in *Boston Globe,* May 18, 1982.

95. Commonwealth of Massachusetts, "A True Bill for the Indictment of Kenneth Edelin," April 11, 1975.

96. The exact date is not noted on her chart, and Dr. Hugh Holtrap testified that he saw her "probably late in September of 1973." For ambiguity about the date of her first visit, see transcript of the trial of *Dr. Kenneth Edelin vs. the Commonwealth of Massachusetts* (hereafter cited as Trial Transcript), direct examination of Holtrap by Flanagan, January 13, 1975, p. 78. Alice Roe's medical chart, which is in possession of the author, confirms that.

97. Trial Transcript, direct examination of Holtrap, January 13 and 14, 1975.

98. Trial Transcript, direct examination of Alan Silberman, February 7, 1975.

99. Trial Transcript, direct examination of Dr. Enrique Gimenez-Jimeno, January 17, 1975.

100. Trial Transcript, direct examination of Holtrap, January 13, 1975.

101. The clearest description of Edelin's actions is in the Supreme Judicial Court of Massachusetts's reversal of the Edelin conviction, Supreme Judicial Court of the Commonwealth of Massachusetts, "Summary Statement of Basic Circumstances," December 17, 1976, Criminal No. S-393. Also see Ramsey, *Ethics at the Edges of Life,* 99–100.

102. William P. Homans, Jr., "Defendant's Motion for an Order of Dismissal of the Indictment," *Commonwealth v. Edelin,* submitted to the Superior Court, No. 81823, October 9, 1974.

103. Newman Flanagan, "Affidavit of the Commonwealth Opposing the Defendant's Motion for an Order of Dismissal of the Indictment," *Commonwealth v. Kenneth Edelin,* submitted to the Superior Court, No. 81823, October 10, 1974.

104. Edelin, *Broken Justice,* 119.

105. Nolen, *The Baby in the Bottle,* 89.

106. For the consultants' analysis of the ideal jury for the defense, see Irwin Harrison, "Report on Edelin Case," excerpted from the Decision Research Corp in Trial Transcript, January 6, 1975.

107. Trial Transcript, January 6, 1975; White, "Edelin Defense Asks Dismissal after New U.S. Ruling on Juries," 1. On January 21, 1975, in the case of *Taylor v. Louisiana,* the U.S Supreme Court found that Louisiana's practice of jury selection, which systematically excluded women from jury service unless they specifically requested in writing to be allowed to serve, violated the Sixth Amendment rights of, in this case, the male defendant to have a "jury drawn from a fair cross section of the community." Homans immediately resubmitted his motion, but was again overruled. See Trial Transcript, January 21, 1975, for submission of the second motion and Trial Transcript, January 29, 1975, for McGuire's dismissal of the motion.

108. White, "Edelin Jury: Their Faces Told Nothing," 8; CBS-TV broadcast, "Newman Flanagan says he is not trying Dr. Kenneth Edelin for performing an abortion which is perfectly legal, but for terminating a human life, which is not," in *Collected Speeches of Kenneth Edelin* (Vincent Voice Library, Michigan State University, January 13, 1975), available online at http://www.lib.msu.edu/digital/vincent/findaids/EdelinK.html (accessed June 17, 2008).

109. Trial Transcript, January 6, 1975, 42.

110. Trial Transcript, January 10, 1975, 7.

111. Ibid., 7.

112. Danet, "'Baby' or 'Fetus'?" 194–197, for analysis of the frequency of these terms, and of which terms were used by which side.

113. Trial Transcript, January 10, 1975, 37.

114. Ibid., 71. For more on Jefferson's background and lack of expertise in obstetrics and gynecology, see "Abortion and Manslaughter: A Boston Doctor Goes on Trial," 334.

115. Trial Transcript, January 10, 1975.

116. Ibid., 37–39.

117. Ibid.

118. Ibid., 66–74.

119. Trial Transcript, January 13, 1975, 63–64.

120. Trial Transcript, January 14, 1975, 4. See White, "Abortion Procedure Explained," 1.

121. Trial Transcript, 14 January 1975, 106.

122. Ibid., 126.

123. On this distinction, see William J. Larsen, *Human Embryology*, 398.

124. Trial Transcript, January 22, 1975, 60. In addition to Dr. Mildred Jefferson, founder of Massachusetts Citizens for Life, and Dr. Gimenez-Jimeno, a doctor who refused to perform abortions, expert witnesses included Dr. Fred E. Mecklenburg, an obstetrician-gynecologist from Minnesota and a member of Minnesota Citizens for Life, and Dr. Denis Cavanagh, an obstetrician-gynecologist from St. Louis who had been appointed guardian *ad litem* for all unborn fetuses in the Missouri case of *Rogers v. Danforth*, and who was a member of Missouri Doctors for Life, a group that had recently taken out an ad in the *St. Louis Democrat* reading "Abortion degrades women, our profession, and our country."

125. Trial Transcript, January 22, 1975, 60.

126. Bruzelius, "Abortion: Problem for the Courts in Boston," 1.

127. Edelin, *Broken Justice*, 63–64.

128. White, "Edelin Colleague Supports Contention of Prosecutor," 1.

129. Goldberg, "Obstetric US Imaging: The Past 40 Years."

130. White, "Curtis Testifies Fetus Can Inhale Intrauterine Fluids," 1.

131. Ibid.

132. Ibid.

133. Trial Transcript, January 23, 1975. See also White, "Medical Examiner Tells Court Fetus Had 'Respiratory Activity,'" 1.

134. Diane White, "Pathologist Says Fetus in Edelin Case Breathed," 1.

135. William P. Homans, Jr., "Defendant's Motion for Directed Verdict," *Commonwealth v. Kenneth Edelin*, Suffolk, SS., Superior Court Criminal Session No. 81823.

136. Newman Flanagan, "Commonwealth's Answer to Defendant's Motion for a Directed Verdict," *Commonwealth v. Kenneth Edelin*, Suffolk, SS., Superior Court No. 81823.

137. White, "Acquittal Motion Denied in Edelin Trial," 1.

138. Trial Transcript, February 4, 1975. Also see Diane White, "2 BCH Nurses Say No Clock on Wall When Edelin Operated," 1.

139. Trial Transcript, February 7, 1975, 52–59.

140. Pritchard and Hellman, eds., *Williams Obstetrics*. Pritchard would go on to author the fifteenth, sixteenth, and seventeenth editions of *Williams Obstetrics*.

141. Trial Transcript, February 11, 1975, 83.

142. Ibid. Also see Diane White, "Fetus Never Breathed, Says Pathologist," *Boston Globe*, 1.

143. White, "Witness Says Fetus 'Very Likely' Dead before Abortion," 8.

144. White, "Survival 'Rare' at 1½ Pounds, Edelin Jury Told," 1.

145. White, "Edelin Delay in Taking Fetus Proper Practice, Expert Says," 1; White, "Edelin's Judgment Sound, Say Experts," 1.

146. Trial Transcript, February 3, 1975, 19–84. Also see White, "Duty to Mother, Not Fetus, Edelin Says," 1.

147. Trial Transcript, February 3, 1975, 20–38.

148. Trial Transcript, February 14, 1975, 35.

149. Ibid., 36.

150. Ibid., 72.

151. Ibid., 111.

152. Ibid., 111.

153. Ibid., 120. Also see Diane White, "Edelin Trial Arguments Conclude, Jury May Get Case Today," 9.

154. *Commonwealth v. Edelin*, "The Charge to the Jury," appendix to Trial Transcript, February 14, 1975, 10:25 A.M., reprinted in *The Edelin Trial, Court Documents* (Boston University; Legal-Medical Studies, Inc., 1975).

155. Diane White, "Jury Convicts Edelin of Manslaughter," 1.

156. Ibid., 1.

157. Ibid., 1.

158. Ibid., 1.

159. Editorial, "Edelin and the Law."

160. Editorial, "The Edelin Trial."

161. Editorial, "Abortion Error."

162. "Edelin Supported," statement signed by twenty-one medical house officers of the New England Deaconess Hospital, as reprinted in the *New England Journal of Medicine.*

163. "Abortion: The Edelin Shock Wave," 54.

164. Ibid.

165. Bruzelius, "Hub Medical Community Is Dismayed," 1; UPI, "Medical Implications of Edelin Verdict Studied," 8; Bruzelius, "Research on Humans an Issue," 9. For other attacks on the decision from the medical community, see "Setback for Abortion," 67; Culliton, "Edelin Trial: Jury Not Persuaded by Scientists for the Defense," 814; Ingelfinger, "The Edelin Trial Fiasco."

166. Altman, "Implications of Abortion Verdict," 41.

167. Kifner, "Women Rally for Doctor Convicted in Abortion," 27; Ross, "African-American Women and Abortion," 184.

168. Breins, *The Trouble between Us,* 123.

169. Proceedings of the 1975 Conference on Women and Health, April 4–7, 1975, Boston, Mass., 11. Available at http://www.ourbodiesourselves.org/about/1975conf.asp (accessed September 25, 2009).

170. Bruzelius, "Research on Humans an Issue," 9.

171. Falkner, "Biomedical Research at Crossroads," sec. 4, 16.

172. "Abortion: The Edelin Shock Wave," 54.

173. House Subcommittee on Civil and Constitutional Rights of the Committee on the Judiciary, *Hearings on Proposed Constitutional Amendments on Abortion,* 94th Cong., 2nd sess. (1976); Senate Subcommittee on Constitutional Amendments of the Committee on the Judiciary, *Hearings on S.J. Res. 119, proposing an amendment to the protection of unborn children and other persons, and S.J. 130, proposing an amendment*

guaranteeing the right of life to the unborn, the ill, the aged, or the incapacitated, 93rd Cong., 2nd sess. (1974).

174. Kifner, "Women Rally for Doctor," 27.

175. Bruzelius, "Hub Medical Community Is Dismayed," 1; CBS-TV Nightly News Broadcast, "Drs. Eisenberg, John Zelenk, and Christopher Tietze express shocked reactions to the abortion conviction of Dr. Kenneth Edelin," in *Collected Speeches of Kenneth Edelin* (Vincent Voice Library, Michigan State University, February 22, 1975), available online at http://www.lib.msu.edu/digital/vincent/findaids/EdelinK.html (accessed June 17, 2008).

176. "Abortion: The Edelin Shock Wave."

177. Clark., "Abortion and the Law," 18.

178. Sheehan, "Edelin Sentenced to Year's Probation," 1.

179. Clark., "Right-to-Life," 29.

180. Clark, "Abortion and the Law," 18.

181. Sheehan, "Edelin Sentenced to Year's Probation," 1; Sheehan, "Edelin Returns to Work at City Hospital," 1.

182. William P. Homans, Jr., "Defendant's Motion that the Court Order the Verdict Set Aside, for Order of the Entry of a Verdict of Not Guilty, or in the Alternative, For a New Trial," *Commonwealth v. Massachusetts,* Suffolk County, SS., Superior Court No. 81823; *Commonwealth v. Gricus,* 317 Mass. 403 (1944). See also Anglin, "Edelin Asks for Verdict to Be Set Aside or Retrial," 9.

183. *Commonwealth of Massachusetts v. Kenneth Edelin,* Supreme Judicial Court of Massachusetts, Criminal Suffolk SS. No. S-393, December 17, 1976. Five of the justices ruled that the verdict should be overturned, and one ruled that a new trial should be ordered. In addition to the majority opinion, which overthrew the verdict on the limited claim that the language of the indictment and the language of McGuire's jury instructions differed, three concurring opinions arguing that McGuire should have issued a directed verdict were offered in support for the majority decision to overthrow the verdict. For an analysis of these three opinions, see Ramsey, *Ethics at the Edges of Life,* 94–143.

184. *Harpers' Weekly,* March 4, 1975. Also see White, "Edelin Jury: Their Faces Told Nothing," 8, for biographical background on the jurors.

185. Robinson and King, "Jurors Say 'Negligence' Was Basis," 1.

186. Ibid.

187. Ibid.

188. Ibid.

189. Ibid.

190. Altman, "Doctor Guilty in Death of a Fetus in Abortion," 1.

191. Ibid.

192. Robinson and King, "Jurors Say 'Negligence' Was Basis," 1.

193. Anglin, "Edelin Asks for Verdict to Be Set Aside or Retrial," 9.

194. Ibid.

195. Clark, "Abortion and the Law," 18.

196. King, "Several Jurors Happy about Light Sentence," 1; and Kifner, "Convicted Boston Doctor Put on Probation for Year," 73.

197. Nolen, *The Baby in the Bottle*, 88.

198. Ibid.

199. UPI, "Doctor, Convicted in Abortion, Charges Prejudice Barred Fair Trial in Boston," 41; Culliton, "Edelin Trial," 814; Margulies, "Dying after Edelin," 48–50.

200. UPI, "Doctor, Convicted in Abortion," 41.

201. Nolen, *The Baby in the Bottle*, 88.

202. Fields, "Edelin's Wife Blames Bias, Religion for Conviction," 46.

203. Anglin, "Edelin Asks for Verdict to Be Set Aside or Retrial," 9. In 1949, the city charter was amended to replace ward-based elections with an at-large system. When Atkins was elected to the city council in 1967, he became the first black member of the council since that change, and the only elected black official in Boston. Lukas, *Common Ground*, 60.

204. "Doctor Asks Judge to Void Conviction in Abortion," 28.

205. "Edelin Returns to Work at City Hospital," 1.

206. Harvey, "Edelin Prosecutor's Aide Loses Hospital-Counsel Job," 6.

207. Pilati, "Edelin Was Not the Only One Who Was on Trial, Pilot Says," 8.

208. Buckley, "Edelin Abortion Verdict."

209. *Roe v. Wade*.

210. Lukas, *Common Ground*, 12.

211. Hillson, *The Battle of Boston*, 123.

212. Ibid.

213. Ibid., 134.

214. "ERA: Yes; Abortion: No," 1.

215. "Women of ROAR v. Edelin supporters," 1.

216. Paige, *The Right-to-Lifers*, 13–14.

217. Ibid.

218. Safire, "What's with Boston?"

219. Ibid.

220. "In the Name of the Father" offers Quindlen's view on how politics have changed since Democrat Joe Moakley spoke about his loyal Catholic base. She describes a service at her Catholic Church in the days preceding the 2000 election: "Our pastor with disguised distaste, informed us from the pulpit that he had been told to read a letter from the archbishop. This said in part: 'In the coming election, in addition to issues of basic human rights, there will also be addressed the questions of parents' rights to decide how their children are to be educated.' After delivering this free advertisement for school vouchers and, by extension, the Republican candidates, Father was expected to dust the dirt of lobbying off his hands and move seamlessly to transubstantiation." The links between abortion and schools that exposed the fissures within the Democratic Party in Boston in the 1970s have remained at the heart of the Catholic shift to the Republican Party.

221. Witcover, *Marathon*, 240–252.

222. Schrag, "The Forgotten American," 28, quoted in Carroll, *It Seemed Like Nothing Happened*; Farrell, *Tip O'Neill and the Democratic Century*, 526.

223. Padgett and Mazo, *The Presidential Campaign, 1976*, 93, 105–106.

224. Lukas, *Common Ground*; Carter, *The Politics of Rage*; O'Connor, *South Boston*; Farrell, *Tip O'Neill and the Democratic Century*; Kazin, *The Populist Persuasion*; and

"The Antiabortion Movement and the Rise of the New Right," ch. 7 in Petchesky, *Abortion and Woman's Choice.*

225. "Killing of Fetus Is Charged on L.I.," 27.

226. Clark et al., "Abortion and the Law," 18.

227. Kifner, "Convicted Boston Doctor Put on Probation for Year," 1.

228. Clark, "Abortion and the Law," 18.

229. Altman, "Implications of Abortion Verdict," 41.

230. Public Law 95–205, 95th Cong., 1st sess. (December 9, 1977). In 1980, the Supreme Court upheld this amendment in the case of *Harris v. McRae*, ruling that although the "government may not place obstacles in the path of a woman's exercise of her freedom of choice, it need not remove those not of its own creation. Indigence falls within the latter category."

231. For case law on these restrictions, see the following: *Committee to Defend Reprod. Rights v. Myers*, 625 P.2d 779 (Cal. 1981); *Doe v. Maher*, 515 A.2d 134 (Conn. Super. Ct. 1986); *Roe v. Harris*, No. 96977 (Idaho Dist. Ct. Feb. 1, 1994); *Doe v. Wright*, No. 91 CH 1958 (Ill. Cir. Ct. Dec. 2, 1994); *Moe v. Secretary of Admin. & Fin.*, 417 N.E.2d 387 (Mass. 1981); *Women of Minnesota v. Gomez*, No. CX-94–1442 (Minn. Dec. 15, 1995); *Jeanette R. v. Ellery*, No. BDV-94–811 (Mont. Dist. Ct. May 22, 1995); *Right to Choose v. Byrne*, 450 A.2d 925 (N.J. 1982); *New Mexico Right to Choose/NARAL v. Danfelser*, No. SF 95–867(c) (N.M. Dist. Ct. June 5, 1995); *appeal argued*, No. 23239 (N.M. Aug. 2, 1995); *Planned Parenthood Ass'n v. Department of Human Resources*, 663 P.2d 1247 (Or. Ct. App. 1983), *aff'd on statutory grounds*, 687 P.2d 785 (Or. 1984); *Doe v. Celani*, No. S81–84CnC (Vt. Super. Ct. May 26, 1986); *Women's Health Center of West Virginia, Inc. v. Panepinto*, 446 S.E.2d 658 (W.Va. 1993), *reh'g denied*, No. 21924 (Jan. 26, 1994); See *Doe v. Childers*, No. 94CI02183 (Ky. Cir. Ct. Aug. 3, 1995), *appeal dismissed* (Ky. Aug. 21, 1996); *Doe v. Department of Soc. Servs.*, 487 N.W.2d 166 (Mich. 1992); *Rosie J. v. North Carolina Department of Human Resources*, 491 S.E.2d 535 (N.C. 1997); *Fischer v. Department of Pub. Welfare*, 502 A.2d 114 (Pa. 1985). For analysis of these laws and their disparate impact on low-income and minority women, see Henshaw and Wallisch, "The Medicaid Cutoff and Abortion Services for the Poor"; James Trussell et al., "The Impact of Restricting Medicaid Financing for Abortion"; and Torres et al., "Public Benefits and Costs of Government Funding for Abortion."

232. Edelin, "Review of *The Dilemma of the Fetus* by Steven Maynard-Moody."

233. *Abortion Rights: Silent No More* (videocassette). As associate dean for Student and Minority Affairs at Boston University School of Medicine, Edelin is a member of the National Board of the NAACP Legal Defense and Educational Fund. He also remains an outspoken advocate for reproductive rights. From 1989 to 1992, Edelin was the chairman of the board of Planned Parenthood Federation of America, and he publishes widely in the field of obstetrics and gynecology, with special emphasis in the areas of teen pregnancy and substance abuse during pregnancy.

Chapter 4

1. Roth, *Making Women Pay.*

2. On bad mothers, see Ladd-Taylor and Umansky, *"Bad" Mothers*; Siegal, "Abortion as Sex Equality: Its Basis in Feminist Theory"; Slaughter, "The Legal

Construction of 'Mother'"; Ashe, "Postmodernism, Legal Ethics, and Representation of 'Bad Mothers,'" ; Ashe, "The 'Bad Mother' in Law and Literature: A Problem of Representation"; and L. Davidoff., "Motherhood, Race, and the State in the Twentieth Century."

3. Chadwick, "Protecting the Unborn"; Davidson, "Drug Babies Push Issue of Fetal Rights"; Jack Foley, "Stillbirth Is Called Murder: Mother Admitted She Used Cocaine"; and Lewin, "Court Acting to Force Care of the Unborn."

4. Bowes and Selgestad, "Fetal versus Maternal Rights"; Shriner, "Maternal versus Fetal Rights: A Clinical Dilemma"; Locke, "Mother v. Her Unborn Child"; King, "Should Mom Be Constrained in the Best Interests of the Fetus?"; and Sherman, "Keeping Baby Safe from Mom," 24.

5. On legal and philosophical theories of rights, see Rawls, A *Theory of Justice*; Michael Sandel, *Liberalism and the Limits of Justice*; Young, *Justice and the Politics of Difference*. On legal theories of rights, see MacKinnon, "Difference and Dominance"; Goldstein, *The Constitutional Rights of Women*; Eisenstein, *The Female Body and the Law*; Minow, *Making All the Difference*; Okin, *Justice, Gender, and the Family*; and Haag, *Consent*.

6. "The Patient within the Patient: Problems in Perinatal Medicine," xi.

7. Zimmerman, *Rh*, 94.

8. See Casper, *The Making of the Unborn Patient*, ch. 2, for biographical information on Liley.

9. Senate Subcommittee on Constitutional Amendments of the Committee on the Judiciary, Hearings on S.J. Res. 119, proposing an amendment to the protection of unborn children and other persons, and S.J. 130, proposing an amendment guaranteeing the right of life to the unborn, the ill, the aged, or the incapacitated, 93rd Cong., 2nd sess., 1974.

10. Liley, "The Fetus as a Personality."

11. Ibid., 10.

12. The women's health movement of the 1970s was part of a larger set of challenges to the previously unassailable authority of doctors, challenges that succeeded in expanding the medical rights of children, the elderly, the mentally ill, the chronically ill, the fatally ill, research subjects, and now fetuses. See Tribe, *American Constitutional Law*; and Gallagher, "The Fetus and the Law," 62, for discussions of the simultaneous expansion of patients' rights and abrogation of pregnant patients' rights. For more on the women's health movement, see also Ehrenreich and English, *For Her Own Good*, 316; Frankfort, *Vaginal Politics*; Boston Women's Health Collective's *Our Bodies, Ourselves*; Dreifus, *Seizing Our Bodies*; and Ehrenreich, *The Cultural Crisis of Modern Medicine*.

13. Arney, *Power and the Profession of Obstetrics*, 135–137.

14. Gallagher, "Fetus as Patient," 191.

15. *Raleigh Fitkin-Paul Morgan Memorial Hospital v. Anderson*, 201 A.2d 537 (N.J. 1964).

16. *Application of the President and Directors of Georgetown College*, 1964, 1007.

17. *In re Melideo*, 390 N.Y.S. 2d 523 (1976).

18. Roth, *Making Women Pay*, 107.

19. Ibid.

20. The first case establishing patients' rights was decided in 1891 when, in the case of *Union Pacific Railway Company v. Botsford*, the U.S. Supreme Court asserted that "no right is held more sacred or is more carefully guarded by the common law, than the right of every individual to the possession and control of his own person," 141 U.S. 250 (1891). In 1914, in the case of *Schloendorff v. Society of New York Hospital* the New York Superior Court found that "every human being of adult years and sound mind has a right to determine what shall be done with his own body," and found that a surgeon operating without the patient's consent was guilty of "trespass," 105 N.E. 2d 92 (1914). Since then, the courts have acknowledged that the state may have a compelling state interest in public health and safety that allows them to override a patient's refusal to seek treatment. See *Prince v. Massachusetts*, 321 U.S. 158 (1944) for a decision that mandated inoculating school children. But courts have agreed that the state cannot subject a competent adult to invasive medical treatment for the benefit of another patient. See *McFall v. Shrimp*, No. 78–17711 (1978) for a decision that refuses to order an unconsenting individual to undergo a marrow transplant for the benefit of another individual. For a full legal commentary on these and other cases, see Clarke, "The Choice to Refuse or Withhold Medical Treatment"; and Gallagher, "Fetus as Patient."

21. *In re Melideo*, 390 N.Y.S. 2d 523 (1976).

22. *In re Jamaica Hospital*, 491 N.Y.S. 2d 898 (Sup. 1985).

23. *Crouse Irving Memorial Hospital, Inc. v. Paddock*, 485 N.Y.S. 2d 443 (Sup. 1985), quoted in Roth, *Making Women Pay*, 111.

24. A 1987 study by the Public Interest Research Group charged that about half of the caesareans performed in 1986 were unnecessary. See Gallagher, "Fetus as Patient," 206, for a discussion of this pattern.

25. Lieberman et al., "The Fetal Right to Live."

26. Asch, "Psychiatric Complications," 461–462.

27. Ibid., 461.

28. Ibid.

29. Ibid.

30. *Jefferson v. Griffin Spalding County Hospital Authority*, 274 S.E. 2d 457 (Ga. 1981).

31. Kolder et al., "Court-Ordered Obstetrical Interventions."

32. Roth, *Making Women Pay*, 95. There is no way to assess the number of court-ordered medical procedures without underestimating the prevalence of the phenomenon because, as Roth explains, "these applications for court orders may be made to juvenile or family courts, whose proceedings are private and decisions unpublished or sealed. Some judges do not put their orders in writing at all. If the cases are not appealed and the media do not somehow learn of them, there will be no discernable record." Also, many women may sign consent forms after presented with the threat of a court order. One example from 1979 is the case of Francis Kenner, a white woman on welfare, who was in her forty-first week of pregnancy when she went into labor and was taken to the emergency room of the University of Colorado Medical Center. Noting signs of fetal distress on the EFM, the physician decided a caesarean was indicated, but Kenner refused to consent to the procedure. The hospital requested, and was granted, an emergency hearing, and a judge

from the juvenile court presided over a hearing in Kenner's hospital room. Kenner and her fetus were represented by two different court-appointed lawyers. The judge ultimately ruled in favor of the hospital, finding that a caesarean was in order. Before the surgery, Kenner signed a consent form. Because of this form, Kenner's case is not counted among statistics of court-imposed medical treatment upon pregnant women, but it indicates the kinds of pressures that women were increasingly subjected to in order to obtain their consent. See also Irwin and Jordan, "Knowledge, Practice, and Power" 34; Ikemoto, "Furthering the Inquiry"; Ikemoto, "The Code of Perfect Pregnancy"; Jorow and Paul, "Caesarean Section for Fetal Distress without Maternal Consent"; Kolder et al., "Court-Ordered Obstetrical Interventions."

33. Daniels, *At Women's Expense*, 33.

34. Dr. Harold Brody's introductory remarks to "Medical Ethics Case Conference: Ethical and Legal Issues in a Court-Ordered Caesarean Section," Medical Humanities Report (Medical Humanities Program, Michigan State University, 1984), quoted in Gallagher, "Fetus as Patient," 202.

35. Kolder et al., "Court-Ordered Obstetrical Interventions," 1192.

36. Sandroff, "Invasion of the Body Snatchers," 331; Gallagher, "The Fetus and the Law," 134–135. For larger discussions of the phenomenon of doctors overriding women's expressed wishes, see Ehrenreich and English, *For Her Own Good*; and Fisher, *In the Patient's Best Interest*.

37. Daniels, *At Women's Expense*, 33.

38. Roth, Making Women Pay, 103. For analyses of the ethical, legal, and medical implications of enforcing medical treatment on pregnant women, see Roth, *Making Women Pay*, ch. 5; Blank, *Mother and Fetus*, 106–123; Gallagher, "Prenatal Invasions and Interventions?"; Gallagher, "Fetus as Patient," 185–216; Merrick, "Caring for the Fetus to Protect the Born Child?"; Robertson, "The Right to Procreate and In Utero Fetal Therapy," 333; Robertson, "Procreative Liberty and the Control of Conception, Pregnancy, and Childbirth," 437; Shaw, "Conditional Prospective Rights of the Fetus"; Kolder et al., "Court-Ordered Obstetrical Interventions"; Steinbock, *Life before Birth*; Daniels, *At Women's Expense*, ch. 2.

39. See Alderman and Kennedy, *The Right to Privacy*; Gorney, "Whose Body Is It, Anyway?"; David Remnick, "Whose Life Is It Anyway?"

40. *In re A.C.*, 533 A.2d 611 (D.C. App. 1987).

41. *In the Matter of A.C.*, 539 A.2d 203 (D.C. App. 1988). *In re A.C.*, 573 A.2d 1235 (D.C. 1990) an appellate court reversed the order authorizing the surgery.

42. Ibid.

43. Rhoden, "The Judge in the Delivery Room," 1959.

44. Rhoden, "Caesarians and Samaritans," 118.

45. Harrison, Golbus, and Filly, *The Unborn Patient*; and Kolata, *The Baby Doctors*.

46. More than 300 genetic traits can now be tested prenatally. Many of them are associated with particular populations, most notably Down syndrome with older women, Tay-Sachs disease with Jews, and sickle cell anemia with blacks. For analyses of the discriminatory impact of prenatal tests, see Hubbard and Henifin, "Genetic Screening of Prospective Parents and Workers: Some Scientific and Social

Issues"; Culliton, "Sickle Cell"; and Kenen and Schmidt, "Social Implications of Screening Programs for Carrier Status." For analyses of the more generalized impact of these tests on the experience of pregnancy for women, see Faden et al., "Prenatal Screening and Pregnant Women's Attitude toward the Abortion of Defective Fetuses"; Rothman, The Tentative Pregnancy; Cowan, "Aspects of the History of Prenatal Diagnosis"; and Rapp, *Testing Women, Testing the Fetus*, for discussions of the pressures of deciding whether and how to treat prenatally diagnosed disorders.

47. Jones, "A Miracle, and Yet...."

48. For one of the earliest analyses of fetal rights that focuses on occupational and reproductive health in the post Roe v. Wade era, see Petchesky, "Workers, Reproductive Hazards, and the Politics of Protection."

49. Minutes of the Environmental Health Committee of the Lead Industries Association, Inc., September 9, 1974, cited in Stellman, *Women's Work, Women's Health*, 178; Bertin, "Reproductive Hazards in the Workplace," 279; and in Hunt, *Occupational Health Problems of Pregnant Women*.

50. Williams, "Firing the Woman to Protect the Fetus," 647; U.S. Congress, Office of Technology Assessment, *Reproductive Hazards in the Workplace*; Paul, Daniels, and Rosofsky, "Corporate Response to Reproductive Hazards in the Workplace."

51. See Chavkin, *Double Exposure*; Blank, *Fetal Protection in the Workplace*; Gonen, "Women's Rights vs. Fetal Rights"; Kenney, For Whose Protection?; Johnsen, "The Creation of Fetal Rights," 599–625; Becker, "From Muller v. Oregon to Fetal Vulnerability Policies," 1219–1273; Williams, "Firing the Woman to Protect the Fetus"; Steinbock, *Life before Birth*, 142–146; Daniels, *At Women's Expense*, ch. 3; and Roth, *Making Women Pay*, chs. 3 and 4.

52. *Muller v. Oregon*, 208 U.S. 412 (1908).

53. Ibid.

54. For a full discussion of the history of protective labor legislation, see Baer, *The Chains of Protection*.

55. Kessler-Harris, *In Pursuit of Equity*, ch. 6, 239–289.

56. For a thorough legal analysis of this argument, see Becker, "From Muller v. Oregon to Fetal Vulnerability Policies." For an analysis of the ways in which the role of federal and state courts, legislatures, administrative agencies, and interest groups navigated this transition, see Samuels, *Fetal Rights, Women's Rights*.

57. For the most thorough analysis of the history of women in the workplace, see Kessler-Harris, *Out to Work*.

58. *Historical Statistics of the United States, Millennial Edition,* online. Statistics are from Table Ba340–354, "Labor Force Participation, Employment, and Unemployment by Sex: 1850–1990," 1900 and 1970. See http://hsus.cambridge.org/HSUSWeb/toc/table-Toc.do?id=Ba340–354 for the table (accessed July 15, 2008).

59. For analyses of fetal protection policies in the context of the history of occupational and industrial health, see Hepler, *Women in Labor*; Hunt, *Occupational Health Problems of Pregnant Women*; Society for Occupational and Environmental Health, *Proceedings: Conference on Women and the Workplace*, Washington, D.C., June 1976. For general overviews of the history of industrial health, see Rosner and

Markowitz, *Dying for Work*; Rosner and Markowitz, *Deadly Dust*; Sellers, *Hazards of the Job*; and Markowitz and Rosner, *Deceit and Denial*.

60. Sicherman, Alice Hamilton; Young, "Interpreting the Dangerous Trades."

61. U.S. Department of Labor, Bureau of Labor Statistics, *Women in the Lead Industries*, quoted in Kessler-Harris, Out to Work, 107. For other historical analyses of the dangers of lead, see Rom, "Effects of Lead on the Female and Reproduction"; Wright, "Reproductive Hazards and 'Protective' Discrimination," 303–309.

62. Hamilton, "Protection for Working Women."

63. Wikander, Lewis, and Kessler-Harris, *Protecting Women*.

64. U.S. Department of Labor, Women's Bureau, The Employment of Women in Hazardous Industries, quoted in Kessler-Harris, "Protection for Women: Trade Unions and Labor Laws."

65. For discussions of the conflicts in the 1920s between the "equality feminists" and "difference feminists" over protective labor legislation and the Equal Rights Amendment, see Cott, *The Grounding of Modern Feminism*, ch. 4; and Kessler-Harris, "Protection for Women," 139–154. For an analysis of Hamilton's position on this dilemma, see Corn, "Alice Hamilton, M.D., and Women's Welfare."

66. Metler, *Divided Citizens*; Kessler-Harris, *In Pursuit of Equity*, ch. 2, 64–116.

67. Kessler-Harris, *In Pursuit of Equity*, 106. By excluding those who worked in domestic service, agriculture, retail and service industries, food processing, and the government, the FLSA disproportionately excluded women and almost entirely excluded African-American men and women.

68. Kessler-Harris, *Out to Work*, chs. 9 and 10.

69. Frosch-Morello, "The Politics of Reproductive Hazards in the Workplace."

70. For a discussion of the events of Bunker Hill, see Randall and Short, "Women in Toxic Work Environments"; Tate, "American Dilemma of Jobs, Health in an Idaho Town."

71. Wampler, Industrial Medicine, 543, quoted in Evanoff, "Reproductive Rights and Occupational Health."

72. Tate, "American Dilemma of Jobs, Health in an Idaho Town," 415.

73. Tate, "Women Shifted from Bunker Hill Smelter Jobs."

74. Anderson, "Bunker Hill: Sterilization Not Required," B1; "Thirty Moved from Smelter," 5; U.S. Department of Labor, "Citation and Notification of Penalty Issued to the Bunker Hill Company," September 11, 1980; *Yoss v. Bunker Hill Co.*, U.S. District Court for the State of Idaho, Civil 77–2030 (June 2, 1977); House Subcommittee on Manpower, Compensation, and Health and Safety of the Committee on Education and Labor, Hearings of the United Steelworkers of America, 94th Cong., 2nd sess., Part 2 (Washington, D.C.: U.S. Government Printing Office, 1976).

75. Quoted in Randall and Short, "Women in Toxic Work Environments," 415.

76. Fraser and Gerstle, *The Rise and Fall of the New Deal Order*; Wolfe, *Impasse*; Levy, *Dollars and Dreams*; Calleo, *The Imperious Economy*, 112–113; Cyert, *The American Economy*.

77. Bluestone and Hanson, *The Deindustrialization of America*; Vietor, *Energy Policy in America Since 1945*; and Yergin, *The Prize*.

78. Camp, *Worker Response to Plant Closings*.

79. Patterson, *Grand Expectations: The United States, 1946–1974*, 783.

80. Peurala, "People in the Plant Looked on Me as a Fighter"; Deaux and Ullman, *Women of Steel.*

81. Goodman, "Women and Jobs in Recoveries."

82. See http://www.eeoc.gov/eeoc/history/35th/milestones/1974.html for details of this settlement.

83. Anderson, "Bunker Hill: Sterilization Not Required," B1.

84. Randall and Short, "Women in Toxic Work Environments," 417.

85. Daniels, *At Women's Expense*, 63. See also Bayer, "Reproductive Hazards in the Workplace."

86. *Secretary of Labor v. American Cyanamid Co.*, OSHRC Docket No. 79–5762 (July 15, 1980). For a discussion of this case, see Scott, "Keeping Women in Their Place: Exclusionary Policies and Reproduction."

87. Faludi, *Backlash*, 441.

88. Harrell, "The Fetus and Workplace Safety."

89. Kenney, "Who Is Protected?"

90. Terry, "Conflict of Interest," quoted in Kenney, *For Whose Protection?* 155.

91. On lead causing birth defects transmitted through men, see Hatch, "Mother, Father, Worker," in Chavkin, *Double Exposure*; Lancreanjan, Popescu, Gavenescu, et al., "Reproductive Ability of Workmen Occupationally Exposed to Lead"; Plechaty, Noll, and Sunderman, "Lead Concentrations in Healthy Men without Occupational Exposure to Lead," 515–518; Kantor, "Occupations of Fathers of Patients with Wilms' Tumour"; Savitz, Sonnenfeld, and Olshan, "Review of Epidemiologic Studies of Paternal Occupational Exposure and Spontaneous Abortion." For a discussion of the absence of interest in the relationship between sperm and birth defects, or in "paternal-fetal" conflicts, see Daniels, "Between Fathers and Fetuses." For paternally transmitted birth defects, see Lindbohm et al., "Effects of Paternal Occupational Exposure in Spontaneous Abortions"; Olsham et al., "Birth Defects among Offspring of Firemen"; Colie, "Male Mediated Teratogenesis"; Davis, "Fathers and Fetuses"; Davis et al., "Male-Mediated Teratogenesis and Other Reproductive Effects"; Friedler, "Developmental Toxicology: Male-Mediated Effects," 52–59; Holly et al., "Ewing's Bone Sarcoma, Paternal Occupational Exposure, and Other Factors"; Merewood, "Studies Reveal Men's Role in Producing Healthy Babies"; Nelson, "Paternal-Fetal Conflict"; and Savitz and Chen, "Paternal Occupation and Childhood Cancer: Review of Epidemiological Studies."

92. Samuels, *Fetal Rights, Women's Rights*, 116.

93. Harrell, "The Fetus and Workplace Safety," A1.

94. Quoted in Scott, "Keeping Women in Their Place," 180.

95. Faludi, *Backlash*, 441–444; Roth, *Making Women Pay*, 47.

96. Roth, *Making Women Pay*, 53.

97. Ibid., 142.

98. *Secretary of Labor v. American Cyanamid*, OSHRC Docket No. 79–5762, 1980, 2.

99. Ibid.

100. *Oil, Chemical and Atomic Workers v. American Cyanamid Co.*, 741 F. 2d. 444 (D.C. Circuit, 1984).

101. Ibid., 448.

102. Ibid., 456.

103. Greenhouse, "The Bork Hearings."

104. Ibid.

105. Terry, "Conflict of Interest," 50.

106. Faludi, *Backlash*, 449; Roth, *Making Women Pay*, 58.

107. Kenney, *For Whose Protection?* 211.

108. Kressen, "Who We Are," 2.

109. American Public Health Association Policy Statement, "Reproductive Health and Rights of Workers," November 7, 1979, reprinted at http://www.apha.org.

110. Kressen, "American Cyanamid Update: No More Willow Islands."

111. For the most thorough collection of these cartoons, see "Pregnancy" file of the Comic Art Collection, Michigan State University Libraries, Special Collections Division. Hollander, *The Best (So Far) of Nicole Hollander*; Hollander, "Ma, Can I Be a Feminist and Still Like Men?"; Musgrave, *Womb with Views: A Contradictionary of the English Language*; Warren, *Women's Glibber: State-of-the-Art Women's Humor*; and Wilkinson, *Abortion (on Demand) Cartoons*.

112. No author, owned by MC/Union Art Services/LNS, printed in Washington Post, op-ed page, January 29, 1980, found at http://www.cartoonweb.com.

113. Nicole Hollander cartoon, reprinted in Kressen, "American Cyanamid Update."

114. Signe Wilkinson, *Philadelphia Daily News*, December 12, 1986, reprinted in Williams, "American Cyanamid: The Fight against Exclusionary Policies."

115. Reprinted in Evanoff, "Reproductive Rights and Occupational Health."

116. On the growing environmental movement in the 1970s, see Brown, *Laying Waste*; Freudenberg, *Not in Our Backyards!*; and Robinson, *Toil and Toxics*. On the particular implications of environmental and industrial hazards for women, see Bale, "Women's Toxic Experience." On Love Canal, see Gibbs, *Love Canal*; Levine, *Love Canal*. On women's grassroots activism surrounding issues of environmental justice, see Tucker, "Women Make It Happen"; Bullard, *Unequal Protection*; Rosenberg, "From Trash to Treasure: Housewife Activists and the Environmental Justice Movement"; Krauss, "Blue-Collar Women and Toxic-Waste Protests." On Agent Orange, see Wilcox, *Waiting for an Army to Die*; Schuck, *Agent Orange on Trial*; Nesmith, "Studies Link Agent Orange to Birth Defects in Children of Vietnam Vets"; Reynolds, "How Soon the Cheering Stops When Veterans Become Ill"; Serrano, "Birth Defects in Gulf Vets' Babies Stir Fear, Debate"; "Birth Defects May Relate to Agent Orange Herbicide."

117. Schlichtmann, "Accommodation of Pregnancy-Related Disabilities on the Job," 357; Blank, *Fetal Protection in the Workplace*; and Daniels, *At Women's Expense*, make this argument. Davis, "The Impact of Workplace Health and Safety on Black Workers"; Eggen, "Toxic Reproduction and Genetic Hazards in the Workplace," 843–864; Randall, "Slavery, Segregation and Racism," 191–223; and Rutherford, "Reproductive Freedoms and African American Women," 255–275. Roth disagrees, concluding that "general statistics do not demonstrate whether any particular group of women is disproportionately affected by fetal protection policies. . . . There is no evidence of [the claim] that fetal protection policies harm women of color more than white women."

118. Roth, *Making Women Pay*, 48; Adler, "Cytomegalovirus and Child Day Care"; Coleman and Dickinson, "The Risk of Healing"; Jasso and Mazorra, "Following the Harvest"; Fleishman, "The Health Hazards of Office Work"; Henifen, "The Particular Problems of Video Display Terminals"; Chavkin, "Closed Office-Building Syndrome."

119. *United Auto Workers v. Johnson Controls, Inc.*, 111 S. Ct. 1196 (1991).

120. Daniels, *At Women's Expense*, 63.

121. All quotes from Daniels, *At Women's Expense*, 64–65.

122. Ibid., 58. See also McNamara, "Factory and Fertility"; and Schmidt, "Risk to Fetus Ruled as Barring Women from Jobs."

123. Daniels, *At Women's Expense*, 88.

124. Ibid., 68.

125. Ibid., 68.

126. Ibid., 71.

127. Quoted in Roth, *Making Women Pay*, 68.

128. Quoted in Kirp, "The Pitfalls of Fetal Protection."

129. Quoted in Kenney, *For Whose Protection?* 163.

130. Rivera, *The Littlest Junkie: A Children's Story*; O'Connor, "TV: Heroin Addiction in the Newborn."

131. A 1992 report to Congress from the National Institute on Drug Use, of the National Institutes of Health, U.S. Department of Health and Human Services found that "little difference in terms of race or ethnicity exists among lifetime heroin users."

132. Chasnoff et al., "Prevalence of Illicit Drug or Alcohol Use During Pregnancy and Discrepancies in Mandatory Reporting in Pinellas County, Florida."

133. Substance Abuse and Mental Health Services Administration, National Household Survey on Drug Abuse Population Estimates, 1997 Series H-7 (Rockville, Md.: Department of Health and Human Services, 1998), quoted in Drucker, "U.S. Drug Policy."

134. Chasnoff, "Prevalence of Illicit Drugs," 1204; Roberts, Killing the Black Body, 172.

135. Roberts, *Killing the Black Body*, 194.

136. Terry and Pellens, *The Opium Problem*; Kandall, *Substance and Shadow*; Grey, *Drug Crazy*; and Campbell, *Using Women*.

137. Quoted in Campbell, *Using Women*, 146.

138. For a history of this problem between the years 1875 and 1934, see Perlstein, "Congenital Morphinism"; and Kunstadter et al., "Narcotic Withdrawal Symptoms in Newborn Infants."

139. Graham-Mulhall, *Opium: The Demon Flower*, 57, 62.

140. Chein, Gerard, Lee, and Rosenfeld, *The Road to H*, 72.

141. Chessick, "The Pharmacogenic Orgasm in the Drug Addict."

142. Chein et al., The Road to H, 313. Affiliated with the Research Center for Human Relations of New York University, Chein et al. were responding the New York City Welfare Council report indicating a 700 percent increase in the number of known addicts from 1946 to 1950. For more on the problem of heroin in New York City, see Fernandez, Heroin; Courtwright, Dark Paradise; and Goldstein, Narcotics.

143. Stern, "The Pregnant Addict," 253–257, publication of a report originally compiled in 1960.

144. Ibid., 254.

145. *Robinson v. California*, 370 U.S. 554 (1962).

146. *Robinson v. California*, quoted in Campbell, Using Women, 160.

147. Cuskey et al., "Survey of Opiate Addiction among Females in the United States between 1850 and 1970," 7.

148. Paltrow, "Criminal Prosecution against Pregnant Women."

149. Roth, *Making Women Pay*, 164.

150. Ibid.

151. Schroedel, *Is the Fetus a Person?* 101–126; Roth, *Making Women Pay*, 145–160.

152. *Reyes v. Superior Court of San Bernardino County*, 75 Cal. App. 3d 214, 141 Cal. Rptr. 912 (Cal. Ct. of Ap., 4th App. Div. 1977).

153. Gomez, *Misconceiving Mothers*, 42–46.

154. Daniels, *At Women's Expense*, ch. 4.

155. For an analysis of the Reyes case, and the history of California's response to prenatal drug exposure, see Gomez, *Misconceiving Mothers*, 85.

156. Gomez, *Misconceiving Mothers*, 84.

157. *Jennifer Clarise Johnson v. State of Florida*, 602 So. 2d 1288 (1992).

158. See Gomez, *Misconceiving Mothers* for a full examination of the different strategies of legislating and prosecuting prenatal behavior.

159. See Schroedel, *Is the Fetus a Person?* 114, for a table comparing state laws on fetal drug exposure as of January 1998. Also see Roth, *Making Women Pay*, 164, for a table on states with/without legislation on women's drug and alcohol use during pregnancy; and Roth, *Making Women Pay*, 166, for a chart summarizing state legislation on women's substance use during pregnancy as of December 31, 1992.

160. Banks and Zerai, "Maternal Drug Abuse and Infant Health," 53–67.

161. Chavkin, "Drug Addiction and Pregnancy"; Jones, "A Casualty of Deficit."

162. Blumner, "Prosecuting the Persecuted."

163. Cohen, "Challenging Pregnancy Discrimination in Drug Treatment," 91–142; Kumpfer, "Treatment Programs for Drug-Abusing Women."

164. Hudson, "With Neglect Charge behind Her, Mother Intent on Staying Clean."

165. *Elaine W. v. Joint Diseases North General Hospital*, 180 A.D.2d 525, 527; *Elaine W. v. Joint Diseases North General Hospital, Inc.*, 613 N.E.2d 523 (N.Y. 1993).

166. Senate Subcommittee on Children, Family, Drugs, and Alcoholism of the Committee on Labor and Human Resources, *Falling through the Crack*, 8. See also House Select Committee on Children, Youth, and Families, *Born Hooked*; Senate Committee on Labor and Human Resources and Committee on the Judiciary, Impact on Children and Families; House Subcommittee on Human Resources of the Committee on Ways and Means, *Impact of Crack Cocaine on the Child Welfare System*; Senate Committee on Governmental Affairs, *Missing Links*; Senate Committee on Labor and Human Resources, *Role of Treatment and Prevention in the National Drug Strategy*; Senate Subcommittee on Children, Family, Drugs, and Alcoholism of the Committee on Labor and Human Resources, *Addicted Babies*; House Select Committee

on Children, Youth, and Families, *Law and Policy Affecting Addicted Women and Their Children*; Senate Committee on Finance, *Infant Victims of Drug Abuse*.

167. "Crack Kids."

168. Dale, "Born on Crack and Coping with Kindergarten."

169. Zuckerman and Frank, "Crack Kids." Most of these articles relied on the 1985 study of fifty infants credited with starting the "crack baby myth." See Chasnoff et al., "Cocaine Use in Pregnancy." Chasnoff has since retracted the conclusions of his 1985 study, finding that the effects of maternal cocaine use are temporary. See Ira J. Chasnoff et al., "The Prevalence of Illicit-Drug or Alcohol Use during Pregnancy and Discrepancies in Mandatory Reporting in Pinellas County, Florida." The second study has received considerably less attention.

170. House Select Committee on Children, Youth, and Families, *Law and Policy Affecting Addicted Women and Their Children*, 22, quoted in Campbell, *Using Women*, 5.

171. Campbell, *Using Women*, 170–171.

172. Ibid., 139.

173. Ibid., 140.

174. Ibid., 183.

175. Baer, *Reinventing Democrats*.

176. The Democratic Leadership Council, "The New Democratic Credo," January 1, 2001, found at http://www.dlc.org/ndol_ci.cfm?kaid=86&subid=194&contentid=3775 (accessed July 7, 2008).

177. Church, "Is Bill Clinton for Real?"

178. House Select Committee on Narcotics Abuse and Control, "On the Edge of the American Dream," 3.

179. Senate Committee on Finance, Infant Victims of Drug Abuse, 38; Moynihan, "The Negro Family: The Case for National Action," also available online at http://www.dol.gov/oasam/programs/history/webid-meynihan.htm (accessed July 10, 2008).

180. See 1994 State of the Union Address, President Bill Clinton, January 23, 1995.

181. Personal Responsibility and Work Opportunity Reconciliation Act of 1996, Public Law No. 104–193.

182. For more on welfare policy under the Clinton administration, see Johnson, Duerst-Lahti, and Norton, *Creating Gender*; DeParle, *American Dream*; Hays, *Flat Broke with Children*; Mink, *Whose Welfare*.

183. "Era of Big Citizen Is Dawning."

184. Bragg, "Defender of God, South, and the Unborn."

185. Donnelly, "The Postpartum Prosecutor."

186. Facts on the case are from *Crystal M. Ferguson, et al., Petitioners v. City of Charleston, South Carolina*, 183 F. 3d 469, No. 99–936, Supreme Court of the United States, October Term 1999, decided on March 21, 2001; and from Motion of the ACLU et al to file brief for Amicus Curiae. Joining the ACLU were the Now Legal Defense and Education Fund; National Organization for Women Foundation Inc.; African American Women Evolving; Americans for Democratic Action, Inc; Center for Constitutional Rights; Center for Women Policy Studies; Chicago Abortion Fund; Choice; Connecticut Women's Education and Legal Fund; Hawaii State Coalition Against Domestic Violence; Hawaii Women Lawyers; Iowa Coalition Against Domestic Violence; Medical Students

for Choice; National Association of Women Lawyers; National Center for Pro-Choice Majority; National Network of Abortion Funds; National Society of Genetic Counselors; Northwest Women's Law Center; South Carolina Against Domestic Violence and Sexual Assault; South Dakota Coalition Against Domestic Violence and Sexual Assault; Women's Law Center of Maryland, Inc.; and Wider Opportunities for Women.

187. Lewin, "Abuse Laws Cover Fetus, a High Court Rules."

188. Cornelia Whitner, "Letter to the Governor of South Carolina."

189. Lewin, "Abuse Laws Cover Fetus"; Bragg, "Defender of God, South, and Unborn"

190. Greenhouse, "Justices Allow Broad Leeway in Police Chases."

191. Bragg, "Defender of God, South, and Unborn."

192. Greenhouse, "Justices Allow Broad Leeway in Police Chases."

193. All quotes and descriptions come from the Center for Reproductive Rights webpage, which provides summaries of the plaintiffs' experiences, available online at http://www.reproductiverights.org/crt_preg_ferguson.html#plaintiff (accessed July 8, 2008).

194. Paltrow, "Our Common Struggle."

195. Paltrow, "Punishing Women for their Behavior during Pregnancy." See Jos et al., "The Charleston Policy on Cocaine Use During Pregnancy"; "Plaintiffs' Memorandum in Support of their Partial Cross-Motion for Summary Judgment and in Opposition to Defendants' Motion for Summary Judgment," Ferguson v. City of Charleston, No. 2:93–2624–2 (D.S.C. filed Oct. 5, 1993); Settlement Agreement between Medical Center of the Medical University of South Carolina and Office for Civil Rights, Department of Health and Human Services, September 8, 1994 (on file with author); Letter from J. Thomas Puglisi, Ph.D., Chief Compliance Oversight Branch, Division of Human Subject Protections, Office for Protection from Research Risk, National Institutes of Health, to Dr. James B. Appel, President, Medical University of South Carolina, September 30, 1994 (on file with author).

196. Condon, "Clinton's Cocaine Babies," 12.

197. Condon, "Clinton's Cocaine Babies."

198. Ferguson v. City of Charleston, 183 F. 3d 469.

199. Ibid.

200. Weiss and Sternberg quoted in "In Victory for Privacy, Supreme Court Rejects State's Drug Testing of Pregnant Women," ACLU Freedom Network, press release, March 21, 2001, http://www.aclu.org/scotus/2000/12685prs20010321.html (accessed July 8, 2008).

201. Frank et al., "Growth, Development, and Behavior in Early Childhood Following Prenatal Cocaine Exposure." The publication of this study received national attention. See Tanner, "Crack Is Major Peril to Infants, but Not the Only Danger." Frank finds that "crack babies" suffer primarily not from maternal crack use, but rather from multiple health and environmental problems, and their development and behavior—if abnormal—are quite remediable. The latest research in which this was found analyzed thirty-six studies in which pregnant women or newborns were drug tested and the babies tracked over the years. "There is no need to assume that [cocaine-exposed babies] are a doomed generation or a biologic underclass, which is what was said about them

initially," according to Frank. "The idea that these children are uniquely 'unteachable' or somehow out of control is simply not supported by the data." The study notes that developmental problems "can be explained in whole or in part by other factors, including prenatal exposure to tobacco, marijuana, or alcohol, and the quality of the child's environment." For earlier studies that reached the same conclusion, see Koren et al., "Bias against the Null Hypothesis"; Mayes et al., "The Problem of Prenatal Cocaine Exposure"; Zuckerman and Frank, "Crack Kids"; Castoffs et al., "Cocaine/Polydrug Use in Pregnancy." Betancourt et al., "Problem-Solving Ability of Inner-City Children with and without In Utero Cocaine Exposure," discusses a study of "crack babies" led by the chairman of the division of neonatology at the Albert Einstein Medical Center in Philadelphia that reported, "The findings are overwhelming and persistent—there may be a drug effect, but it's totally overshadowed by poverty." The researchers found that poor children tracked to 4.5 years of age performed poorly on cognitive tests compared with other children, whether or not the poor children had been exposed to cocaine prenatally.

202. Zuckerman and Frank, "Crack Kids," 338.

203. The American Medical Association, the American Academy of Pediatrics, the Association of Reproductive Health Professionals, the American Medical Women's Association, the American College of Obstetricians and Gynecologists, the American Public Health Association, the American Nurses Association, the American Society on Addiction Medicine, the National Council on Alcoholism and Drug Dependence, the National Association of Social Workers, and the March of Dimes.

204. Frank et al., "Growth, Development, and Behavior in Early Childhood following Prenatal Cocaine Exposure."

205. Roberts, *Killing the Black Body*, 192.

206. *Brenda Kay Peppers v. The State of South Carolina.*

207. Pressley, "S.C. Verdict Fuels Debate over Rights of the Unborn," A3.

208. The Lindesmith Center, Delegation to the United Nation's World Conference Against Racism, "The War on Drugs Is a War on Women of Color," (Durban, South Africa: August 28–September 7, 2001).

209. Pressley, "S.C. Verdict Fuels Debate over Rights of the Unborn."

210. S.C. Code Ann. 20–7–50 (1985).

211. Hartz, *The Liberal Tradition in America*; Pateman, *The Sexual Contract*; Rawls, *A Theory of Justice*; Minow, *Making All the Difference*; Fraser, *Unruly Practices*; Poovey, "The Abortion Question and the Death of Man"; Rawls, *Political Liberalism*; Rodgers, "Republicanism," in Fox and Kloppenberg, *A Companion to American Thought*, 585; Sara Ahmed, "Beyond Humanism and Postmodernism: Theorizing a Feminist Practice" 93; Brinkley, *Liberalism and Its Discontents*; Haag, *Consent*; Greenberg, "Twentieth-Century Liberalisms."

Chapter 5

1. On March 6, 2006, the South Dakota legislature passed HB 1215, the South Dakota Women's Health and Human Life Protection Act, which, as SD Codified Laws § 22–17, was a ballot measure in the November 6, 2006 election, when 56 percent of voters voted against it.

2. December 5, 2006, H.R. 6099, "Unborn Child Pain Awareness Act," 109th Cong., 1st sess. The 250–162 vote in favor of the bill fell short of the two-thirds majority required in order to pass a bill by ending debate.

3. *Alberto R. Gonzales, Attorney General, Petitioner v. Planned Parenthood Federation of America, Inc., et al.,* Docket #05–1382 [on the decision in *Gonzales v. Planned Parenthood, Inc.,* 443 F.3d. 1163 (9th Cir.), 2006]; *Alberto R. Gonzales, Attorney General, Petitioner v. Leroy Carhart, et al.,* Docket #: 05–380 [on the decision in *Carhart v. Gonzales,* 413 F. 3d. 791 (8th Cir.), 2005]; Partial-Birth Abortion Ban Act § 2(14)(O).

4. *The Silent Scream,* a 28-min. film, produced by Donald S. Smith (American Portrait Films, 1984), script and visuals at http://www.silentscream.org (accessed July 14, 2008).

5. For a discussion of the rise of woman-protective antiabortion arguments, see Siegel, "The New Politics of Abortion"; and Siegel, "The Right's Reasons."

6. Brownlee and Graham, eds., *The Reagan Presidency;* Critchlow, *Phyllis Schlafly and Grassroots Conservatism;* Rymph, *Republican Women;* Diamond, *Roads to Dominion;* Schoenwald, *A Time for Choosing;* Tomasi and Velona, "All the President's Men? A Study of Ronald Reagan's Appointments to the U.S. Court of Appeals," 766–796.

7. Garrow, *Liberty and Sexuality;* Luker, *Abortion and the Politics of Motherhood;* Petchesky, *Abortion and Woman's Choice,* 217–244; Tribe, *Abortion;* Solinger, *The Abortionist;* Joffe, *Doctors of Conscience;* Kaplan, *The Story of Jane;* Ginsburg, *Contested Lives;* Petchesky, *Abortion and Woman's Choice;* and Solinger, *Abortion Wars.*

8. See chapter 4 of Corner, *Ourselves Unborn,* for a full discussion of maternal-fetal conflicts.

9. National Abortion Foundation, "NAF Violence and Disruption Statistics," available at http://www.prochoice.org/about_abortion/violence (accessed July 19, 2008).

10. This strategy has posed unique challenges to the antiabortion movement. Agreeing with Paul Weyrich, founding president of the Heritage Foundation and chair and CEO of the Free Congress Research and Education Foundation, that fetal pain is the "next step" of the pro-life movement, organizations including the National Right to Life Committee, the Family Research Council, Concerned Women for America, the U.S. Conference of Catholic Bishops, and the Christian Medical Society actively lobby for fetal pain legislation. Some opponents of abortion argue that focusing on the means, rather than the fact, of abortion, is not in keeping with pro-life principles. Jim Rudd, National Director of the Christian Street Preachers Association and editor of *The Covenant News,* calls the bill a "shocking example of genocidal thinking...out-doing even the Nazi's 'more efficient' and 'humane' extermination projects [that] sets forth a completely new set of definitions in how 'abortion providers' (the State's Willing Executioners) are to anesthetize children in the womb before killing them." Douglas R. Scott, president of Life Decisions International, argues that "allowing a mother to choose anesthesia for her preborn child will make it easier for her to choose abortion....Anesthesia will make abortion more palatable, not less. The legislation allows a mother to anesthetize her baby. It also allows her to anesthetize her own conscience." And Reverend Flip Benham of Operation Save America characterizes the "bogus" bill as "the typical

National Right to Life 'incremental' approach to end abortion." See Paul Weyrich, "Unborn Pain"; Rudd, "Fetal Pain Legislation Is Bogus"; Scott, "Unborn Child Pain Awareness Act Could Backfire"; Benham, "Fetal Pain Legislation Is Bogus."

11. Forsythe, "Our Philosophy: The Cultural Yearning for Human Dignity," on the Americans United for Life website. AUL was the first national pro-life organization in America, founded in 1971.

12. Forsythe, "Our Philosophy." The other six objectives are to "protect the rights of conscience of all healthcare professionals; protect parental rights, ensuring parents and guardians are involved in medical decisions of children; protect unborn victims from criminal violence, including homicide; ban all forms of human cloning; promote adult stem cell, cord blood, and other forms of life-affirming stem cell research; prevent euthanasia and assisted suicide."

13. Anonymous, "Life Is Sacred".

14. "Abortion's Psycho-Social Consequences," National Right to Life Educational Trust Fund, December 2006.

15. "Is Abortion Safe? Physical Complications."

16. "Concerns and Goals."

17. In his 1988 inaugural address, George H. W. Bush used the phrase "kinder, gentler nation."

18. For foundational work on the paradigm of separate spheres, see Cott, *Bonds of Womanhood*; Linda Kerber, "Separate Spheres, Female Worlds, and Women's Place"; Rosenberg, *Beyond Separate Spheres*; Smith-Rosenberg, "The Female World of Love and Ritual"; Barbara Welter, "The Cult of True Womanhood." For more on family values, see Coontz, *The Way We Never Were*; and Lassiter, "Inventing Family Values," chapter 1 in Schulman, *Rightward Bound*.

19. Tabor, "Believe It or Not: Abortion Causes Illegal Immigration." Tabor's argument is that abortion has contributed to a labor shortage which in turn lures illegal immigrants: "We have killed off almost 12 million potential workers in the U.S.A who would now be between the ages of 26 and 35. Nature abhors a vacuum, economic or otherwise."

20. Quoted in Huang, "Which Babies Are Real Americans?" Willke further describes this strategy in J "Twenty Five Years of Loving Them Both."

21. Schlafly, "American Citizenship Is Precious."

22. Republican National Coalition for Life website, http://www.rnclife.org (accessed July 14, 2008).

23. Quoted in Alexander Zaitchik, "'Christian' Nativism."; Gary Bauer, www.bauer2k.com/html/indepthissues.html, May 24, 1999.

24. Buchanan, *The Death of the West*, 8.

25. Reagan, "Remarks at the National Religious Broadcasters Convention"; Unborn Child Pain Awareness Act, S. 51, 109th Congress and H.R. 356, 109th Cong. (2005).

26. "Letter to the President, Signed by 26 Eminent Physicians," February 13, 1984, reprinted in *Fetal Pain: Hearing before the Subcommittee on the Constitution of the Committee on the Judiciary*, 55. Also see Collins et al., "Fetal Pain and Abortion"; Clines, "Reagan Appeal on Abortion Is Made to Fundamentalists"; "Charges Disputed"; American College of Obstetricians & Gynecologists, "Statement on Pain of the Fetus."

27. The medical and scientific literature, primarily in the fields of neurology, psychology, and anesthesiology, does not disagree about the developmental stages of the anatomical and physiological structures that make pain possible, but about whether pain is best understood as an objective function that can be measured and assessed mechanistically, or as a subjective experience that must be experienced and perceived cognitively. The foundation medical text on pain is Melzack, *The Puzzle of Pain*. For examples of medical literature supporting the existence of fetal pain, see Anand et al., "Pain and Its Effects in the Human Neonate and Fetus"; Glover and Fisk, "Do Fetuses Feel Pain?" 96; Giannakoulopoulos et al., "Fetal Plasma Cortisol and (beta)-Endorphin Response to Intrauterine Needling"; M. Fitzgerald, "Neurobiology of Fetal and Neonatal Pain," in Wall and Melzack, *The Textbook of Pain*, 153–163; Derbyshire, "Locating the Beginnings of Pain"; Derbyshire, "Fetal Pain: An Infantile Debate"; Griffith, "Fetal Death, Fetal Pain, and the Moral Standing of a Fetus." For examples of historical, anthropological, and cultural analyses of the meaning of pain, see Rey, *The History of Pain*; Elkins, *Pictures of the Body*; Sontag, *Regarding the Pain of Others*; Scarry, *The Body in Pain*; DelVecchio et al., *Pain as Human Experience*; Wall, *Pain*; Morris, *The Culture of Pain*. For the most recent and thorough scholarship on theories of pain, see Aydede, *Pain*.

28. Noonan, "The Experience of Pain by the Unborn." John Noonan has served on the Ninth Circuit Court since 1986. Prior to his appointment by Ronald Reagan, he was a law professor at the University of California at Berkeley and the University of Notre Dame. He has a doctorate in philosophy from the Catholic University of America and in 1995 received the Aquinas Medal from the American Catholic Philosophical Association. He has been a member of the editorial boards of the *American Journal of Jurisprudence, Human Life Review, Law and Society Review,* and *Harvard Law Review.*

29. Scarry, *The Body in Pain*, 14.

30. Hall, "The First Ache"; Clark, "'The Sacred Rights of the Weak.'"

31. Pernick, *A Calculus of Suffering*.

32. Scarry, *The Body in Pain*, 14.

33. Incorporated in 1971, Americans United for Life describes itself as the "first national pro-life organization to counter, through national education, the growing threat of disrespect for human life. Americans United for Life (AUL) defends human life through vigorous legislative, judicial, and educational efforts, state by state," http://www.aul.org (accessed July 14, 2008).

34. Collins, Zielinski, and Marzen, "Fetal Pain and Abortion."

35. Nathanson, *The Hand of God*; Nathanson, *Aborting America*.

36. *The Silent Scream*.

37. *The Silent Scream*.

38. Willis, "Silent Scream."

39. Ibid.

40. Vrazo, "Causing an Outcry with a 'Silent Scream.'"

41. Clark, "Inquiry: Topic: 'The Silent Scream.'"

42. Planned Parenthood Federation of America, *The Facts Speak Louder: Planned Parenthood's Critique of "The Silent Scream"* (pamphlet, 1985). Also see Faye Wattleton, "Memorandum to House and Senate Staff on 'The Silent Scream,'" March 1, 1985; and Patricia Jaworski, "Thinking About *The Silent Scream*," audiotape interview with

physicians who challenge Nathanson's interpretation of what is happening in the ultrasound, and neurologists who challenge the premise that a twelve-week fetus can experience pain (New York: Jaworski Productions, 1986).

43. Planned Parenthood, *The Facts Speak Louder.*

44. Ibid.

45. Ibid.

46. Ibid.

47. Ibid.

48. *The Silent Scream.*

49. *Abortion and Family Relations,* Testimony Presented before the Subcommittee on the Constitution, U.S. Senate Judiciary Committee, U.S. Senate, 97th Congress, Washington, D.C., 1981. Vincent Rue holds a PhD in family relations and in 1981 was a consultant to Surgeon General C. Everett Koop. He is a Fellow of the American Academy of Experts in Traumatic Stress, a member of the International Society for Traumatic Stress Studies, and the codirector of the Institute for Pregnancy Loss.

50. In 1987, David Reardon published *Aborted Women: Silent No More,* a collection of testimonies from women who had undergone postabortion religious conversions. In 1988 he founded the Elliot Institute for Social Science Research, dedicated to the study of postabortion trauma. For an article debunking Reardon's credentials, motives, and evidence, see Mooney, "Research and Destroy." For a recent article focusing on Reardon's role in the debate about postabortion syndrome, see Bazelon, "Is There a Post-Abortion Syndrome?" 43.

51. Reardon et al., "Deaths Associated with Abortion Compared to Childbirth"; Coleman et al., "Substance Abuse among Pregnant Women in the Context of Previous Reproductive Loss and Desire for Current Pregnancy," 10, 264.

52. Rachel's Vineyard Ministries, http://rachelsvineyard.org (accessed July 14, 2008); Safe Haven, http://www.safehavenministries.com (accessed July 14, 2008); Healing Hearts, http://www.healinghearts.org/index.php (accessed July 14, 2008); Victim's of Choice, http://www.victimsofchoice.com (accessed July 14, 2008).

53. In 1983, Speckhard was a Public Health Service Fellow in the United States Department of Health and Human Services Offices of Family Planning and Adolescent Pregnancy Programs. She subsequently published her research in *Psycho-Social Stress following Abortion.*

54. Reardon, "Their Deepest Wound."

55. "Bobbitt Mutilation and Abortion."

56. Brind, "Induced Abortion as an Independent Risk Factor for Breast Cancer," 209.

57. "Online Publications" and "Fact Sheets," The Breast Cancer Prevention Institute, http://www.bcpinstitute.org (accessed July 14, 2008).

58. Coalition on Abortion/Breast Cancer, http://www.abortionbreastcancer.com/abc.html (accessed July 14, 2008).

59. The Breast Cancer Prevention Institute homepage, www.bcpinstitute.org (accessed July 14, 2008).

60. Melbye, "Induced Abortion and the Risk of Breast Cancer"; Jensen, "Breast Cancer and the Politics of Abortion in the United States"; National Cancer Institute "Fact Sheet: Abortion, Miscarriage, and Breast Cancer."

61. American Psychological Association, "APA Research Review Finds No Evidence of 'Post-Abortion Syndrome' but Research Studies on Psychological Effects of Abortion Inconclusive," press release, January 18, 1989.

62. Stotland, "The Myth of the Abortion Trauma Syndrome."

63. Kleiman, "Debate on Abortion Focuses on Graphic Film."

64. *Fetal Pain: Hearing before the Subcommittee on the Constitution of the Committee on the Judiciary* (hereafter cited as *Fetal Pain*).

65. Orrin Hatch, "Opening Statement," in *Fetal Pain*, 1.

66. Sobran, "The Averted Gaze: Liberalism and Fetal Pain." Sobran was fired from the *National Review* following a conflict with Norman Podhoretz, in which Podhoretz attacked Sobran's positions toward Holocaust revisionism and Zionism, calling them anti-Semitic.

67. Ibid., 7.

68. Ibid.

69. Ibid., 10.

70. Saletin, *Bearing Right*; Olasky, *Renewing American Compassion* and *Compassionate Conservatism*. The phrase was popularized when George W. Bush adopted it as one of his key slogans during his 2000 presidential campaign against Al Gore. Also see Cavanaugh, "Secularization and the Politics of Traditionalism"; Lake, "The Metaethical Framework of Anti-Abortion Rhetoric."

71. Prescott, "The Abortion of 'The Silent Scream.'"

72. In the 2006 case of *Hudson v. Michigan*, the U.S. Supreme Court ruled that a violation of the "knock-and-announce" rule, based on a centuries-old idea of home privacy and the Fourth Amendment protection against unreasonable searches and requiring police to knock, announce themselves and wait a 'reasonable time' before entering, does not require suppression of evidence found in a search. The decision expanded the legality of "no-knock" laws that allow the police to forcibly enter a private residence without first knocking and announcing that they're the police.

73. Prescott, "The Abortion of 'The Silent Scream,'" 11.

74. Ibid.

75. Ibid.

76. Prepared statement of Richard L. Berkowitz, M.D., *Fetal Pain*, 27.

77. Prepared statement of Jeremiah Mahoney, M.D., *Fetal Pain*, 33.

78. *Fetal Pain*, 49.

79. *Fetal Pain*, 49.

80. *Fetal Pain*, 50.

81. DeCamp, *Common Ground—Occasional Papers from Presbyterians Pro-Life*.

82. *Charles v. Carey*, 627 F.2d 772 (7th Cir. 1980), 784. For a discussion of this case, see Collett, "Fetal Pain Legislation," 135.

83. *Charles v. Carey*.

84. *Planned Parenthood of Southeastern Pennsylvania v. Casey*, 505 U.S. 833 (1992).

85. *Planned Parenthood v. Casey*, 882. Sandra Day O'Connor had introduced the "undue burden" standard in *Webster v. Reproductive Health Services*, 492 U.S. 490 (1989). In a 5–4 decision, *Webster* upheld a Missouri regulation that barred public facilities and public employees in from performing abortions and required physicians to test for the viability of any fetus believed to be more than twenty weeks old.

86. By 2006, thirty-one states had established mandatory counseling and/or twenty-four-hour waiting periods, seventeen states prohibited state-funded insurance plans from providing abortions, twenty-eight states required parental consent, and sixteen states required parental notification. As of January 2007, five states required that women be told that the fetus may be able to feel pain, and thirteen more states are considering similar legislation; see NARAL Pro Choice America website, http://www.prochoiceamerica.org/choice-action-center/in_your_state/who-decides (accessed July 15, 2008). And by 2000, 87 percent of counties in the United States had no abortion provider, and 34 percent of women lived in counties with no abortion provider; see http://www.guttmacher.org/tablemaker/page4.mhtml (accessed January 17, 2007); and Guttmacher Institute, "State Policies in Brief: As of January 1, 2007," http://www.guttmacher.org/statecenter/updates/2006/april.html#FetalPain (accessed July 15, 2008).

87. Interview: Peter Samuelson, "The Last Abortion Clinic," *Frontline*, September 1, 2005, http://www.pbs.org/wgbh/pages/frontline/clinic/interviews/samuelson.html#casey (accessed July 15, 2008).

88. Martin Haskell, "Dilation and Extraction for Late Second Trimester Abortion."

89. The methods involve dilating a woman's cervix to allow most of the fetus to emerge into the vagina intact, rather than dismembering the fetus in the uterus by using forceps and other instruments. In the intact method, a doctor then suctions out the fetus' brain to collapse the head and allow delivery.

90. Jenny Westberg, "Grim Technology for Abortion's Older Victims."

91. Gorney, "Gambling with Abortion."

92. Ibid.

93. Ibid.

94. H.R.1833. To amend title 18, United States Code, to ban partial-birth abortions, June 4, 1995.

95. H.R. 1833, Calendar No. 224, 104th Cong., 1st sess.

96. Letter from Dr. Robinson to Representative Charles Canady, June 28, 1995, in *Congressional Record*, October 30, 1995, H11786.

97. The vote was 332–38.

98. Letter from Robinson to Canady, H11429.

99. Letter from Robinson to Canady, H11431.

100. Testimony of Vikki Stella, November 17, 1995, Senate Judiciary Committee Hearing: Partial-Birth Abortions.

101. Testimony of Tammy Watts, November 17, 1995, Senate Judiciary Committee Hearing: Partial Birth Abortions.

102. Testimony of Claudia Crown Ades, November 17, 1995, Senate Judiciary Committee Hearing: Partial-Birth Abortions.

103. Letter from Robinson to Canady, H11596.

104. For a legislative history of the bill, see Gordon, "The Partial-Birth Abortion Ban Act of 2003."

105. *Congressional Record*, November 7, 1995, S16734.

106. Ibid., S16735.

107. In May 1997, the bill was reintroduced, and approved in the Senate, by a vote of 64–36; in October 1997, the bill was passed in the House by a vote of 295–136; and on October 10, 1997, President Clinton vetoed it for the second time.

108. H.R. 1833, the Partial-Birth Abortion Ban Act of 1995, "subjects any physician who knowingly performs a partial-birth abortion in or affecting interstate or foreign commerce to a fine or imprisonment for not more than two years or both, except where such an abortion is necessary to save the life of a mother endangered by a physical disorder, illness, or injury, provided that no other medical procedure would suffice," summary from http://www.congress.gov/cgi-bin/bdquery/z?d104:HR01833: @@@D&summ2=3& (accessed July 11, 2008); Subcommittee on the Constitution, Committee on the Constitution, U.S. House of Representatives, Oversight Hearing: Fetal Death or Dangerous Deception: The Effects of Anesthesia During a Partial-Birth Abortion, March 21, 1996.

109. Prepared Statement by Norig Ellison, M.D., President, American Society of Anesthesiologists, *Hearing on the Effects of Anesthesia,* and Prepared Statement by Jean A. Wright, M.D., M.B.A., Associate Professor Pediatrics and Anesthesia, Emory University, *Hearing on the Effects of Anesthesia;* Prepared Statement by David J. Birnbach, M.D., Director of Obstetric Anesthesiology, St. Luke's-Roosevelt Hospital Center, *Hearing on the Effects of Anesthesia;* Prepared Statement by David H. Chestnut, M.D., Professor and Chairman of the Department of Anesthesiology, University of Alabama at Birmingham, *Hearing on the Effects of Anesthesia;* Marilyn Rauber, "Leading Doc Tells Congress Pro-Choicers 'Misinformed,'" *New York Post,* March 22, 1996.

110. Brenda P. Shafer, *Hearing on the Effects of Anesthesia.*

111. Prepared Testimony of Mary-Dorothy Line before the House Judiciary Committee, Subcommittee on the Constitution, March 21, 1996.

112. Ibid.

113. Prepared Statement by Coreen Costello before the Subcommittee on the Constitution, Committee on the Constitution, U.S. House of Representatives, Oversight Hearing: Fetal Death or Dangerous Deception: The Effects of Anesthesia During a Partial-Birth Abortion, March 21, 1996.

114. Ibid.

115. Ibid.

116. Ibid.

117. Center for Reproductive Rights, "So-Called 'Partial-Birth Abortion' Ban Legislation: By State," briefing paper, February 2004 (on file with author).

118. *Stenberg v. Carhart,* 530 U.S. 914 (2000).

119. 149 Congressional Record, H9146 (October 2, 2003)

120. Johnsen, "Functional Departmentalism and Nonjudicial Interpretation," 105.

121. 149 Congressional Record, H9146 (October 2, 2003). The 2003 Act states that Congress "is entitled to reach its own factual findings…that the Supreme Court accords great deference." It states further that Congress may "enact legislation based upon these findings so long as it seeks to pursue a legitimate interest that is within the scope of the Constitution, and draws reasonable inferences based upon substantial evidence." In support of this assertion, the Act's authors cite *Katzenbach v. Morgan,* http://www.law.harvard.edu/students/orgs/jol/vol41_2/gordon.php—fn85#fn85, as

providing evidence of the Supreme Court's "highly deferential review of congressional factual findings." The act also cites *Turner Broadcasting System, Inc. v. Federal Communications Commission (Turner I)*, and a case between the same parties three years later. Partial-Birth Abortion Ban Act of 2003, Pub. L. No. 108–105, § 2(8), 117 Stat. 1201, 1202 (2003); 384 U.S. 641, 653 (1966) ("It is not for us to review the congressional resolution of these factors. It is enough that we be able to perceive a basis upon which the Congress might resolve the conflict as it did."); 512 U.S. 622 (1994).

122. 149 Congressional Record, H.4925 (June 4, 2003).

123. Ibid.

124. Ibid.

125. 149 *Congressional Record*, S3457.

126. Holsinger, "The Partial-Birth Abortion Ban Act of 2003"; *Planned Parenthood Federation of America v. Ashcroft*, U.S. District Court for the Northern District of California on June 1, 2004; *National Abortion Federation v. Ashcroft*, U.S. District Court for the Southern District of New York, *Carhart v. Ashcroft*, U.S. District Court for the District of Nebraska.

127. Dailard, "Court Strike 'Partial-Birth' Abortion Ban."

128. *Carhart v. Ashcroft*, 331 F. Supp. 2d 805 (D. Neb. 2004), 1017 and 1031.

129. Dailard, "Court Strike 'Partial-Birth' Abortion Ban," 3.

130. Ibid. Also see Collett, "Fetal Pain Legislation: Is It Viable?" 127; Kolenc, "Easing Abortion's Pain: Can Fetal Pain Legislation Survive the New Judicial Scrutiny of Legislative Fact-Finding?" 171; Kolenc, "The Science, Law, and Politics of Fetal Pain Legislation."

131. Lee et al., "Fetal Pain: A Systematic Multidisciplinary Review of Evidence," 947.

132. Ibid.

133. See also Saletan, "I Feel Your Fetus' Pain: Compassionate Conservatism Enters the Womb"; Colb, "The *Journal of the American Medical Association* Says Fetuses Under 29 Weeks Do Not Feel Pain" Findlaw, September 7, 2005, http://writ.news.findlaw.com/colb/20050907.html; and Minkoff and Paltrow, "The Rights of 'Unborn Children' and the Value of Pregnant Women."

134. Lee et al., "Fetal Pain," 952.

135. Grady, "Study Finds Six-Week Fetuses Feel No Pain and Need No Abortion Anesthesia."

136. Grady, "Study Authors Didn't Report Abortion Ties."

137. Quoted in Cynthia L. Cooper, "'Fetal Pain' Bill New Item on Anti-Choice Agenda."

138. Quoted in *Karlin v. Foust*, 188 F. 3d 446, 491 (7th Cir. 1999). The Supreme Court has held that the government can require information to be made available to a woman seeking an abortion "[i]f the information the State provides requires to be made available to the woman *is truthful and not misleading*," *Planned Parenthood v. Casey*, 505 U.S. 833, 882 (1992). Also see Weisman, "House to Consider Abortion Anesthesia Bill: Conservatives Vow More Tests for Democrats on Social Issues When Congress Returns."

139. Lois Capps quoted in Levey, "The Nation; Antiabortion Measure Falls Short in House," A23. Phil Gingrey quoted in "Gingrey: Women Should Be Fully Informed

about Pain to Unborn Babies," webpage of Congressman Phil Gingrey, M.D., 11th District of Georgia, http://gingrey.house.gov/news/DocumentSingle.aspx?Document ID=54033 (accessed July 11, 2008).

140. H.R. 6099 (109th): Unborn Child Pain Awareness Act of 2006, last action taken on December 6, http://www.govtrack.us/congress/bill.xpd?bill=h109-6099 (accessed July 20, 2008).

141. Guttmacher Institute, "State Policies in Brief: An Overview of Abortion Laws."

142. *Planned Parenthood Federation of America v. Ashcroft,* 320 F. Supp. 2d 957 (N.D. Cal. 2004); *NAF v. Ashcroft,* 330 F. Supp. 2d. 436 (S.D.N.Y. 2004); *Carhart v. Ashcroft,* 331 F. Supp. 2d 805 (D. Neb. 2004). On July 8, 2005, the Eighth Circuit unanimously affirmed the judgment of the district court finding the ban unconstitutional in *Carhart v. Gonzalez,* 413 F.3d 791 (8th Cir. 2005). Concluding that the government presented no "new evidence which would serve to distinguish this record from the record reviewed by the Supreme Court in Stenberg," the Eighth Circuit decided that the ban was unconstitutional for failing to provide a health exception. Id. at 803. The circuit court did not reach the issue of whether the ban prohibits D&E procedures. The Eighth Circuit panel consisted of Judge James B. Loken (appointed by President George H. W. Bush), Kermit E. Bye (appointed by President Clinton), and George G. Fagg (appointed by President Ronald Reagan). On September 23, 2005, the attorney general petitioned the United States Supreme Court for review of the Eighth Circuit's decision. On January 31, 2006, the Courts of Appeals for the Ninth and Second Circuits affirmed the lower court rulings in both *Planned Parenthood Federation v. Gonzalez,* 04–16621 (9th Cir.2006) and *National Abortion Federation v. Gonzalez,* 04–5201-CV (2d Cir.2006), respectively. On February 21, 2006, the Supreme Court granted review in *Gonzalez v. Carhart.*

143. Oral Arguments, p. 5.

144. Ibid., 17.

145. Ibid., 13.

146. Ibid., 20.

147. *Gonzales v. Carhart* 8.

148. Ibid.

149. Congressional Findings (14) (N) in notes following U.S.C. §1531 (2000 ed., Supp. IV, 769), quoted in *Gonzales v. Carhart,* 26.

150. *Gonzales v. Carhart,* 28.

151. Ibid., 30.

152. Ginsburg, *Gonzales v. Carhart,* 21.

153. Ibid., 19.

154. Ibid., 15.

155. Ibid., 15.

156. Ibid., 18.

Chapter 6

1. Pear, "Abortion Proposal Sets Condition on Aid"; Department of Health and Human Services, 45 C.F.R. Part ___, RIN ___, [Title], Agency: Office of the Secretary, Action: Proposed Rule (in possession of author). The proposal clearly says, "This is a

confidential, deliberative, pre-decisional document and does not necessarily reflect current policy efforts or plans. For official use only."

2. This particular policy had become a symbol—albeit one with very material consequences—for whoever came into office: Ronald Reagan had first imposed this ban in 1984; Bill Clinton lifted it in 1993; George W. Bush restored it in 2001.

3. See http://www.personhoodusa.com/ (accessed September 30, 2009).

4. "How Personhood USA and the Bills They Support Will Hurt ALL Pregnant Women," National Advocates for Pregnant Women, video available at http://vimeo.com/3726108.

5. "North Dakota Personhood Bill Passes, First in U.S. History," Standard Newswire, February 18, 2009, http://www.standardnewswire.com/news/22733892.html.

6. Gilbert, "North Dakota Personhood Bill Defeated in Senate, Informed Consent and Ultrasound Bills Pass."

7. Ibid.

8. Brewer, *Super Baby;* Van De Carr et al., *While You Are Expecting.*

9. Mullen, "A Work in (and of) Progress," 1.

10. Ellenbogen and Foutz, "Prenatal Development Exhibition.

11. Ibid.

12. Ellenbogen and Foutz, "Prenatal Development Exhibit," 15.

13. Dave Andrusko, "An Update on Umbert the Unborn.." Readership numbers provided on http://www.catholic.net, "Culture of Life: Pro-Life Comic Umbert the Unborn" (accessed July 22, 2006).

14. Cangemi, *Umbert the Unborn: A Womb with a View.*

15. "Culture of Life: Pro-Life Comic Umbert the Unborn," http://www.catholic.net.

16. See http://www.prolifebillboards for images of the billboards (accessed July 27, 2006); Taylor, "The Public Fetus and the Family Car."

17. Petchesky, "Fetal Images," 263–288. Quote is from Petchesky, *Abortion and Woman's Choice,* xiv.

18. Newman, *Fetal Positions,* 68; Duden, *Disembodying Women,* 50–55; Corea, *The Mother Machine;* Theriot, "Women's Voices in Nineteenth-Century Medical Discourse."

19. Cangemi, *Umbert the Unborn,* 39.

20. Ibid., 40.

21. Ibid, 51.

22. Ibid., 75.

23. Ibid.

24. Ibid., 7.

25. Ibid., 75.

26. Risen and Thomas, *Wrath of Angels;* Maxwell, *Pro-Life Activists in America;* Mason, "Minority Unborn," 159–174.

27. Cangemi, *Umbert the Unborn,* 62.

28. See http://www.ohsaratoga.com/.

29. Ibid.

30. Mason, *Killing for Life.*

BIBLIOGRAPHY

Library and Archival Collections

American Civil Liberties Union. Reproductive Freedom Project. Papers. Correspondence, Publications, Legal Briefs. New York.

American College of Obstetricians and Gynecologists. Papers. Conference Notes and Correspondence. Washington, D.C.

American Medical Association, 1866–1890. Annual Meetings Collection. National Library of Medicine, History of Medicine Division. Bethesda, Md.

Guttmacher, Alan F. Papers. Countway Library of Medicine, Harvard University, Boston, Mass.

National Abortion and Reproductive Rights Action League. Silent No More Campaign Files. Washington, D.C.

Pilpel, Harriet F. Papers, 1930s–1980s. Unprocessed. Transcript of the trial of *Dr. Kenneth Edelin vs. the Commonwealth of Massachusetts*. Sophia Smith Collection, Smith College, Northampton, Mass.

Storer, Horatio R. Papers. Countway Library of Medicine, Harvard University, Boston, Mass.

Court Cases

Dietrich v. Inhabitants of Northampton 138 Mass. 14 (1884).

Union Pacific Railway Co. v. Botsford 141 U.S. 250 (1891).

Walker v. Gt. Northern Railway Co. 28 L.R. 69 (1891).

Allaire v. St. Luke's Hospital 56 N.E. 638 (1900).

Gorman v. Budlong 23 R.I. 169 (1901).

Muller v. Oregon 208 U.S. 412 (1908).

Schloendorff v. Society of New York Hospital 105 N.E. 2d 92 (1914).

Drobner v. Peters 133 N.E. 657 (1921).

Buck v. Bell 274 U.S. 207 (1927).

Dunlap v. Dunlap 84 N.H. 352 (1930).

Smith v. Luckhardt 19 N.E. 2d 446 (1938).

Stemmer v. Kline 128 N.J.L. 455 (1942).

Prince v. Massachusetts 321 U.S. 158 (1944).

Commonwealth v. Gricus 317 Mass. 403 (1944).

Bonbrest v. Kotz 65 F. Supp. 138 (1946).

Verkennes v. Corniea 38 N.W. 2d 838 (1949).

Williams v. Marion Rapid Transit Inc. Supreme Court of Ohio 87 N.E. 2d 334 (1949).

Woods v. Lancet 102 N.E. 2d 691 (1951).

Mitchell v. Crouch 285 S.W. 2d 901 (1955).

Hornbuckle v. Plantation Pipe Line, Co. 23 S.E. 2d 727 (1956).

Application of Donald L. Clarke, for a Writ of Habeas Corpus 309 P.2d. 142 (1957).

Brennecke v. Kilpatrick 336 S.W. 2d 68 (1960).

Hastings v. Hastings 33 N.J. 247, 163 A.2d 147 (1960).

Smith v. Brennan 31 N.J. 353, 157 A.2d 497 (1960).

Robinson v. California 370 U.S. 554 (1962).

Goller v. White 122 N.W. 2d 193 (1963).

Trevarton v. Trevarton 151 Clo. 418, 378 P.2d 640 (1963).

Application of the President and Directors of Georgetown College 1007 (1964).

Raleigh Fitkin-Paul Morgan Memorial Hospital v. Anderson 201 A.2d 537 (1964).

Tucker v. Tucker 395 P.2d 67 (1964).

Teramano v. Teramano 216 N.E. 2d 375 (1966).

Roe v. Wade 410 U.S. 113 (1973).

Burns v. Alcala 420 U.S. 575 (1975).

In re Melideo 390 N.Y.S. 2d 523 (1976).

Renslow v. Mennonite Hospital 367 N.E. 2d 1250 (1977).

Reyes v. Superior Court of San Bernardino County 141 Cal. Rptr. 912 (1977).

Yoss v. Bunker Hill Co. U.S. District Court for the State of Idaho, Civil 77–2030 (1977).

McFall v. Shrimp No. 78–17711 (1978).

Charles v. Carey 627 F.2d 772 (7 Cir. 1980).

Grodin v. Grodin 102 Mich. App. 396, 301 N.W. 2d 389 (1980).

Secretary of Labor v. American Cyanamid Co. OSHRC Docket No. 79–5762 (1980).

Committee to Defend Reprod. Rights v. Myers 625 P. 2d 779 (1981).

Jefferson v. Griffin Spalding Country Hospital Authority 274 S.E. 2d 457 (1981).

Moe v. Secretary of Admin & Fin. 417 N.E. 2d 387 (1981).

Right to Choose v. Byrne 450 A. 2d 925 (1982).

Wright v. Olin Corp 697 F.2d 986 (1982).

Zuniga v. Kleberg County Hospital 692 F.2d 986 (1982).

Planned Parenthood Ass'n v. Department of Human Resources 663 P. 2d 1247 (1983).

Hayes v. Shelby Memorial Hospital 726 F.2d 1543 (1984).

Oil, Chemical and Atomic Workers v. American Cyanamid Co. 741 F. 2d 444 (1984).

Crouse Irving Memorial Hospital, Inc. v. Paddock 485 N.Y.S. 2d 443 (1985).

Fischer v. Department of Pub. Welfare 502 A.2d 114 (1985).

In re Jamaica Hospital 491 N.Y.S. 2d 898 (1985).

Doe v. Celani No. S81–84CnC (1986).

Doe v. Maher 515 A. 2d 134 (1986).

In re Madyun 114 Daily Wash. L. Rptr. 2233 (1986).

In re A.C. 533 A.2d 611 (1987).

In the Matter of A.C. 539 A.2d 203 (1988).

Webster v. Reproductive Health Services 492 U.S. 49 (1989).

In re A.C. 573 A.2d 1235 (1990).

United Auto Workers v. Johnson Controls, Inc. 111 S. Ct. 1196 (1991).

Doe v. Department of Soc. Servs. 487 N.W. 2d 166 (1992).

Planned Parenthood v. Casey 505 U.S. 833 (1992).

Elaine W. v. Joint Diseases North General Hospital, Inc. 613 N.E. 2d 523 (1993).

Women's Health Center of West Virginia, Inc. v. Panepinto 446 S.E. 2d 658 (1993).

Doe v. Wright No. 91 CH 1958 (1994).

Roe v. Harris No. 96977 (1994).

Doe v. Childers No. 94C102183 (1995).

Jeanette R. v. Ellery No. Bdv-94–811 (1995).

Women of Minnesota v. Gomez No. Cx-94–1442 (1995).

Rosie J. v. North Carolina Department of Human Resource 491 S.E. 2d 535 (1997).

Stenberg v. Carhart 192 F.3d 1142 (2000).

Brenda Kay Peppers v. The State of South Carolina 552 S.E. 2d 288 (2001).

Ferguson v. City of Charleston 183 F. 3d 469 (2001).

Carhart v. Gonzalez 413 F. 3d (2005).

Gonzalez v. Planned Parenthood 443 F.3d (2006).

Gonzalez v. Carhart 550 U.S. __ (2007).

Planned Parenthood Minnesota, North Dakota, South Dakota; Carol E. Ball, M.D. v. Governor Mike Rounds, Attorney General Larry Long, Alpha Center; Black Hills Crisi Pregnancy Center, Appeal from the U.S. District Court for the District of South Dakota, filed on June 27, 2008.

Government Documents

U.S. Department of Labor, Bureau of Labor Statistics. *Women in the Lead Industries*. Special report prepared by Alice Hamilton. Bulletin No. 263. Washington, D.C.: Government Printing Office, 1919.

U.S. Department of Labor, Women's Bureau. *The Employment of Women in Hazardous Industries*. Special report prepared by Alice Hamilton. Bulletin No. 6. Washington, D.C.: Government Printing Office, 1921.

U.S. Department of Health, Education, and Welfare. *Protecting the Unborn Baby*, Public Health Service, Publication No. 430, Health Information Series 85, 1950.

U.S. Congress. Senate Subcommittee on Government Research of the Committee on Government Operations. *Hearings on S.J. Resolution 145*. 90th Congress, 2d sess., 1968.

U.S. Congress. Senate. Subcommittee on Health of the Committee on Labor and Public Welfare. *Joint Hearing of the National Advisory Commission on Health Science and Society*. 92d. Cong., 1st sess., 1971.

U.S. Congress. House. Committee on Ways and Means. *Report on the Social Security Amendments of 1971*. 92d Cong., 1st sess., 1971.

U.S. Congress. Senate. Committee on Finance. *Report on the Social Security Amendments of 1972*. 92d. Cong. 2d sess., September 26, 1972.

U.S. Congress. Senate. Committee on Labor and Public Policy. *Hearings on the National Research Act*. 92d. Cong., 1st sess., 1973.

U.S. Department of Health, Education, and Welfare. National Institutes of Health. *Protection of Human Subjects: Policies and Procedures*. 38 Fed. Reg. 221, 1973.

U.S. Department of Health, Education, and Welfare, National Institutes of Health. *Protection of Human Subjects: Policies and Procedures*. 39 Fed. Reg. 30, 1974.

U.S. Department of Health, Education, and Welfare. National Commission for the Protection of Human Subjects of Biomedical and Behavioral Research. *Report and Recommendations: Research on the Fetus*. DHEW Publication No. (OS) 76–128. Washington, D.C.: Government Printing Office, 1974.

U.S. Congress. House. Committee on the Judiciary. Subcommittee on Civil and Constitutional Rights of the Committee on the Judiciary, *Hearings on Proposed Constitutional Amendments on Abortion*, 94th Cong., 2d sess., 1976.

U.S. Congress. Senate. Committee on the Judiciary. Subcommittee on Constitutional Amendments. *Hearings on S.J. Res. 119, Proposing an Amendment to the Protection of Unborn Children and Other Persons, and S.J. 130, Proposing an Amendment Guaranteeing the Right of Life to the Unborn, the Ill, the Aged, or the Incapacitated.* 93d Cong., 2d sess., 1974.

U.S. Congress. House. Committee on Education and Labor, Subcommittee on Manpower, Compensation, and Health and Safety. *Testimony from the United Steelworkers of America.* 94th Cong., 2d sess., 1976.

U.S. Congress. Senate. Committee on the Judiciary, Subcommittee on the Constitution. *Abortion and Family Relations.* 97th Cong., 1st sess., 1981.

U.S. Congress. Senate. Committee on the Judiciary. Subcommittee on Separation of Powers. *Hearings on S.J. 158, a Bill to Provide that Human Life Shall Be Deemed to Exist from Conception.* 97th Cong., 1st sess., 1981.

U.S. Congress. Office of Technology Assessment. *Reproductive Hazards in the Workplace.* 1985.

U.S. Congress. Senate. Committee on the Judiciary. *The Medical Evidence Concerning Fetal Pain: Hearing before the Subcommittee on the Constitution.* 99th Cong., 1st sess., 1985.

U.S. Congress. Senate. Committee on Governmental Affairs. *Missing Links: Coordinating Federal Drug Policy for Women, Infants, and Children.* 101st Cong., 1st sess., 1989.

U.S. Congress. Senate Subcommittee on Children, Family, Drugs, and Alcoholism of the Committee on Labor and Human Resources. *Addicted Babies: What Can Be Done?* 101st Cong., 1st sess., 1989.

U.S. Congress. Senate Subcommittee on Children, Family, Drugs, and Alcoholism of the Committee on Labor and Human Resources. *Falling through the Crack: The Impact of Drug-Exposed Children on the Child Welfare System.* 101st Cong., 2d. sess., 1990.

U.S. Congress. House Subcommittee on Human Resources of the Committee on Ways and Means. *Impact of Crack Cocaine on the Child Welfare System*, 101st Cong., 2d. sess., 1990.

U.S. Congress. Senate Committee on Labor and Human Resources. *Role of Treatment and Prevention in the National Drug Strategy.* 101st Cong., 2d sess., 1990.

U.S. Congress. House Select Committee on Children, Youth, and Families. *Law and Policy Affecting Addicted Women and Their Children.* 101st Cong., 2d sess., 1990.

U.S. Congress. Senate. Committee on Finance. *Infant Victims of Drug Abuse.* 101st Cong., 2d sess., 1990.

U.S. Congress. Senate. Committee on Labor and Human Resources. *On Finding Medical Cures: The Promise of Fetal Tissue Transplantation Research.* 102d Cong., 1st sess., 1991.

U.S. Congress. House. *Report of the Select Committee on Narcotics Abuse and Control, "On the Edge of the American Dream": A Social and Economic Profile in 1992.* 102d Cong., 2d sess, 1992.

Department of Health and Human Services. Memorandum for the Secretary. *Federal Funding of Fetal Tissue Transplantation Research*. 58 Fed. Reg. 7457, 1993.

U.S. Congress. House. Committee on the Judiciary. Subcommittee on Crime and Criminal Justice. *Hearings on Abortion clinic violence*. 103d Cong., 1st. sess., 1993.

H.R. 1833. *To Amend Title 18, United States Code, To Ban Partial-Birth Abortions*, 4. June 1995.

U.S. Congress. Senate. Committee on the Judiciary. *Hearing on Partial Birth Abortion*. 1995.

U.S. Congress. House. Committee on the Judiciary. Subcommittee on the Constitution. *Oversight Hearing: Fetal Death or Dangerous Deception: The Effects of Anesthesia During a Partial-Birth Abortion*. March 21, 1996.

U.S. Congress. House Select Committee on Children, Youth, and Families. *Born Hooked: Confronting the Impact of Perinatal Substance Abuse*. 101st Cong., 1st sess., 1999.

U.S. Congress. Senate Committee on Labor and Human Resources and Committee on the Judiciary. *Impact on Children and Families*. 101st Cong., 1st sess., 1999.

U.S. Department of Health and Human Services, National Institutes of Health. "Fact Sheet: Pluripotent Stem Cells: A Primer." 1999.

U.S. Department of Health and Human Services, National Institutes of Health. "Fact Sheet: Stem Cell Research." 1999.

U.S. Congress. Senate. Committee on Labor and Human Resources. *Finding Medical Cures: The Promise of Fetal Tissue Transplantation Research: Hearings on S. 1902*. 102d Cong., 1st sess., 1999.

State Children's Health Insurance Program; Eligibility for Prenatal Care and Other Health Services for Unborn Children; Final Rule, 67 Fed. Reg. 61955–61974 (2002) (to be codified at 42 C.F.R. pt. 457).

Books, Articles, and Films

"Abortion and Manslaughter: A Boston Doctor Goes on Trial." *Science*, January 31, 1975, 334.

"Abortion Error." *New York Times*, February 19, 1975, 31.

"Abortion Reform Bill Passes." *New York Times*, July 15, 1970, 2.

"Abortion Rights: Silent No More." Documentary produced by Tom Goodwin and Gerardine Wurzburg, Planned Parenthood of America, 1985.

"Abortion: The Edelin Shock Wave." *Time*, March 3, 1975, 54–55.

"Abortion's Psycho-Social Consequences: Factsheet." National Right to Life Education Trust Fund, December 2006, www.nrlc.org/factsheets/FS18_AbtnPsychoSocial.pdf (accessed June 8, 2010).

Abram, Ruth J. ed. *Send Us a Lady Physician: Women Doctors in America, 1835–1920*. New York: Norton, 1985.

Adams, Alice E. *Reproducing the Womb: Images of Childbirth in Science, Feminist Theory, and Literature*. Ithaca, N.Y.: Cornell University Press, 1994.

Ad Hoc Committee to Examine the Definition of Death, Harvard Medical School. "A Definition of Irreversible Coma." *Journal of American Medical Association* 205 (1968): 337–340.

Adler, Stuart. "Cytomegelovirus and Child Day Care: Evidence for an Increased Infection Rate among Day-Care Workers." *New England Journal of Medicine* 321 (November 9, 1989): 1290–1296.

Ahmed, Sara. "Beyond Humanism and Postmodernism: Theorizing a Feminist Practice." *Hypatia* 11, no. 2 (Spring 1996): 71–93.

"Aid to Families with Unborn Dependent Children: May the States Withhold Benefits?" *Michigan Law Review* 73, no. 3 (January 1975): 561–583.

"Aid for the Unborn." *Time*, October 1, 1973, http://www.time.com/time/magazine/article/0,9171,942739,00.html (accessed June 13, 2010).

Aiken, Katherine G. *Idaho's Bunker Hill: The Rise and Fall of a Great Mining Company, 1885–1981.* Norman: University of Oklahoma Press, 2005.

Alderman, Ellen, and Caroline Kennedy. *The Right to Privacy*. New York: Knopf, 1995.

Alsop, Gulielma. "The Right to Be Well Born." *Women Citizen*, February 9, 1924, 30.

Althusser, Louis. "Ideology and Ideological State Apparatuses." *Lenin and Philosophy and Other Essays*. Translated by Ben Brewster. New York: Monthly Review Press, 1971.

Altman, Lawrence K. "Doctor Guilty in Death of Fetus in Abortion." *New York Times*, February 16, 1975, 1.

———. "Implications of Abortion Verdict," *New York Times*, February 17, 1975, 41.

Alton, Jack R. "Torts: Action by Child for Prenatal Injuries." *Ohio State Law Journal* 10 (1949): 411.

Ambert, Didier. "The Graphic Sphere: Images and Civic Conscience in the Progressive Era." Unpublished paper presented at "Public Spheres and America Cultures," Brown University, June 15, 2004.

American College of Obstetricians and Gynecologists. "Statement of Pain of the Fetus." Washington, D.C.: ACOG, February 13, 1984.

American Medical Association. "Medical Applications of Fetal Tissue Transplantation." *Journal of the American Medical Association* 263 (1900): 565–570.

American Psychological Association. "APA Research Review Finds No Evidence of 'Post-Abortion Syndrome' But Research Studies on Psychological Effects of Abortion Inconclusive." Press release, January 18, 1989.

Anand, K., et al. "Pain and Its Effects in the Human Neonate and Fetus," *New England Journal of Medicine* 317 (1987): 1321–1329.

Anderson, Steven. "Bunker Hill: Sterilization Not Required." *Idaho Statesmen*, September 17, 1975, 1.

Anderson, Walter H. "Rights of Action in an Unborn Child." *Tennessee Law Review* 14 (1962): 632–634.

Andrews, Lori. *Future Perfect*. New York: Columbia University Press, 2001.

Andrusko, Dave. "An Update on Umbert the Unborn," *Today's News and Views*, National Right to Life, http://www.nrlc.org/News_and_Views/Aug09/nv082509part2.html (accessed October 1, 2009).

Angell, Marcia. *Science on Trial: The Clash of Medical Evidence and the Law in the Breast Implant Case*. New York: W. W. Norton, 1997.

Anglin, Robert J. "Edelin Asks for Verdict to Be Set Aside or Retrial." *Boston Globe*, February 22, 1975, 9.

Annas, George J., and Michael A. Grodin, eds. *The Nazi Doctors and the Nuremberg Code: Human Rights in Human Experimentation*. New York: Oxford University Press, 1992.

Anonymous. "Life Is Sacred." *Focus on the Family*, 2002, http://www.family.org/lifechallenges/A000000129.cfm (accessed July 14, 2008).

Apple, Rima D. "Postmodernism, Legal Ethics, and Representation of 'Bad Mothers.'" In *Mothers in Law: Feminist Theory and the Legal Regulation of Motherhood*, edited by Martha Albertson Fineman and Isabel Karpin. New York: Columbia University Press, 1995.

———, ed. *Women, Health, and Medicine in America: A Historical Handbook*. New Brunswick, N.J.: Rutgers University Press, 1992. First published in 1990, Garland.

Appleman, Herman. *When Two Become Three*. New York: Henry Holt, 1958.

Aprison, Barry. "The Prenatal Exhibit at the Museum of Science and Industry." *Visitor Behavior*. 12, nos. 1 and 2 (1997): 25.

Arendt, Hannah. *Human Condition*. Chicago: University of Chicago Press, 1958.

Armstrong, Elizabeth Mitchell. "Conceiving Risk, Bearing Responsibility: Ideas about Alcohol and Offspring in the Modern Era." PhD diss., University of Pennsylvania, 1998.

Arney, William Ray. *Power and the Profession of Obstetrics*. Chicago: University of Chicago Press, 1982.

Arnold, John D., and Thomas F. Zimmerman, and Daniel C. Martin. "Public Attitudes and the Diagnosis of Death." *Journal of American Medical Association* 209 (1969): 1505–1509.

Asch, Stuart S. "Psychiatric Complications: Mental and Emotional Problems." *Rovinsky & Guttmacher's Medical, Surgical, and Gynecological Complications of Pregnancy*, 3rd ed. Baltimore: Williams and Wilkins, Co., 1985.

Ashe, Marie. "The 'Bad Mother' in Law and Literature: A Problem of Representation." *Hastings Law Journal* 43 (1992): 1017.

———. "Postmodernism, Legal Ethics, and Representations of 'Bad Mothers'." In *Mothers in Law: Feminist Theory and the Legal Regulation of Motherhood*, edited by Martha Fineman and Isabel Karpin. New York: Columbia University Press, 1995.

Atchison, C. J. "*Ard. v. Ard.*: Limiting The Parent-Child Immunity Doctrine." *University of Pittsburgh Law Review* 10 (1976): 977–1033.

Athey, Stephanie. "Eugenic Feminisms in Late Nineteenth-Century America: Reading Race in Victoria Woodhull, Frances Willard, Anna Julia Cooper, and Ida B. Wells." *Genders* 31 (2000), http://www.genders.org/g31/g31_athey.html (accessed June 8, 2010).

Aud, C. J. "In What Per Cent, Is the Regular Profession Responsible for Criminal Abortions, and What Is the Remedy?" *Kentucky Medical Journal* 2 (September 1904): 100.

Aydede, Murat, ed. *Pain: New Essays on Its Nature and the Methodology of Study*. Cambridge: MIT Press, 2005.

"Babies before Birth: Excerpt from the First Nine Months of Life." *Look*, June 5, 1962, 19.

"Baby May Be Neurotic if Mother Is Disturbed." *Science News Letter*, June 20, 1953, 376.

Baer, Judith A. *The Chains of Protection: The Judicial Response to Women's Labor Legislation*. Westport: Greenwood Press, 1978.

Baer, Kenneth S. *Reinventing Democrats: The Politics of Liberalism from Reagan to Clinton*. Lawrence: University of Kansas Press, 2000.

Baker, Lee. *From Savage to Negro: Anthropology and the Construction of Race, 1896–1954*. Los Angeles: University of California Press, 1998.

Bale, Anthony. "Women's Toxic Experience." In *Women, Health, and Medicine in America*, edited by Rima Apple. New York: Garland, 1990.

Ballantyne, John William. *Manual of Antenatal Pathology and Hygiene: The Embryo*, vol. 2. Edinburgh: William Green & Sons, 1904.

Bancroft, Hubert Howe. *The Book of the Fair: An Historical and Description Presentation of the World's Science, Art, and Industry, as Viewed through the Columbian Exposition in Chicago in 1893, Designed to Set Forth the Display Made by the Congress of Nations, of Human Achievement in Material Form, so as to More Effectually Illustrate the Progress of Mankind in All the Departments of Civilized Life*. Chicago: Bancroft, 1893.

Banks, Rae, and Assata Zerai. "Maternal Drug Abuse and Infant Health: A Proposal for a Multilevel Model." In *African-Americans and the Public Agenda: The Paradoxes of Public Policy*, edited by Sedrick Herring. Newbury Park, Calif.: Sage, 1997.

Barber, Bernard, et al. *Research on Human Subjects*. New York: Russell Sage Foundation, 1973.

Bayer, Charles J. *Maternal Impressions: A Study of Child Life before and after Birth, and Their Effect upon Individual Life and Character*. Minnesota: Jones & Kroeger, 1897.

Bayer, Ronald. "Reproductive Hazards in the Workplace: Bearing the Burden of Fetal Risk." *Millbank Memorial Fund Quarterly Health and Safety* 60 (Fall 1982): 633–656.

Bazelon, Emily. "Is There a Post-Abortion Syndrome?" *New York Times Magazine*, January 21, 2007.

———. "Telling Doctors What to Think: South Dakota's Unbelievable New Abortion Law." *Slate*, June 27, 2008, http://www.slate.com/id/2194605/ (accessed June 8, 2010).

Becker, Mary. "From *Muller v. Oregon* to Fetal Vulnerability Policies." *University of Chicago Law Review* 53 (1986): 1217–1273.

Beckett, Katherine. "Managing Motherhood: The Civil Regulation of Prenatal Drug Users." *Studies in Law, Politics and Society* 16 (1997): 299–325.

Bederman, Gail. *Manliness and Civilization: A Cultural History of Gender and Race in the United States, 1880–1917*. Chicago: University of Chicago Press, 1995.

Beecher, Henry. "After the Definition of Irreversible Coma." *New England Journal of Medicine* 281 (1969): 1070–1071.

Beisel, Nicole Kay. *Imperiled Innocents: Anthony Comstock and Family Reproduction in Victorian America*. Princeton: Princeton University Press, 1997.

Beller, Fritz K., and Robert F. Weir, eds. *The Beginning of Human Life*. Dordrecht, The Netherlands: Kluwer Academic, 1994.

Benham, Flip. "Fetal Pain Legislation Is Bogus." *Christian Newswire*, December 2, 2006, http://www.christiannewswire.com/index.php?module=releases&task=view&releaseID=1640 (accessed July 14, 2008).

Benson, Keith B., Jane Maienschein, and Ronald Rainger, eds. *Expansion of American Biology*. New Brunswick, N.J.: Rutgers University Press, 1991.

Berlant, Lauren. *The Queen of America Goes to Washington City: Essays on Sex and Citizenship*. Durham, N.C.: Duke University Press, 1997.

Bermudez, Jose Luis, Anthony Marcel, and Naomi Eilan, eds. *The Body and the Self*. Cambridge: Massachusetts Institute of Technology Press, 1998.

Berrian, Jacqueline. "Pregnancy and Drug Use: The Dangerous and Unequal Use of Punitive Measures." *Yale Law and Feminism* 2 (1990): 239–250.

Berrill, Norman J. *The Person in the Womb*. New York: Dodd, Mead, 1958.

Bertin, Joan. "Reproductive Hazards in the Workplace." In *Reproductive Laws for the 1990s*, edited by Sherrill Cohen and Nadine Taub. Clifton, N.J.: Human Press; New Brunswick, N.J.: Rutgers University Press, 1989.

Betancourt, L., et al. "Problem-Solving Ability of Inner-City Children with and without In Utero Cocaine Exposure." *Journal of Developmental and Behavioral Pediatrics* 20 (1999): 418–424.

Bhargava, Shalini. "Challenging Punishment and Privatization: A Response to the Conviction of Regina McKnight." *Harvard Civil Rights-Civil Liberties Law Review* 39, no. 2 (Summer 2004): 1–29.

Bibby, Cyril. *How Life Is Handed On*. London: Thomas Nelson and Sons, 1946.

Bingham, Eula, ed. "Proceedings: Conference on Women and the Workplace, June 17–19, 1976," Washington, D.C., Society for Occupational and Environmental Health, 1977.

"Birth Defects May Relate to Agent Orange Herbicide." *Wall Street Journal*, March 15, 1996, 15.

Blanchard, Dallas. *The Anti-Abortion Movement and the Rise of the Religious Right: From Polite to Fiery Protest*. New York: Twayne, 1994.

Blank, Robert H. *Fetal Protection in the Workplace: Women's Rights, Business Interests, and the Unborn*. New York: Columbia University Press, 1993.

———. *Mother and Fetus: Changing Notions of Maternal Responsibility*. New York: Greenwood Press, 1992.

Blee, Kathleen, ed. *No Middle Ground: Women and Radical Protest*. New York, NY: NYU Press, 1997.

Bluestone, Barry and Bennett, Hanson. *The Deindustrialization of America: Plant Closings, Community Abandonment, and the Dismantling of Basic Industry*. New York: Basic Books, 1980.

Blumberg, Lisa. "The Politics of Prenatal Testing and Selective Abortion." In "Women with Disabilities: Reproduction and Motherhood," a special issue of *Sexuality and Disability Journal* 12, no. 2 (Summer 1994): 135–153.

Blumner, Robyn E. "Prosecuting the Persecuted: Addicted Mothers-to-Be." *Miami Herald*, April 18, 1991, 1.

"Bobbitt Mutilation and Abortion." January 2004, Physicians for Life website, http://www.physiciansforlife.org/content/view/323/26 (accessed July 14, 2008).

Bolotin, Norman, and Laing, Christine. *The Chicago World's Fair of 1893: The World's Columbian Exposition*. Washington, D.C.: Preservation Press, 1992.

Bolter, Sidney. "The Psychiatrist's Role in Therapeutic Abortion: The Unwitting Accomplice." *American Journal of Psychiatry* 119 (September 1962): 315.

Bondeson, William B, ed. *Abortion and the Status of the Fetus*. Dordrecht, Holland: D. Reidel, 1983.

Bordo, Susan. "Are Mothers Persons? Reproductive Rights and the Politics of Subjectivity." In *Unbearable Weight: Feminism, Western Culture, and the Body*. Berkeley, Calif.: University of California Press, 1993.

Borstelmann, Thomas. *The Cold War and the Color Line: American Race Relations in the Global Arena*. Cambridge: Harvard University Press, 2001.

Boston Women's Health Collective. *Our Bodies, Ourselves*. New York: Simon and Schuster, 1976.

Bowes, Watson A., and Brad Selgestad. "Fetal versus Maternal Rights: Medical and Legal Perspectives." *Obstetrics & Gynecology* 58, no. 2 (August 1982): 209–214.

Boyer, Paul. *By the Bomb's Early Light: American Thought and Culture at the Dawn of the Atomic Age*. Chapel Hill: University of North Carolina Press, 1984.

———. *Urban Masses and Moral Order in America, 1820–1920*. Cambridge: Harvard University Press, 1978.

Bragg, Rick. "Defender of God, South, and Unborn: Prosecutor Fighting Pregnant Addicts All the Way to High Court." *New York Times*, January 13, 1998, A10.

Braude, Ann. *Radical Spirits: Spiritualism and Women's Rights in Nineteenth-Century America*, 2nd ed. Bloomington: Indiana University Press, 2001.

Braude, Peter R., and Martin H. Johnson. "The Embryo in Contemporary Science." In *The Human Embryo: Aristotle and the Arabic and European Tradition*, edited by G. R. Dunston. Exeter: University of Exeter Press, 1990.

Breines, Winifred. *The Trouble between Us: An Uneasy History of White and Black Women in the Feminist Movement*. New York: Oxford University Press, 2006.

Brewer, Sarah. *Super Baby: Boost Your Baby's Potential from Conception to Year One*. Thorson's, 1998.

Brind, Joel. "Induced Abortion as an Independent Risk Factor for Breast Cancer: A Comprehensive Review and Meta-Analysis." *Journal of American Physicians and Surgeons* 10, no. 4 (Winter 2009): 209.

Brinkley, Alan. *Liberalism and Its Discontents*. Cambridge, MA: Harvard University Press, 2000.

Brodie, Janet Farrell. *Contraception and Abortion in Nineteenth-Century America*. Ithaca, N.Y.: Cornell University Press, 1994.

Brown, Donald D. "The Department of Embryology of the Carnegie Institution of Washington." *BioEssays* (1997): 92–96.

Brown, Michael H. *Laying Waste: The Poisoning of America by Toxic Chemicals*. New York: Pantheon, 1979.

Brownlee, W. Elliot, and Hugh Davis Graham, eds. *The Reagan Presidency: Pragmatic Conservatism and Its Legacies*. Lawrence: University of Kansas Press, 2003.

Bruce, Robert V. *The Launching of Modern American Science, 1846–1876*. NY: Knopf, 1987.

Brundrett, Rick. "Woman Challenges Court's Views of Fetus." *State*, June 21, 2001, A3.

Bruzelius, Nils J. "Abortion: Problem for the Courts in Boston." *Boston Globe*, January 19, 1975, 1.

———. "BCH to Resume Abortion When Way Is Clear." *Boston Globe*, May 15, 1974, 4.

———. "Edelin: A Dedicated Doctor." *Boston Globe*, February 16, 1975, 2.

———. "Hub Medical Community Is Dismayed." *Boston Globe*, February 16, 1975, 1.

———. "Research on Humans an Issue." *Boston Globe* February 23, 1975, 9.

Buchanan, Patrick J. *The Death of the West: How Dying Populations and Immigrant Invasions Imperil Our Country and Civilization*. New York: St. Martin's Press, 2002.

Buck, Pearl S. *Johnny Jack and His Beginnings*. New York: John Day, 1954.

Buckley, William. "Edelin Abortion Verdict." *National Review* 27, no. 9 (March 14, 1975): 261–262.

Bullard, Robert D., ed. *Unequal Protection: Environmental Justice & Communities of Color*. San Francisco: Sierra Club Books, 1994.

Burke, Theresa Karminski. *Rachel's Vineyard: A Psychological and Spiritual Journey of Post-Abortion Healing*. New York: Alba House, 1995.

Burnham, Daniel H. *The Final Official Report of the Director of Works of the World's Columbian Exposition, Parts One and Two*. New York: Garland. 1989.

Burtt, Shelley. "Reproductive Responsibilities: Rethinking the Fetal Rights Debate." *Policy Sciences* 27, nos. 2–3 (1994): 179–196.

Butler, Judith. *Bodies That Matter: On the Discursive Limits of "Sex."* New York: Routledge, 1993.

Calderone, Mary S. ed. *Abortion in the United States*. New York: Harper and Brothers, 1958.

Callahan, Joan C., ed. *Reproduction, Ethics, and the Law: Feminist Perspectives*. Bloomington: Indiana University Press, 1995.

Calleo, David. *The Imperious Economy*. Cambridge: Harvard University Press, 1983.

Camp, Scott D. *Worker Response to Plant Closings: Steelworkers in Johnstown and Youngstown*. New York: Garland, 1995.

Campbell, Nancy D. *Using Women: Gender, Drug Policy, and Social Justice*. New York: Routledge, 2000.

Cangemi, Gary. *Umbert the Unborn: A Womb with a View*. Washington, D.C.: Circle Press, 2003.

"Can Predict Sex of Baby." *Science News Letter* (April 14, 1956), 226,

Carey, Eben James. "Health Education at the Exposition." *Hygeia* 11 (June 1934): 490.

———. *Medical Science Exhibits: A Century of Progress, Chicago World's Fair, 1933 and 1934*. Chicago: A Century of Progress, 1936.

Carlisle, Norman, and Madeline Carlisle. "Secrets of Life before Birth." *Coronet* (March 1952), 85–88.

Carlson, Elof Axel. *The Unfit: A History of a Bad Idea*. New York: Cold Spring Harbor Laboratory Press, 20001.

Carnes, Mark. *Meanings for Manhood: Construction of Masculinity in Victorian America*. Chicago: University of Chicago, 1990.

Carrithers, Michael, Steven Collins, and Steven Lukes, eds. *The Category of Person: Anthropology, Philosophy, History*. New York: Cambridge University Press, 1985.

Carroll, Peter N. *It Seemed Like Nothing Happened: America in the 1970s*. New Brunswick, N.J.: Rutgers University Press, 1982.

Carter, Dan T. *The Politics of Rage: George Wallace, the Origins of the New Conservatism, and the Transformation of American Culture*. Baton Rouge: Louisiana State University Press, 2000.

Elizabeth, Cartwright. "The Logic of Heartbeats." In *Cyborgs and Citadels*. Edited by Joseph Dumit and Gary Lee Downey. Santa Fe, NM: School of American Research Press, 1998.

Cartwright, Lisa. *Screening the Body: Tracing Medicine's Visual Culture*. Minneapolis, MN: University of Minnesota Press, 1995.

Casper, Monica J. *The Making of the Unborn Patient: A Social Anatomy of Fetal Surgery*. New Brunswick, NJ: Rutgers University Press, 1998.

Casper, Monica J., and Lynn M. Morgan. "Constructing Fetal Citizens," *Anthropology News*, December 2004, http://www.aaanet.org/press/an/infocus/reprorights/Casper.htm (accessed June 10, 2010).

Cavanaugh, Michael A. "Secularization and the Politics of Traditionalism: The Case of the Right-to-Life Movement." *Sociological Forum* 1, no. 2 (Spring 1986), 251–283.

Chadwick, David. "Protecting the Unborn: The Problems of Expectant Mothers on Drugs," *Los Angeles Times*, October 19, 1986, SD2.

Champness, E. I. "Heredity versus the Power of Thought." *The Westminster Review* (July 1907): 59–63.

"Charges Disputed: MD Group Claims That Fetuses Suffer Pain." *American Medical News* February 24, 1984.

Charo, R. Alta. "Embryo Research: An Argument for Federal Funding." *Journal of Women's Health* 4:6 (1995): 603–604.

Chasnoff, Ira J., et al. "Cocaine Use in Pregnancy." *New England Journal of Medicine* 313 (September 12, 1985): 666–669.

———. "Cocaine/Polydrug Use in Pregnancy: Two-Year Follow-Up." *Pediatrics* 89 (1992): 284–289.

———. "The Prevalence of Illicit Drug or Alcohol Use during Pregnancy and Discrepancies in Mandatory Reporting in Pinellas County, Florida." *New England Journal of Medicine* 332 (1990): 1202–1206.

Chavkin, Wendy. "Closed Office-Building Syndrome." In *Double Exposure*, edited by Wendy Chavkin. New York: Monthly Review Press, 1984.

———, ed. *Double Exposure: Women's Health Hazards on the Job and at Home*. New York: Monthly Review Press, 1984.

———. "Drug Addiction and Pregnancy: Policy Crossroads." *American Journal of Public Health* 80, no. 4 (April 1990): 483–487.

Chein, Isodor, Donald L. Gerard, Robert S. Lee, and Eva Rosenfeld. *The Road to H: Narcotics, Delinquency, and Social Policy*. New York: Basic Books, 1964.

Chernaik, B. I. "Recovery for Prenatal Injuries: The Right of a Child against Its Mother." *Suffolk University Law Review* 10 (1976): 582–609.

Chessik, Robert J. "The Pharmacogenic Orgasm in the Drug Addict." *Archives of General Psychiatry* 3, no. 5 (1960).

"A Child Is to Be Born." *Hygeia* (May–October 1926): 367–369.

Choulant, Loudwig. *History and Bibliography of Anatomic Illustration*. Leipzig: 1852. Translated and edited by Frank Mortimer. Chicago: University of Chicago Press, 1920.

Church, George J. "Is Bill Clinton for Real?" *Time*, January 1992, 14–18.

Church, Louise Randall. "Parents: Architects of Peace." *American Home*, November 1946, 18–19.

Clark, Elizabeth. "The Sacred Rights of the Weak: Pain, Sympathy, and the Culture of Individual Rights in Antebellum America." *Journal of American History* 82, no. 2 (September 1995): 463–493.

Clark, Kristin. "Inquiry Topic: 'The Silent Scream.'" *USA Today*, March 21, 1985, 13A.

Clark, Matt. "Abortion and the Law." *Newsweek*, March 3, 1975, 18.

Clarke, Adele. "The Choice to Refuse or Withhold Medical Treatment: The Emerging Technology and Medical-Ethical Consensus." *Creighton Law Review* 13 (1980): 795.

———. *Disciplining Reproduction: Modernity, American Life, and the Problems of Sex.* Berkeley: University of California Press, 1998.

———. "Money, Sex, and Legitimacy at Chicago, circa 1892–1940: Lillie's Center of Reproductive Biology." *Perspectives on Science* 1, no. 3 (1993): 367–415.

———. "Research Materials and Reproductive Science in the United States, 1910–1940." In *Physiology in the American Context, 1850–1940*, edited by Gerald L. Geitson. Baltimore: Williams & Wilkins, 1987.

Clarke, Robert. *Ellen Swallow: The Woman Who Founded Ecology.* Chicago: Follett, 1973.

Clift, Eleanor, and Evan Thomas. "Battle for Bush's Soul: President Is Trapped Between Religion and Science over Stem Cells." *Newsweek*, July 9, 2001, 28–30.

Clines, Francis X. "Reagan Appeal on Abortion Is Made to Fundamentalists." *New York Times*, January 31, 2004.

Clymer, Swinburne R. *By Means of the Art or Science Known as Stirpiculture, or Prenatal Culture and Influence, in the Development of a More Perfect Race.* Chicago: College of Medicine and Surgery, 1902.

Coady, Regina M. "Extending Child Abuse Protection to the Viable Fetus: *Whitner v. State of South Carolina.*" *St. John's Law Review*, vol. 71 (Summer 1997): 667–668.

Cobb, Matthew. *Generation: The Seventeenth-Century Scientists Who Unraveled the Secrets of Sex, Life, and Growth.* New York: Bloomsbury, 2006.

"Cocaine-Using Fathers Linked to Birth Defects." *New York Times*, October 15, 1991, C5.

Cockefair, Edgar A., and Ada Milam Cockefair. *The Story of You.* Madison, Wis.: Milam, 1955.

Cohen, Alys I. "Challenging Pregnancy Discrimination in Drug Treatment: Does the ADAMHA Reorganization Act Provide an Answer?" *Yale Journal of Law and Feminism* 6 (1994): 91–142.

Cohen, Peter J. *Drugs, Addiction and the Law: Policy, Politics, and Public Health.* Durham, N.C.: Carolina Academic Press, 2004.

Cohen, Sherrill, and Nadine Taub, eds. *New Reproductive Laws for the 1990s.* New Brunswick, N.J.: Rutgers University Press, 1989.

Cohen, Victor. "Live Fetal Research Debated." *Washington Post*, April 10, 1973, A1.

———. "NIH Vows Not to Fund Fetus Work." *Washington Post*, April 13, 1973, A1.

———. "Scientists and Fetal Research." *Washington Post*, April 15, 1973, A1.

Colb, Sherry F. "The *Journal of the American Medical Association* Says Fetuses under 29 Weeks Do Not Feel Pain: The Legal Implications for Mandatory Information

Sessions." Findlaw, September 7, 2005, http://writ.news.findlaw.com/colb/20050907.html.

Cole, Catherine. "Sex and Death on Display: Women, Reproduction, and Fetuses at Chicago's Museum of Science and Industry." *Drama Review* 37, no. 1 (1993): 48.

Coleman, Linda, and Dickinson, Cindy. "The Risk of Healing: The Hazards of the Nursing Profession." In *Double Exposure*, edited by Wendy Chavkin. New York: Monthly Review Press, 1984.

Coleman, Priscilla, et al. "Substance Abuse among Pregnant Women in the Context of Previous Reproductive Loss and Desire for Current Pregnancy." *British Journal of Health Psychology* 10 (2005): 255–268.

Colie, Christine. "Male Mediated Teratogenesis." *Reproductive Toxicology* 7 (1993): 3–9.

Collett, Teresa A. "Fetal Pain Legislation: Is It Viable?" *Pepperdine Law Review*. 30, no. 161 (2003): 161–184.

Collins, Vincent J., Steven R. Zielinski, and Thomas J. Marzen. "Fetal Pain and Abortion: The Medical Evidence," *Studies in Law and Medicine* 18. Chicago: Americans United for Life, 1984.

Commager, Henry Steele. *The American Mind: An Interpretation of American Thought and Character since the 1980s*. New Haven: Yale University Press, 1950.

Conboy, Katie, Nadia Media, and Sarah Stenburg, eds. *Writing on the Body*. New York: Columbia University Press, 1997.

"Conception in a Watch Glass," *New England Journal of Medicine* 217, no. 17 (October 21, 1937): 678.

"Concerns and Goals." Sanctity of Life, sec. 2, *Concerned Women for America*, http://www.cwfa.org/goals-concerns.asp (accessed July 14, 2008).

Condit, Celeste Michelle. *Decoding Abortion Rhetoric: Communicating Social Change*. Urbana: University of Illinois Press, 1990.

Condon, Charles M. "Clinton's Cocaine Babies: Why Won't the Administration Let Us Save Our Children?" *Policy Review* 72 (spring 1995): 12–13.

Conklin, Beth A. and Lynn Morgan. "Babies, Bodies, and the Production of Personhood in North America and a Native Amazonian Society." *Ethos* 24, no. 4 (1996): 657–694.

Cooke, Joseph Brown. *The Baby before and after Arrival: Intimate Talks with Prospective Mothers in Plain Non-Technical Language*. Philadelphia: Lippincott, 1916.

Cooke, Kathy. "Non-Sense and Anti-Sentimentality: Home Economics, Euthenics, and the 'Threat' to Race Betterment Efforts in America." Paper delivered at Cornell University, Department of Human Ecology, September 20, 2001.

Coontz, Stephanie. *The Way We Never Were: American Families and the Nostalgia Trap*. New York: Basic Books, 1992.

Cooper, Cynthia L. "'Fetal Pain' Bill New Item on Anti-Choice Agenda." *Women's eNews*, August 16, 2004, http://www.womensenews.org/article.cfm/dyn/aid/1951 (accessed July 11, 2008).

Corea, Gena. *The Hidden Malpractice*. New York: Harper & Row, 1985.

———. *The Mother Machine: Reproductive Technologies from Artificial Insemination to Artificial Wombs*. London: Women's Press, 1988.

Corn, Jacqueline Karnell. "Alice Hamilton, M.D., and Women's Welfare." *New England Journal of Medicine* 294 (February 5, 1976): 316–318.

"Cornell Education Heads New Yale Child Center." *New York Times*, November 1, 1948, 30.

Corner, George Washington. *Ourselves Unborn: An Embryologists Essay on Man.* New Haven: Yale University Press, 1944.

———. *The Seven Ages of a Medical Scientist: An Autobiography.* Philadelphia: University of Pennsylvania Press, 1981.

Cott, Nancy. *Bonds of Womanhood: Woman's Sphere in New England, 1780–1835.* Cambridge: Cambridge University Press, 1977.

———. *The Grounding of Modern Feminism.* New Haven: Yale University Press, 1986.

Courtwright, David T. *Dark Paradise: A History of Opiate Addiction in America.* Cambridge: Harvard University Press, 2001.

Coutts, Mary Carrington. "Ethical Issues in In Vitro Fertilization." *Scope Note* 10. Kennedy Institute of Ethics, 1988.

———. "Fetal Tissue Research." *Kennedy Institute of Ethics Journal* 31 (March 1993): 81–101.

Cowan, Ruth Schwartz. "Aspects of the History of Prenatal Diagnosis." *Fetal Diagnosis and Therapy* 8, no. 1 (1993): 10–17.

Creed, Barbara. *The Monstrous-Feminine: Film, Feminism, Psychoanalysis.* New York: Routledge, 1993.

Critchlow, Donald T. *Phyllis Schlafly and Grassroots Conservatism: A Woman's Crusade.* Princeton: Princeton University Press, 2005.

Crosby, John F. "The Personhood of the Human Embryo." *The Journal of Medicine and Philosophy* 18, no. 4 (1993): 399–418.

Csordas, Thomas J., ed. *Embodiment and Experience: The Existential Ground of Culture and Self.* Cambridge: Cambridge University Press, 1994.

Culliton, Barbara J. "Edelin Trial: Jury Not Persuaded by Scientists for Defense." *Science* 187 (March 7, 1975): 814–816.

———. "Fetal Research: The Case History of a Massachusetts Law." *Science* 187 (January 24, 1975): 237–238.

———. "Grave-Robbing: The Charge against Four from Boston City," *Science* 186 (November 1, 1974): 420–421.

———. "Sickle Cell Anemia: The Route from Obscurity to Prominence, " *Science* 178 (1972): 138.

Cumming, J.B. "Right-to-Life: Two Crusaders," *Newsweek*, March 3, 1975, 29.

Curran, William J. "The Approach of Two Federal Agencies." In *Experimentation with Human Subjects*, edited by Paul A. Freund. New York: George Braziller, 1969.

———. "The Law and Human Experimentation." *New England Journal of Medicine* 275, no. 6 (August 11, 1966): 323–325.

Cushman, Philip. *Constructing the Self, Constructing America: A Cultural History of Psychotherapy.* Boston: Addison-Wesley, 1995.

Cuskey, Walter R., T. Premkumar, and Lois Sigel. "Survey of Opiate Addiction among Females in the United States between 1850 and 1970." *Public Health Reviews* 1 (1972): 6–39.

Cyert, Richard Michael. *The American Economy.* New York: Free Press, 1983.

Dailard, Cynthia. "Court Strike 'Partial Birth Abortion Ban: Decisions Presage Future Debates." *Guttmacher Report on Public Policy*, October 2004, http://www.guttmacher.org/pubs/tgr/07/4/gr070401.html (accessed June 8, 2010).

Dale, Suzanne. "Born on Crack and Coping with Kindergarten." *New York Times*, February 7, 1991, A1.

Danet, Brenda. "'Baby' or 'Fetus'?: Language and the Construction of Reality in a Manslaughter Trial." *Semiotica* 32 nos. 3–4 (1980): 187–219.

Daniels, Cynthia. *At Women's Expense: State Power and the Politics of Fetal Rights*. Cambridge: Harvard University Press, 1993.

———. "Between Fathers and Fetuses: The Social Construction of Male Reproduction and the Politics of Fetal Harm." *Signs: Journal of Women and Culture in Society* 22, no. 31 (1997): 579–616.

David, Morris E. "The Impact of Workplace Health and Safety on Black Workers: Assessment and Prognosis." *Labor Law Journal* 31 (1980): 723–732.

Davidoff, L., ed. "Motherhood, Race, and the State in the Twentieth Century." Special issue, *Gender and History* 4, no. 2 (1992).

Davidson, Jean. "Drug Babies Push Issue of Fetal Rights." *Los Angeles Times*, April 15, 1989, 11.

Davis, Devra Lee. "Fathers and Fetuses." *New York Times*, March 1, 1991, A27.

———. "Paternal Smoking and Fetal Health." *Lancet* 337 (January 12, 1991): 123.

Davis, Devra Lee, Gladys Friedler, Donald Mattison, and Robert Morrison. "Male-Mediated Teratogenesis and Other Reproductive Effects: Biological and Epidemiologic Findings and Plea for Clinical Research." *Reproductive Toxicology* 6 (1992): 289–292.

Davis, Edward P. *A Treatise on Obstetrics for Students and Practitioners*. Philadelphia: Lea Brothers, 1896.

Davis, Morris E. "The Impact of Workplace Health and Safety on Black Workers: Assessment and Prognosis." *Labor Law Journal* 31 (1980): 723–732.

Dawson, George E. *The Right of the Child to Be Well Born*. New York: Funk & Wagnalls, 1912.

Dayton, Cornelia Hughes. "Taking the Trade: Abortion and Gender Relations in Eighteenth Century New England Village." *William and Mary Quarterly* 3rd series, 48 (1991): 19–49.

Deaux, Kay, and Joseph C. Ullman. *Women of Steel: Female Blue-Collar Workers in the Basic Steel Industry*. New York: Praeger Press, 1983.

DeCamp, James A. *Common Ground—Occasional Papers from Presbyterians Pro-Life*. No. 3 (May 1988).

Degler, Carl N. *At Odds: Women and the Family in America from the Revolution to the Present*. New York: Oxford University Press, 1980.

———. *In Search of Human Nature: The Decline and Revival of Darwinism in American Social Thought*. New York: Oxford University Press, 1991.

DelVecchio, Mary-Jo, et al., eds. *Pain as a Human Experience: An Anthropological Perspective*. Berkeley: University of California Press, 2000.

Dempsey, David. *The Way We Die: An Investigation of Death and Dying in America Today*. New York: Macmillan, 1975.

Denson-Gerber, Judianne, M. Wiender, and R. Hochstedler. "Sexual Behavior, Abortion and Birth Control in Heroin Addicts." *Contemporary Drug Problems* 1, no. 4 (1972): 72.

DeParle, Jason. *American Dream: Three Women, Ten Kids, and a Nation's Drive to End Welfare.* New York: Viking, 2004.

Derbyshire, S. W. G. "Fetal Pain: An Infantile Debate." *Bioethics* 5, no. 1 (2001): 77–84.

———. "Locating the Beginnings of Pain." *Bioethics* 13, no. 1 (1999): 1–31.

Dettwyler, Katherine A. *Dancing Skeletons: Life and Death in West Africa.* Prospect Heights, Ill.: Waveland, 1994.

Dewey, Evelyn. *Behavior Development in Infants: A Survey of the Literature on Prenatal and Postnatal Activity, 1920–1934.* New York: Columbia University Press, 1935.

Diamond, Sara. *Roads to Dominion: Right-Wing Movements and Political Power in the United States.* New York: Guilford Press, 1995.

Dicker, Marvin, and Eldin Leighton. "Trends in Diagnosed Drug Problems among Newborns: United States, 1979–1987." Paper presented at the annual meeting of the American Public Health Association, New York City, November 1990.

Dietrich, John H. "The Melting Pot: A Plea for the Unborn Children of America." Published by St. Mark's Memorial Reformed Church, Pittsburgh, PA: 1910.

Diggins, John Patrick. *The Promise of Pragmatism: Modernism and the Crisis of Knowledge and Authority.* Chicago: University of Chicago Press, 1994.

Dixon-Jones, Mary A. "Criminal Abortion—Its Evils and Its Sad Consequences." *Women's Medical Journal* (August and September 1894): 3.

"Doctor Asks Judge to Void Conviction in Abortion." *New York Times,* February 21, 1975, 28.

Doerr, Ed, and James W. Prescott, eds. *Abortion Rights and Fetal 'Personhood.'* Long Beach, Calif.: Centerline Press, 1990.

"Does the Greater Understanding of Man and Nature Increase the Scientist's Social Responsibility?" *Science,* June 26, 1953, 701–703.

Doniger, Wendy, and Gregory Spinner. "Misconceptions: Female Imaginations and Male Fantasies in Parental Imprintings." *Daedalus* 127 (1998): 97–129.

Donnelly, Sally B. "The Postpartum Prosecutor." *Time,* December 15, 1997, 4.

Doran, Kevin. *What Is a Person: The Concept and the Implications for Ethics.* Lewiston, N.Y.: Edwin Mellen Press, 1989.

Dorland, William A. Newman. *A Manual of Obstetrics.* Philadelphia: W. B. Saunders, 1896.

———. *X-Ray in Embryology and Obstetrics.* Philadelphia: W.B. Saunders, 1926.

Dougherty, Charles. "The Right to Begin Life with a Sound Body and Mind: Fetal Patients and Conflicts with Their Mother." *University of Detroit Law Review* 63 (1985): 89–117.

Drachman, Virginia G. "The Limits of Progress: The Professional Lives of Women Doctors, 1881–1926." *Bulletin of the History of Medicine* 60 (1986): 58–72.

Dreifus, Claudia. *Seizing Our Bodies: The Politics of Women's Health Care.* New York: Vintage, 1978.

Dresser, Horatio Willis. *A History of the New Thought Movement.* New York: T. Y. Crowell Company, 1919.

Drucker, Ernest, "U.S. Drug Policy." *Public Health Reports* 114 (January/February 1999): 23.

Drug Addiction: Crime or Disease? Interim and Final Reports on the Joint Committee of the American Bar Association and the American Medical Association on Narcotic Drugs. Bloomington: Indiana University Press, 1961.

Duden, Barbara. *Disembodying Women: Perspectives on Pregnancy and the Unborn.* Cambridge: Harvard University Press, 1993.

Dudziak, Mary L. *Cold War Civil Rights: Race and the Image of American Democracy.* Princeton: Princeton University Press, 2000.

Dunstan, Gordon R., ed. *The Human Embryo: Aristotle and the Arabic and European Tradition.* Exeter: University of Exeter Press, 1990.

Duster, Troy. *Backdoor to Eugenics.* New York: Routledge, 1990.

Dyer, Frederick N. *Champion of Women and the Unborn: Horatio Robinson Storer, M.D.* Canton, Mass.: Science History, 1999.

Eastman Nicholas Joseph, ed. *Williams Obstetrics.* New York: Appleton-Century-Crofts, 1945.

———. *Williams Obstetrics.* New York: Appleton-Century-Crofts, 1956.

Edelin, Kenneth C. *Broken Justice: A True Story of Race, Sex, and Revenge in a Boston Courtroom.* Martha's Vineyard, Mass.: Pondview Press, 2007.

———. "Review of *The Dilemma of the Fetus,* by Stephen Maynard Moody." *New England Journal of Medicine* 334, no. 9 (February 29, 1996): 610–611.

"Edelin and the Law." *Boston Globe,* February 19, 1975, 1.

"Edelin Returns to Work at City Hospital." *Boston Globe,* February 19, 1975, 1.

"Edelin Supported." *New England Journal of Medicine* 292, no. 13 (March 27, 1975): 705.

"The Edelin Trial." *Washington Post,* February 18, 1975, A14.

Edsall, Thomas Byrne, and Mary D. Edsall. *Chain Reaction: The Impact of Race, Rights, and Taxes on American Politics.* New York: W. W. Norton, 1991.

"The Effect of Alcohol upon the Foetus through the Blood of the Mother." *Maryland Medical Journal* 10 (1883): 15.

Eggen, Jean Macchiaroli. "Toxic Reproduction and Genetic Hazards in the Workplace: Challenging the Myth of Tort and Workers' Compensation Systems." *Fordham Law Review* 60 (1992): 843–864.

Ehrenfest, Hugo. *Fetal, Newborn, and Maternal Mortality: Report of the Subcommittee to the White House Conference on Child Health and Protection.* New York: D. Appleton-Century, 1933.

Ehrenreich, Barbara, and Deirdre English. *For Her Own Good: 150 Years of the Experts' Advice to Women.* New York: Anchor Books, 1978.

Ehrenreich, John. *The Cultural Crisis of Modern Medicine.* New York: Monthly Review Press, 1978.

Eisenstein, Zillah. *The Female Body and the Law.* Berkeley: University of California Press, 1988.

El-Gothamy, Zenab, and May El-Samahy. "Ultrastructure Sperm Defects in Addicts." *Fertility and Sterility* 57, no. 3 (1992): 699–702.

Elkins, James. *The Object Stares Back: On the Nature of Seeing.* New York: Harvest Books, 1997.

————. *Pictures of the Body: Pain and Metamorphosis*. California: Stanford University Press, 1999.

Ellenbogen, Kirsten M., and Foutz, Susan G. "Prenatal Development Exhibition: Front-End Evaluation." Report prepared by the Institute for Learning Innovation, for the Museum of Science and Industry, June 2004.

"Embryo's Face." *Life*, March 30, 1950, 115.

Enders, John F., Thomas H. Weller, and Frederick C. Robbins. "Cultivation of the Lansing Strain of Poliomyelitis Virus in Cultures of Various Human Embryonic Tissues." *Science* 109 (1949): 85–86.

"Era of Big Citizen Is Dawning." *Philadelphia Daily News*, January 28, 1997, 1.

"ERA: Yes; Abortion: No." *Boston Phoenix*, April 15, 1975, 1.

Erickson, Robert A. "'The Books of Generation': Some Observations on the Style of British Midwife Books, 1671–1764." In *Sexuality in Eighteenth-Century Britain*, edited by Paul-Gabriel Bouce. Manchester: University of Manchester Press, 1982.

Evanoff, Ruthann. "Reproductive Rights and Occupational Health." *New Women's Times*, August 16, 1979.

Evans, Roscoe C. *My Future Child and Yours: An Intelligent Program of Improving Life at Its Source, Before Conception and in the Womb, Written in a Simple Style to Be Understood by All*. N.p., 1931.

"Expectant Mothers' Emotions May Have Bearing on Child." *Science Digest*, September 1953, 30.

"Expert Worrying," *Time*, May 31, 1948, 54.

Faden, Ruth R., et al. "Prenatal Screening and Pregnant Women's Attitude toward the Abortion of Defective Fetuses." *American Journal of Public Health* 77 (1987): 288.

Faegre, Marion L. *Your Own Story*. Minneapolis: Minnesota Department of Health, 1943.

Faigman, David C. *Laboratory of Justice: The Supreme Court's 200-Year Struggle to Integrate Science and the Law*. New York: Holt, 2005.

Falkner, Frank. "Biomedical Research at Crossroads," letter to the editor. *New York Times*, March 2, 1975, 184.

Faludi, Susan. *Backlash*. New York: Crown, 1991.

Farquar, Dion. *The Other Machine: Discourse and Reproductive Technologies*. New York: Routledge, 1996.

Farrell, John Aloysius. *Tip O'Neill and the Democratic Century: A Biography*. Boston: Little Brown, 2001.

Fasten, Nathan. "The Myth of Prenatal Influences?" *Today's Health* 28 (October 1950): 27, 43.

"Father's Smoking May Damage Sperm." *Washington Post*, January 25, 1991, A8.

Faux, Marian. *Roe v. Wade: The Untold Story of the Landmark Supreme Court Decision that Made Abortion Legal*. New York: Macmillan, 1988.

"Fears and Babies." *Newsweek*, December 28, 1953, 49.

Feen, Richard. "Abortion and Exposure in Ancient Greece: Assessing the Status of the Fetus and 'Newborn' from Classical Sources." In *Abortion and the State of the Fetus*, edited by William B. Bondeson et. al. New York: Springer-Verlag, LLC, 1983.

Fernandez, Humberto. *Heroin*. Center City, Minn.: Hazelden Information Education, 1998.

"Fetal Position." *Time*, July 30, 1973, 71–72.

"Fetal Rights." *Time*, February 7, 1938, 47.

Fields, Carmen. "Edelin's Wife Blames Bias, Religion for Conviction." *Boston Globe*, February 20, 1975, 46.

Filene, Peter G. *In the Arms of Others: A Cultural History of the Right-to-Die in America*. Chicago: Ivan R. Dee, 1998.

"Film Examines Right to Life of a Mentally Retarded Infant." *New York Times*, October 15, 1971, 31.

Findlay, Palmer. "The Slaughter of the Innocents," *American Journal of Obstetrics and Gynecology* 3 (1922): 35.

Fine, R. A. *The Great Drug Deception*. New York: Stein and Day, 1972.

Fineman, Martha, and Isabel Karpin, eds. *Mothers in Law: Feminist Theory and the Legal Regulation of Motherhood*. New York: Columbia University Press, 1995.

"First Breath of Life." *Newsweek*, August 19, 1946, 56.

Fisher, Sue. *In The Patient's Best Interest: Women and Politics of Medical Decisions*. New Brunswick, N.J.: Rutgers University Press, 1986.

Flanagan, Geraldine Lux. *The First Nine Months of Life: The Baby's Development from Conception through Birth*. New York: Simon & Schuster, 1962.

Fleishman, Jane. "The Health Hazards of Office Work." In *Double Exposure*, edited by Wendy Chavkin. New York: Monthly Review Press, 1984.

Fleishman, Ned A. "Torts: Rights of a Viable Infant to Maintain an Action for Negligent Prenatal Injuries." *University of Illinois Law Forum* (Fall 1949): 541.

Fodor, Nandor. *The Search for the Beloved*. New York: W. W. Norton, 1949.

Foley, Jack. "Stillbirth Is Called Murder: Mother Admitted She Used Cocaine." *San Jose Mercury News*, February 7, 1992, 1.

Foner, Eric. *The Story of American Freedom*. New York: W. W. Norton, 1999.

Formisano, Ronald. *Boston against Busing: Race, Class, and Ethnicity in the 1960s and 1970s*. Chapel Hill: University of North Carolina Press, 1991.

Ford, Norman. *When Did I Begin? Conception of the Human Individual in History, Philosophy and Science*. Cambridge: Cambridge University Press, 1986.

Forsythe, Clarke D. "Our Philosophy: The Cultural Yearning for Human Dignity." *Americans United for Life*, http://www.aul.org/Philosophy (accessed July 14, 2008).

Foster, Lawrence. *Women, Family, and Utopia: Communal Experiments of the Shakers, the Oneida Community, and the Mormons*. Syracuse, N.Y.: 1991.

Fowler, Orson Squier. *Sexual Science: Including Manhood, Womanhood, and Their Sexual Interrelations*. Philadelphia: National, 1870.

Fox, Richard Wightman, and James T. Kloppenberg, eds. *A Companion to American Thought*. New York: Blackwell, 1995.

Frank, Deborah, et al. "Growth, Development and Behavior in Early Childhood following Prenatal Cocaine Exposure: A Systematic Review." *Journal of American Medical Association* 285 (2001): 1613–1625.

Frank, Pat. *Mr. Adam*. New York: J. B. Lippincott, 1946.

Frankfort, Ellen. *Vaginal Politics*. New York: Quadrangle Press, 1972.

Franklin, Sarah. "Fetal Fascinations: New Dimensions to the Medical-Scientific Construction of Fetal Personhood." In *Off Centre: Feminism and Cultural Studies*, edited by Sarah Franklin, Celia Lury, and Jackie Stacey. London: Harper Collins, 1991.

Franklin, Sarah, Celia Lury, and Jackie, Stacey, eds. *Off Centre: Feminism and Cultural Studies*. London: Harper Collins, 1991.

Franklin, Sarah, and Helena Ragone, eds. *Reproducing Reproduction: Kinship, Power and Technological Innovation*. Philadelphia: University of Pennsylvania Press, 1998.

Fraser, Nancy. *Unruly Practices: Power, Discourse, and Gender in Contemporary Social Theory*. Minneapolis: University of Minnesota Press, 1989.

Fraser, Steve, and Gary Gerstle, eds. *The Rise and Fall of the New Deal Order, 1930–1980*. Princeton: Princeton University Press, 1989.

Freudenberg, Nicholas. *Not in Our Backyards! Community Action for Health and the Environment*. New York: Monthly Review Press, 1984.

Fried, Marlene Gerber. "Abortion in the United States—Legal but Inaccessible." In *Abortion Wars: A Half Century of Struggle, 1950–2000*, edited by Rickie Solinger. Berkeley: University of California Press, 1998.

Fried, Marlene Gerber, ed. *From Abortion to Reproductive Freedom: Transforming a Movement*. Boston: South End Press, 1990.

Friedler, Gladys. "Development Toxicology: Male-Mediated Effects." In *Occupational and Environmental Reproductive Hazards*, edited by Maureen Paul. Baltimore: Williams & Wilkins, 1993.

Friedman, Daniel J. *White Militancy in Boston*. Massachusetts: Lexington, Mass.: Lexington Books, 1973.

Frosch-Morello, Rachel. "The Politics of Reproductive Hazards in the Workplace: Class, Gender, and the History of Occupational Lead Exposure." *International Journal of Health Services* 27, no. 3 (1997): 501–521.

"Frozen Sperm Pregnancies." *Science News Letter*, November 7, 1953, 292.

Gallagher, Janet. "The Fetus and the Law: Whose Life Is It Anyway?" *Ms*, September 1984.

———. "Fetus as Patient." In *Reproductive Laws for the 1990s*, edited by Sherrill Cohen and Nadine Taub. New Brunswick, N.J.: Rutgers University Press, 1989.

———. "Prenatal Invasions and Interventions: What's Wrong with Fetal Rights?" *Harvard Women's Law Journal* 10 (Spring 1987): 9–58.

Galland, W. H. *Maternity and Child Care*. Chicago: Frederick J. Drake, 1920.

Galton, Francis Sir. *Eugenics: Its Definition, Scope, and Aims*. London: Macmillan, 1905.

Gardner, Carole Brooks. "The Social Construction of Pregnancy and Fetal Development: Notes on a Nineteenth Century Rhetoric of Endangerment." In *Constructing the Social*, edited by Theodore R. Sarbin and John I. Kitsuse. London: Sage, 1994.

Garrow, David J. *Liberty and Sexuality: The Right to Privacy and the Making of Roe v. Wade*. New York: Macmillan, 1994.

Georges, Eugenia and Lisa Mitchell. "Baby's First Picture: The Cyborg Fetus of Ultrasound Imaging." In *Cyborg Babies: From Techno-Sex to Techno-Tots*, edited by Robbie Davis-Floyd and Joseph Dumit. NY: Routledge, 1998.

"German Measles Menace." *Time*, March 5, 1945, 57.

Gesell, Arnold. *The Embryology of Behavior: The Beginnings of the Human Mind*. New York: Harper & Brothers, 1945.

Giannakoulopoulus, W., et al. "Fetal Plasma Cortisol and (beta)-Endorphin Response to Interuterine Needling." *Lancet* 344 (1994): 77–81.

Gibbs, Lois Marie, as told to Murray Levine. *Love Canal: My Story*. Albany: State University of New York, 1982.

Gibbs, Nancy. "Cloning: Where Do You Draw the Line?" *Time*, August 7, 2001, http://www.time.com/time/magazine/article/0,9171,1101010813-170041,00.html (accessed June 8, 2010).

Gilbert, James. *Redeeming Culture: American Religion in an Age of Science*. Chicago: University of Chicago Press, 1997.

Gilbert, Kathleen. "North Dakota Personhood Bill Defeated in Senate, Informed Consent and Ultrasound Bills Pass." *LifeSiteNews.com*, April 6, 2009, http://www.lifesitenews.com/ldn/2009/apr/09040602.html.

Gilbert, Margaret Shea. *Biography of the Unborn: The First IX Months*. Baltimore: Williams & Wilkins, 1938.

Gilbert, Scott F., ed. *A Conceptual History of Modern Embryology*. New York: Plenum Press, 1991.

Gilbert Scott F., Anna L. Tyler, and Emily J. Zackin, eds. *Bioethics and the New Embryology: Springboards for Debate*. Sunderland, Mass.: Sinauer Associates, 2005.

Gillham, Nicholas Wright. *A Life of Sir Francis Galton: From African Exploration to the Birth of Eugenics*. New York: Oxford University Press, 2001.

Gillis, Justin, and Rick Weiss. "Stem Cell Research Not Yet Booming." *Washington Post*, August 6, 2002, A1.

Ginsburg, Faye D. *Contested Lives: The Abortion Debate in an American Community*. Berkeley: California University Press, 1989.

———. "Rescuing the Nation: Operation Rescue and the Rise of Anti-Abortion Militance." In *Abortion Wars: A Half Century of Struggle, 1950–2000*, edited by Rickie Solinger. Berkeley: University of California Press, 1998.

Ginsburg, Faye, and Rayna Rapp, eds. *Conceiving the New World Order*. Berkeley: University of California Press, 1995.

Glenn, Evelyn Nakano, Grace Chang, and Linda Rennie Forcey, eds. *Mothering: Ideology, Experience, Agency*. New York: Routledge, 1994.

Glover, Katherine. "Making America Safe for Mothers." *Good Housekeeping*, May 1926, 98.

Glover, V., and N. Fisk. "Do Fetuses Feel Pain? We Don't Know; Better to err on the safe side from mid-gestation." *British Medical Journal*, September 28, 1996, vol. 313, no. 7060: 796.

Gold, Rachel B., and Dorothy Lehrman. "Fetal Research under Fire: The Influence of Abortion Politics." *Family Planning Perspectives* 21, no. 1 (January/February 1989): 7.

Goldberg, Barry. "Obstetric US Imaging: The Past 40 Years." *Radiology* 215 (June 2000): 622–629.

Goldstein, Leslie Friedman. *The Constitutional Rights of Women: Cases in Law and Social Change*. 2nd ed. New York: Longman, 1988.

Goldstein, Nathaniel L. *Narcotics: A Growing Problem, a Public Challenge, a Plan for Action, Report to the Legislature Pursuant to Chapter 528 of the Laws of 1951, 175th Session*. Albany, N.Y.: Legislature of the State of New York, 1952.

Gomez, Laura. *Misconceiving Mothers: Legislators, Prosecutors, ad the Politics of Prenatal Drug Exposure*. Philadelphia: Temple University Press, 1997.

Gonen, Julianna. "Women's Rights vs. Fetal Rights: Politics, Law and Reproductive Hazards in the Workplace." *Women and Politics* 13 (1993): 175–190.

Good, Mary-Jo Delvecchio, et al. *Pain as Human Experience: An Anthropological Perspective*. Berkeley: University of California Press, 1992.

"Good-Bye: One Woman Drug War Victim Dies, Another Is About To.' *Drug War Chronicle*, June 15, 2007.

Goodman, William. "Women and Jobs in Recoveries, 1970–93." *Monthly Labor Review*, July 1994, 28.

Gordon, Alex. "The Partial-Birth Abortion Ban Act of 2003." *Harvard Journal on Legislation*. 41, no. 2 (Summer 2004): 501–512.

Gordon, Linda. *Pitied but Not Entitled: Single Mothers and the History of Welfare, 1890–1935*. New York: Free Press, 1994.

———. *Woman's Body, Woman's Right: A Social History of Birth Control in America*. New York: Penguin, 1990.

Gorney, Cynthia. "Gambling with Abortion: Why Both Sides Think They Have Everything to Lose." *Harpers Magazine*, November 2004, 33–46.

———. "Whose Body Is It, Anyway? The Legal Maelstrom That Rages When the Rights of Mother and Fetus Collide." *Washington Post*, December 13, 1988.

Gosden, Roger. *Designing Babies: The Brave New World of Reproductive Technology*. New York: W. H. Freeman, 1999.

Gossett, Thomas F. *Race: The History of an Idea in America*. Dallas: Southern Methodist University Press, 1963.

Gould, Stephen Jay. *The Mismeasure of Man*. New York: W. W. Norton, 1985.

———. *Ontogeny and Phylogeny*. Cambridge: Harvard University Press, 1991.

Grady, Denise. "Study Authors Didn't Report Abortion Ties." *New York Times*, August 26, 2005, A15.

———. "Study Finds Six-Week Fetuses Feel No Pain and Need No Abortion Anesthesia." *New York Times*, August 24, 2005, A10.

Grant, Madison. *The Passing of the Great Race, or the Racial Basis of European History*. New York: Scribners and Sons, 1916.

Greeley, H. T., et al. "The Ethical Use of Human Fetal Tissue in Medicine." *New England Journal of Medicine* 320 (1989): 1093–1096.

Green, Valerie. *Doped Up, Knocked Up, and...Locked Up? The Criminal Prosecution of Women Who Use Drugs During Pregnancy*. New York: Garland, 1993.

Greenberg, Cheryl. "Twentieth-Century Liberalisms: Transformations of an Ideology." In *Perspectives on Modern America: Making Sense of the Twentieth Century*, edited by Harvard Sitkoff. New York: Oxford University Press, 2001, 55–79.

Greenberg, Julie. "Reconceptualizing Preconception Torts." 2006 Research Paper Series, Thomas Jefferson School of Law. Available at http://ssrn.com/abstract_id+897585.

Greenhouse, Linda. "The Bork Hearings: Bork Sets Forth Spirited Defense of His Integrity." *New York Times*, September 19, 1987, 1.

———. "Justices Allow Broad Leeway in Policy Chases." *New York Times*, May 27, 1998, A18.

Greg, Patricia. "The Carnegie Human Embryo Collection: A Brief History." Washington, D.C.: National Museum of Health and Medicine, Human Developmental Anatomy Center. Available at http://www.natmedmuse.afip.org/collections/hdac.index.html.

Grey, Mike. *Drug Crazy*. New York: Random House, 1998.

Griffith, S. "Fetal Death, Fetal Pain, and the Moral Standing of a Fetus." *Public Affairs Quarterly* 9, no. 2 (1995): 115–126.

Grossinger, Richard. *Embryogenesis: Species, Gender, and Identity*. Berkeley: North Atlantic Books, 2000.

Grosz, Elizabeth. *Volatile Bodies: Toward a Corporeal Feminism*. Bloomington: Indiana University Press, 1994.

Gruenberg, Sidonie Matsner. *The Wonderful Story of How You Were Born*. New York: Doubleday, 1952.

Guinn, Melani Gail. "Figuring the Fetus: A Rhetorical Analysis of American Antiabortion Discourse in the Nineteenth and Twentieth Centuries." PhD diss., University of California Press, 1996.

Gustafson, James. "Mongolism, Parental Desires, and the Right to Life." *Perspectives in Biology and Medicine* 16 (1972–1973): 529–537.

Guttmacher, Alan Frank. *In this Universe: The Story of Human Birth*. New York: Viking Press, 1937.

———. *Life in the Making*. New York: Viking Press, 1933.

Guttmacher Institute. "State Policies in Brief: An Overview of Abortion Laws," October 2009. Available at http://www.guttmacher.org/sections/abortion/php.

Guyer, M. F. *Being Well-Born: An Introduction to Eugenics*. Indianapolis: Bobbs-Merrill, 1916.

Haag, Pamela. *Consent: Sexual Rights and the Transformation of American Liberalism*. Ithaca, N.Y.: Cornell University Press, 1990.

Haarsager, Sandra L. *Bertha Knight Landes of Seattle: Big City Mayor and Organized Womanhood: Cultural Politics in the Pacific Northwest, 1840–1920*. Norman: University of Oklahoma Press, 1994.

Hague, W. Grant. *The Eugenic Marriage: A Personal Guide to the New Science of Better Living and Better Babies in Four Volumes*. New York: Review of Books, 1914.

Haller, Mark. *Eugenics: Hereditarian Attitudes in American Thought*. New Brunswick, N.J.: Rutgers University Press, 1963.

Hamilton, Alice. "Protection for Working Women." *International Suffrage News*, May 1924.

Hanna, Kathi E., ed. *Biomedical Politics*. Washington D.C.: National Academy Press, 1991.

Hanson, J. W. *The World's Congress of Religions: The Addresses and Papers Delivered before the Parliament, and Abstract of the Congresses Held in the Art Institute*. Chicago: World's Columbian Exposition, 1893.

Haraway, Donna. *Modest_Witness@Second_Millennium.Femaleman©_Meets_Oncomouse™: Feminism and Technoscience.*. New York: Routledge, 1997.

———. *Simians, Cyborgs, and Women: The Reinvention of Nature.* London: Free Association Books, 1996.

Hardacre, Helen. *Marketing the Menacing Fetus in Japan.* Berkeley: University of California Press, 1999.

Harding, Sandra. *The Science Question in Feminism.* London: Taylor & Francis Group, 1986.

———. *Whose Science? Whose Knowledge? Thinking From Women's Lives.* Ithaca, NY: Cornell University Press, 1991.

Harman, Moses. *The Right to Be Born Well: Most Important of All Human Rights.* Chicago: M. Harmon, 1905.

Harrell, Deborah Carlton. "The Fetus and Workplace Safety: A Court Battleground Opens Up." *Seattle Post-Intelligencer.* (October 27, 1990), A1.

Harris, George W. "Fathers and Fetuses." *Ethics* 96 (3): 594–603.

Harrison, Michael. "Unborn: Historical Perspectives of the Fetus as a Patient." *Pharos of Alpha Omega Alpha Honor Medical Society* 45, no. 1 (1982).

Harrison, Michael, Mitchell S. Golbus, and Roy A. Filly, eds. *The Unborn Patient: Prenatal Diagnosis and Treatment.* Philadelphia: Saunders, 1991.

Hartouni, Valerie. *Cultural Conceptions: On Reproductive Technologies + Remaking of Life.* Minneapolis: University of Minnesota Press, 1997.

———. "Fetal Exposures: Abortion Politics and the Optics of Allusion." *Camera Obscura* 29 (1993): 131–149.

Hartz, Louis. *The Liberal Tradition in America.* New York: Harcourt Brace, 1955.

Harvey, Joseph. "Edelin's Prosecutor's Aide Loses Hospital-Counsel Job." *Boston Globe,* February 26, 1975, 6.

Hasian, Marouf Arif. *The Rhetoric of Eugenic in Anglo-American Thought.* Athens: University of Georgia Press, 1996.

Haskell, Martin. "Dilation and Extraction for Late Second Trimester Abortion." Paper presented at the National Abortion Federation Risk Management Seminar, September 13, 1992.

Hatch, Maureen. "Mother, Father, Worker: Men and Women and the Reproduction Risks of Work." In *Double Exposure,* edited by Wendy Chavkin. New York: Monthly Review Press, 1984.

Hayes, Samuel P. *The Response to Industrialization, 1885–1914.* Chicago: University of Chicago Press, 1957.

Hayes, Sharon. *Flat Broke with Children: Women in the Age of Welfare Reform.* New York: Oxford University Press, 2004.

Hellegers, Andre E. "Fetal Research." In *Encyclopedia of Bioethics,* vol. 2, edited by Warren T. Reich. New York: Free Press, 1978.

Henifen, Mary Sue. "The Particular Problems of Video Display Terminals." In *Double Exposure,* edited by Wendy Chavkin. New York: Monthly Review Press, 1984.

Henriksen, Margot A. *Dr. Strangelove's America: Society and Culture in the Atomic Age.* Berkeley: University of California Press, 1997.

Henshaw, Stanley K., and Lynn S. Wallisch. "The Medicaid Cutoff and Abortion Services for the Poor." *Family Planning Perspectives* 16 (1984): 170, 178–179.

Hepler, Allison. *Women in Labor: Mothers, Medicine, and Occupational Health in the United States*. Columbus: Ohio State University Press, 2000.

Herald, Eve. *Stem Cell Wars: Inside Stories from the Frontlines*. Basingstoke: Palgrave Macmillan, 2007.

Herman, Ellen. *The Romance of American Psychology: Political Culture in the Age of Experts*. Berkeley: University of California Press, 1995.

Hern, Warren M. "Life on the Front Lines." In *Abortion Wars: A Half Century of Struggle, 1950–2000*, edited by Rickie Solinger. Berkeley: University of California Press, 1998.

Hertig, Arthur T. and John Rock. "Some Aspects of Early Human Development." *American Journal Obstetrical Gynecology* 44 (1942): 6–17.

———. "Two Human Ova of the Previllious Stage, Having an Ovulation Age of About Eleven and Twelve Days Respectively." *Carnegie Institution of Washington Publications* 525, *Contributions to Embryology* 29 (1941).

Hertwig, Oscar. *The Biological Problem of today*, trans. P. Chalmers Mitchell. Oceanside, N. J.: Dabor Scientific, 1977.

"HEW's Power to Grant AFDC Benefits to Technically Ineligible Individuals." *University of Pennsylvania Law Review* 124, no. 6 (June 1976): 1359–1384.

Hildebrand, Kit. "How to Tell the Story of Birth." *Parents* 24 (August 1949): 32.

Hillson, Jon. *The Battle of Boston*. New York: Pathfinder Press, 1977.

Hilts, Philip J. "U.S. Urged to End Ban on In Vitro Birth Research." *New York Times*, December 3, 1989, 37.

Hirsch, Charlotte. *The Diary of an Expectant Mother*. Chicago: A. C. McClurg, 1917.

His, Wilhem. *Anatomie Menschlicher Embryonen*. Vogel: Leipzig, 1880–1885.

Historical Statistics of the United States, Millennial Edition Online, http://hsus.cambridge.org/HSUSWeb/toc/tableToc.do?id+Ba340–354.

Hitt, Jack. "Who Will Do Abortions Here?" *New York Times Sunday Magazine*, January 18, 1998. 10–27, 42, 45, 54–55.

Hodes, Devon L. *Renaissance Fictions of Anatomy*. Amherst: University of Massachusetts Press, 1985.

Hodge, Hugh L. *Foeticide, or Criminal Abortion: A Lecture Introductory to the Course of Obstetrics, and Diseases of Women and Children*. Philadelphia: Lindsay & Blakiston, 1839.

———. *Foeticide, or Criminal Abortion*. Philadelphia: Livingston and Blake, 1972.

Hodgson, Jane E. "The Twentieth-Century Gender Battle: Difficulties in Perception." In *Abortion Wars: A Half Century of Struggle, 1950–2000*, edited by Rickie Solinger. Berkeley: University of California Press, 1998.

Hoffman, Anna. *A Young Mother's Tokology: A Twentieth Century Book for Mothers and Nurses*. Chicago: M. A. Donohue, 1906.

Hofstadter, Richard. *Social Darwinism in American Thought*. Boston: Beacon Press, 1944.

Holbo, Christine. "The Home-Making of Americans: Pragmatism and the Construction of the American Way of Life." PhD diss., Yale University, 1999.

Holland, Susanne. *The Human Embryonic Stem Cell Debate: Science, Ethics, and Public Policy*. Cambridge: MIT Press, 2001.

Hollander, Nicole. *The Best (So Far) of Nicole Hollander*. San Francisco: Mother Jones Magazine, 1989.

———. *"Ma, Can I Be a Feminist and Still Like Men?" Lyrics from Life*. New York: St. Martin's Press, 1980.

Hollinger, David A. *In the American Province: Studies in the History and Historiography of Ideas*. Baltimore: Johns Hopkins University Press, 1989.

Hollinger, David A., and Charles Capper, eds. *American Intellectual Tradition: A Sourcebook, 1865 to the Present*. New York: Oxford University Press, 2001.

Holly, Elizabeth, Diana Aston, David Ahn, and Jennifer Kristiansen. "Ewing's Bone Sarcoma, Paternal Occupational Exposure, and Other Factors." *American Journal of Epidemiology* 135 (1992): 122–129.

Holmes, Rudolph. "The Methods of the Professional Abortionist." *Journal of Surgery, Gynecology, and Obstetrics* 10 (1910): 542.

Holsinger, Melissa A. "The Partial-Birth Abortion Ban Act of 2003: The Congressional Reaction to *Stenberg v. Carhart*." *New York University Journal of Legislation and Public Policy* 6 (2003): 603–613.

Hooker, Davenport. *A Preliminary Atlas of Early Human Fetal Activity*. Pittsburgh: Ladd Laboratory of the Department of Anatomy, University of Pittsburgh School of Medicine, 1939.

Hopwood, Nick. *Embryos in Wax: Models from the Ziegler Studio*. Cambridge: University of Cambridge Press, 2002.

———. "'Giving Body' to Embryos: Modelling, Mechanism, and the Microtome in Late Nineteenth Century Anatomy." *Isis* 90 (1999): 462–496.

———. "Pictures of Evolution and Charges of Fraud: Ernst Haeckel's Embryological Illustrations." *Isis* 97 (2006): 260–301.

———. "Producing Development: The Anatomy of Human Embryos and the Norms of Wilhelm His." *Bulletin of the History of Medicine* 74 (2000): 29–79.

Horowitz, Maryanne Cline. "The 'Science' of Embryology before the Discovery of the Ovum." In *Connecting Spheres: European Women in a Globalizing World, 1500 to the Present*, 2nd ed. New York: Oxford University Press, 2000.

Horowitz, Morton J. *The Transformation of American Law, 1870–1960: The Crisis of Legal Orthodoxy*. New York: Oxford University Press, 1992.

Howard, William Lee. "The Child That Is to Be: What Mental Attitudes Can Do to the Unborn Child." *Ladies Home Journal*, October 1912, 32.

Huang, Priscilla. "Which Babies Are Real Americans?" TomPaine.com, February 20, 2007, http://www.tompaine.com/articles/2007/02/20/which_babies_are_real_americans. php (accessed July 14, 2008).

Hubbard, Ruth. *The Politics of Women's Biology*. New Brunswick, N.J.: Rutgers University Press, 1990.

Hubbard, Ruth, and May Sue Henifin. "Genetic Screening of Prospective Parents and Workers: Some Scientific and Social Issues." In *Biomedical Ethics Reviews*, edited by James Humber and Robert Almeder. Clifton, N.J.: Humana Press, 1984.

Hudson, Mike. "With Neglect Charge behind Her, Mother Intent on Staying Clean." *Roanoke Times*, September 17, 1991.

"The Human Embryo." *Life*, July 3, 1950, 79–81.

Humphries, Drew. "Crack Mothers, Drug Wars, and the Politics of Resentment." In *Political Crime in Contemporary Society: A Critical Approach*, edited by Kenneth D. Tunnell. New York: Garland, 1993.

———. *Crack Mothers: Pregnancy, Drugs and the Media*. Columbus: Ohio State University Press, 1999.

———. "Mothers and Children, Drugs and Crack: Reactions to Maternal Drug Dependency." In *The Criminalization of a Woman's Body*, edited by Clarice Feinman. Binghamton, N.Y.: Harrington Park Press, 1992.

Hunt, Caroline L. *The Life of Ellen H. Richards*. Boston: Whitcomb & Hunt, 1912.

Hunt, Vilma. *Occupational Health Problems of Pregnant Women*. Washington, D.C.: U.S. Department of Health, Education, and Welfare, 1975.

Ikemoto, Lisa. "The Code of Pregnancy: At the Intersection of Motherhood, the Practice of Defaulting to Science, and the Interventionist Mindset of Law." *Ohio State Law Journal* 53 (1992): 1205–1306.

———. "Furthering the Inquiry: Race, Class and Culture in the Forced Medical Treatment of Pregnant Women." *Tennessee Law Review* 59 (1992): 487–517.

"Injuries to Infants *en ventre sa mere*." *Central Law Journal* 58 (1904): 143.

"In the Sixth Week of Life." *Time*, October 10, 1949, 83.

"Infants—Prenatal Injuries—Right of Action in Tort." *Tulane Law Review* XIII (1939): 632–634.

"Influence of Scientists." *Science News Letter*, October 2, 1954, 218.

Ingelfinger, F. J. "The Edelin Trial Fiasco." *New England Journal of Medicine* 292, no. 13 (March 27, 1975): 697.

"Injuries to Infants *en ventre sa mere*." *Central Law Review* 58 (1904): 143.

Institute of Medicine, Conference Committee on Fetal Research and Applications, Division of Health Promotion and Disease Prevention. *Fetal Research and Applications: A Conference Summary*. Washington, D.C.: National Academy Press, 1994.

Irwin, Joyce. "Embryology and the Incarnation: A Sixteenth-Century Debate." *Sixteenth Century Journal* 9, no. 3 (1978): 93–104.

Irwin, Susan, and Brigitte Jordan. "Knowledge, Practice, and Power: Court-Ordered Caesarian Sections." *Medical Anthropology Quarterly* 1, no. 3 (1987): 319–334.

"Is Abortion Safe? Physical Complications." Abortion: *Some Medical Facts*, National Right to Life pamphlet, http://www.nrlc.org/abortion/ASMF/asmf13.html (accessed July 14, 2008).

Jackson, E. W. "Infants: Actions: Whether or Not a Cause of Action Exists in Favor of Child for Prenatal Injuries Inflicted upon It." *Chicago-Kent Law Review* 25 (1947): 162–165.

Jaconi, Kristen. "Inez Milholland: A Thanatography of the Suffrage Martyr." Paper written for Professor Barbara Babcock's Women's Legal History Project, Stanford University, April 3, 2000.

Jasanoff, Sheila. *Science at the Bar: Law, Science, and Technology in America*. Cambridge: Harvard University Press, 1995.

Jasen, Patricia. "Breast Cancer and the Politics of Abortion in the United States." *Medical History* 49 (2005): 423–444.

Jasso, Sonio, and Maria Mazorra. "Following the Harvest: The Health Hazards of Migrant and Seasonal Farmworking Women." In *Double Exposure*, edited by Wendy Chavkin. New York: Monthly Review Press, 1984.

Jastrow, Joseph. "The Section of Psychology." In *Official Catalogue of the World's Columbian Exposition*, edited by M. P. Hardy, 50–60. Chicago: W. B. Conkey, 1893.

Jelliffe, Smith Ely, ed. *The Medical News: A Weekly Medical Journal* 86 (January–June 1905).

Jensen, Patricia. "Breast Cancer and the Politics of Abortion in the United States." *Medical History* 49 (2005): 425.

Jetter, Alexis, Annelise Orleck, and Diana Taylor, eds. *The Politics of Motherhood: Activist Voices from Left to Right*. Hanover, N.H.: Dartmouth College Press, 1997.

Joffe, Carole. *Doctors of Conscious: The Struggle to Provide Abortions before and after Roe v. Wade*. Boston: Beacon, 1995.

Joffe, Carole, Patricia Anderson, and Jody Steinauer. "The Crisis in Abortion Provision and Pro-Choice Medical Activism in the 1990s." In *Abortion Wars: A Half Century of Struggle, 1950–2000*, edited by Rickie Solinger. Berkeley: University of California Press, 1998.

Johnsen, Dawn. "The Creation of Fetal Rights: Conflicts with Women's Constitutional Rights to Liberty, Privacy, and Equal Protection." *Yale Law Journal* 95 (1986): 599–635.

———. "Functional Departmentalism and Nonjudicial Interpretation: Who Determines Constitutional Meaning?" *Law and Contemporary Problems* 67 (2004): 105.

Johnson, Cathy Marie, Georgia Duerst-Lahti, and Noelle H. Norton. *Creating Gender: The Sexual Politics of Welfare Policy*. Boulder, Colorado: Lynn Rienner, 2007.

Johnson, Rossiter. *A History of the World's Columbian Exposition Held in Chicago in 1893*, vols. 1–4. New York: D. Appleton, 1897.

Jones, Charisse. "A Casualty of Deficit: Center for Addicts." *New York Times*, January 14, 1996, A27.

Jones, David Albert. *The Soul of the Embryo: An Enquiry into the Status of the Human Embryo in the Christian Tradition*. London: Continuum International, 2005.

Jones, James. *Bad Blood: The Tuskegee Syphilis Experiment*. New York: Free Press, 1981.

Jones, Maggie. "A Miracle, and Yet . . . ." *New York Times Magazine*, July 15, 2001, 38.

Jonsen, Albert R. *The Birth of Bioethics*. New York: Oxford University Press, 1998.

Jonsen, Albert, ed. *Sourcebook in Bioethics: A Documentary History*. Washington, DC: Georgetown University Press, 1998.

Jonsson, Patrik. "South Carolina Tests the Bounds of a Fetus's Rights." *Christian Science Monitor*, June 28, 2001, 1.

Jordan, Robert L. "Constitutional Law: 'Person' Within the Meaning of Section 16, Article I of the Constitution: Unborn Viable Child as Such Person." *University of Cincinnati Law Review* (November 1949): 532–535.

Jordanova, Ludmilla. "Gender, Generation, and Science: William Hunter's Obstetrical Atlas." In *William Hunter and the Eighteenth-Century Medical World*, edited by W. F. Bynum and Roy Porter. Cambridge: University of Cambridge Press, 1985.

Jorow, Ronna, and Richard H. Paul. "Caesarian Section for Fetal Distress without Maternal Consent." *Obstetrics & Gynecology* 63, no. 4 (April 1984): 596–598.

Jos, Philip H., et al. "The Charleston Policy on Cocaine Use during Pregnancy: A Cautionary Tale." *Journal of Medicine & Ethics* 120 (1995): 1–9.

Julkay, Michael. *The Embryo Research Debate: Science and the Politics of Reproduction.* Cambridge: Cambridge University Press, 1997.

Kahn, Robbie. *Bearing Meaning: The Language of Birth.* Urbana-Champaign: University of Illinois Press, 1995.

Kalman, Laura. *The Strange Career of Legal Liberalism.* New Haven, CT: Yale University Press, 1998.

Kandall, Stephen R. *Substance and Shadow: Women and Addiction in the United States.* Cambridge: Harvard University Press, 1996.

Kanner, Leo. *In Defense of Mothers: How to Bring Up Children in Spite of More Zealous Psychologists.* New York: Dodd, Mean, 1944.

Kantor, Arlene F. "Occupations of Fathers of Patients with Wilms' Tumour." *Journal of Epidemiology and Community Health* 33 (1979): 253–256.

Kaplan, Ann E. "Look Who's Talking Indeed: Fetal Images in Recent North American Visual Culture." In *Mothering: Ideology, Experience, Agency,* edited by Evelyn Nakano Glenn, Grace Chang, and Linda Rennie Forcey. New York: Routledge, 1994.

Kaplan, Laura. *The Story of Jane: The Legendary Underground Feminist Abortion Service.* New York: Pantheon, 1995.

Kaplan, Temma. *Crazy for Democracy: Women in Grassroots Movements.* New York: Routledge, 1996.

Karlin, Elizabeth. "'We Called It Kindness': Establishing a Feminist Abortion Practice." In *Abortion Wars: A Half Century of Struggle, 1950–2000,* edited by Rickie Solinger. Berkeley: University of California Press, 1998.

Karp, Laurence E. "Past Perfect: John Humphrey Noyes, Stirpiculture, and the Oneida Community." *American Journal of Medical Genetics* 12, no. 2 (1982): 127–130.

Kazin, Michael. *The Populist Persuasion: An American History.* Ithaca, N.Y.: Cornell University Press, 1998.

Keibel, Franz, and Franklin Mall. *Manual of Human Embryology,* vol. 1. Philadelphia: Lippincott, 1910.

———. *Manual of Human Embryology,* vol. 2. Philadelphia: Lippincott, 1912.

Kelly, James E., "The Ethics of Abortion as a Method of Treatment in Legitimate Practice," *Transactions of the Gynecological Society of Boston* 1 (1889): 25–45.

Kenen, Regina, and Robert Schmidt. "Social Implications of Screening Programs for Carrier Status: Genetic Disease in the 1970s and AIDS in the 1980s." In *Dominant Issues in Medical Sociology,* edited by Howard Schwartz. New York: McGraw Hill, 1987.

Kenney, Sally. *For Whose Protection? Reproductive Hazards and Exclusionary Policies in the United States and Britain.* Ann Arbor: University of Michigan Press, 1992.

———. "Who Is Protected? What's Wrong with Exclusionary Policies." *Women & Politics* 13: 3–4 (1993): 153–173.

Kerber, Linda. "Separate Spheres, Female Worlds, and Women's Place: The Rhetoric of Women's History." *Journal of American History* 75, no. 1 (June 1988): 9–39.

Kern, Louis J. *An Ordered Love: Sex Roles and Sexuality in Victorian Utopias*. Chapel Hill: University of North Carolina Press, 1981.

Kessler-Harris, Alice. *In Pursuit of Equity: Women, Men, and the Quest for Economic Citizenship in 20th-Century America*. New York: Oxford University Press, 2001.

———. *Out to Work: A Work of Wage Earning Women in the United States*. New York: Oxford University Press, 1982.

———. "Protection for Women: Trade Unions and Labor Laws." In *Double Exposure*, edited by Wendy Chavkin. New York: Monthly Review Press, 1984.

Kevles, Bettyann Holtzman. *Naked to the Bone: Medical Imaging in the Twentieth Century*. Reading, Mass.: Addison Wesley, 1997.

Kevles, Daniel. *In the Name of Eugenics: Genetics and the Uses of Human Heredity*. New York: Alfred A. Knopf, 1996.

Kifner, John. "Women Rally for Doctor Convicted in Abortion." *New York Times*, February 18, 1975, 27,

———. "Killing of Fetus Is Charged on L.I." *New York Times*, February 18, 1975, 27.

———. "Convicted Boston Doctor Put on Probation for Year." *New York Times*, February 19, 1975, 73.

King, Nick. "Several Jurors Happy about Light Sentence." *Boston Globe*, February 19, 1975, 1.

King, P. "Should Mom Be Constrained in the Best Interests of the Fetus?" *Nova Law Review* 13, no. 2 (Spring 1989): 393–404.

Kinsey, Alfred. *Sexual Behavior in the Human Female*. Philadelphia: W. B. Saunders, 1953.

Kinsey, Alfred, et al., *Sexual Behavior in the Human Female*. Philadelphia: W. B. Saunders, 1953.

Kirp, David L. "The Pitfalls of Fetal Protection." *Society* 28 (March/April 1991): 71.

Kleiman, Dena. "Debate on Abortion Focuses on Graphic Film." *New York Times*, January 25, 1985, B8.

Kline, Wendy. *Building a Better Race: Gender, Sexuality, & Eugenics from the Turn of the Century to the Baby Boom*. Berkeley: University of California Press, 2001.

Kloppenberg, James. *Uncertain Victory: Social Democracy and Progressivism in European and American Thought, 1870–1920*. New York: Oxford University Press, 1986.

Knox, Richard A. "BCH Trustees Reinstate 3 Indicted Doctors," *Boston Globe*, April 19, 1974, 3.

———. "Citizens' Groups to Push BCH to Resume Abortion Services." *Boston Globe*, May 14, 1974, 3.

Kogan, Herman. *A Continuing Marvel: The Story of the Museum of Science and Industry*. New York: Doubleday, 1973.

Kolata, Gina. *The Baby Doctors: Probing the Limits of Fetal Medicine*. New York: Delacorte Press, 1990.

Kolder, Veronica, Janet Gallagher, and Michael Parsons. "Court-Ordered Obstetrical Interventions." *New England Journal of Medicine* 316 (May 7, 1987): 1192–1196.

Kolenc, Anthony B. "Easing Abortion's Pain: Can Fetal Pain Legislation Survive the New Judicial Scrutiny of Legislative Fact-Finding?" *Texas Review of Law & Politics* 10, no. 1 (Fall 2005): 171.

————. "The Science, Law, and Politics of Fetal Pain Legislation." *Harvard Law Review* 115, no. 7 (May 2002): 2010–2033.

Koren, Gideon, et al. "Bias against the Null Hypothesis: The Reproductive Hazards of Cocaine." *Lancet* 334, no, 8677 (December 16, 1989): 1440–1442.

Krauss, Celine. "Blue-Collar Women and Toxic-Waste Protests: The Process of Politicization." In *Toxic Struggles: The Theory and Practice of Environmental Justice*, edited by Richard Hofrichter. Philadelphia: New Society, 1993.

Kress, D. H. "The Use of Narcotics as Related to the Declining Birth Rate and Race Suicide." *Journal of Inebriety* 15, no. 1 (1911): 62–71.

Kressen, Julie. "American Cyanamid Update: No More Willow Islands." *CCROW Newsletter*, spring 1981, 1.

————. "Who We Are." *CRROW Newsletter*, Spring 1981.

Kübler-Ross, Elisabeth. *On Death and Dying*. New York: Macmillan, 1969.

Kumpfer, Karol. "Treatment Programs for Drug-Abusing Women." *Future of Children* 1, no. 1 (Spring 1991): 50–60.

Kunstadter, Ralph A., Reuben I. Klein, Evelyn C. Lundeen, Winifred Witz, and Mary Morrison. "Narcotic Withdrawal Symptoms in Newborn Infants." *Journal of the American Medical Association* 165 (October 25, 1958): 1008–1010.

Kunzel, Regina. "White Neurosis, Black Pathology: Constructing Out-of-Wedlock Pregnancy in the Wartime and Postwar United States." In *Not June Cleaver: Women and Gender in Postwar America, 1945–1960*, edited by Joanne Meyerowitz. Philadelphia: Temple University Press, 1994.

"Laboratory Conception." *Newsweek*, August 14, 1944, 85.

Lacey, Michael James. *Religion and Twentieth-Century American Intellectual Life*. Cambridge: Cambridge University Press, 1991.

Ladd-Taylor, Molly. *Mother-Work: Women, Child Welfare, and the State, 1890–1930*. Urbana Champaign, IL: University of Illinois Press, 1995.

Ladd-Taylor, Molly, and Lauri Umansky, eds. *"Bad" Mothers: The Politics of Blame in Twentieth-Century American*. New York: New York University Press, 1998.

LaFleur, William R. *Liquid Life: Abortion and Buddhism in Japan*. Princeton: Princeton University Press, 1994.

Lake, Randall A. "The Metaethical Framework of Anti-Abortion Rhetoric." *Signs* 11, no. 3 (Spring 1986): 478–499.

Lamson, Armenouhie Tashjian. *How I Came to Be: The Autobiography of an Unborn Infant*. New York: Macmillan, 1926.

————. *My Birth: The Autobiography of an Unborn Infant*. New York: Macmillan, 1916.

Lancreanjan, I., H. I. Popescu, O. Gavenescu, et al. "Reproductive Ability of Workmen Occupationally Exposed to Lead." *Archives of Environmental Health* 30 (1975): 396–416.

Laqueur, Thomas. *Making Sex: Body and Gender from the Greeks to Freud*. Cambridge: Harvard University Press, 1990.

Larmer, Robert. "Abortion, Personhood and the Potential for Consciousness." *Journal of Applied Philosophy* 12, no. 3 (1995): 241–251.

Larson, Edward J. "Tailored Genes." *Legal Affairs: The Magazine at the Intersection of Law and Life*, November/December 2003, http://www.legalaffairs.org/issues/November-December-2003/review_larson_novdec03.msp (accessed June 8, 2010).

Larsen, William J. *Human Embryology*. New York: Churchill Livingstone, 1993.

Laughlin, Harry H. "Report of the Committee to Study and to Report on the Best Practical Means of Cutting Off the Defective Germ-Plasm in the American Population: The Scope of the Committee's Work." College of Law Faculty Publications, Georgia State University, 2009, http://digitalarchive.gsu.edu/col_facpub/10 (accessed June 8, 2010).

"Law on Abortion Called Too Strict." *New York Times*, June 17, 1960, 38.

Lears, T. J. Jackson. *No Place of Grace: Antimodernism and the Transformation of American Culture, 1880–1920*. New York: Pantheon Books, 1981.

Lederer, Susan E. *Subjected to Science: Human Experimentation in America Before the Second World War*. Baltimore: Johns Hopkins University, 1997.

Lee, Susan J., et al. "Fetal Pain: A Systematic Multidisciplinary Review of Evidence." *Journal of the American Medical Association* 294 (2005): 947–954.

"Legal Protection to Unborn Children." *Harvard Law Review* 15 (1904): 313.

Leinberger, Paul, and Bruce Tucker, ed. *The New Individualists: The Generation after the Organization Man*. New York: Harper-Collins, 1991.

Lerrigo, Marion O., and Helen Southard. *A Story about You*. New York: E. P. Dutton, 1955.

Leslie, Robert L., ed. *The Science of Eugenics and Sex Life, Love, Marriage, Maternity: The Regeneration of the Human Race*. New York: Martin & Murray, 1917.

Levey, Noam M. "The Nation; Antiabortion Measure Falls Short in House; Conservatives Hoped for a Symbolic 'Yes' Vote on Fetal Pain Bill," *Los Angeles Times* December 7, 2006, A23.

Levine, Adeline Gordon. *Love Canal: Science, Politics, and People*. Lexington: D. C. Heath, 1982.

Levy, David. *Maternal Overprotection*. New York: Norton, 1943.

Levy, Frank. *Dollars and Dreams: The Changing American Income Distribution*. New York: Russell Sage Foundation, 1987.

Lewin, Tamar. "Abuse Laws Cover Fetus, a High Court Rules." *New York Times*, October 30, 1997, A22.

———. "Court Acting to Force Care of the Unborn." *New York Times*, November 28, 1988, A1.

Lewotin, Richard C. *Biology as Ideology: The Doctrine of DNA*. New York: Harper Perennial, 1991.

Lieberman, J. R., et al. "The Fetal Right to Live." *Obstetrics and Gynecology* 53 (1979): 515–517.

Liebling, A. J. "Masters of the Midway: Dufour & Rogers." *New Yorker*, August 19, 1939, 25.

———. *The Telephone Booth Indian*. NY: Broadway Books, 2004.

"Life's Beginning." *Science News Letter*, December 16, 1939, 387.

Liley, Margaret, and Beth Day. *Modern Motherhood: Pregnancy, Childbirth, and the Newborn Baby*. New York: Random House, 1966.

Liley, William. "The Fetus as a Personality." *Fetal Therapy* 1 (1986): 8–17.

———. "The Unborn Child." *Health* (1971): 12–13.).

Lindbohhm, Marja-Lusa., et al. "Effects of Paternal Occupational Exposure in Spontaneous Abortions." *American Journal of Public Health* (August 1991): 1029–1033.

Lindenmeyer, Kriste. *A Right to Childhood: The United States Children's Bureau and Child Welfare, 1912–1946.* Urbana: University of Illinois Press, 1997.

Liotta, Mathew A. *The Unborn Child.* N.p., 1931.

Lippincott, Gail. "Something in Motion and Something to Eat Attract the Crowd: Cooking with Science at the 1893 World's Fair." *Journal of Technical Writing and Communication.* 33:2 (2003): 141–164.

Lippmann, Walter. *Drift and Mastery: An Attempt to Diagnose the Current Unrest.* Madison: University of Wisconsin Press, 1914.

Livingston, James. *Pragmatism, Feminism, and Democracy: Rethinking the Politics of American History.* New York: Routledge, 2001.

Locke, N. G. "Mother v. Her Unborn Child: Where Should Texas Draw the Line?" *Houston Law Review* 24 (1987): 549–576.

Long, H. W. *Motherhood: A Practical Guide for the Newly Married, Including Determination of Sex, Intercourse during Pregnancy, and Prenatal Influence.* Boston: Richard G. Badger, 1921.

Longino, Helen. *Science as Social Knowledge.* Princeton: Princeton University Press, 1990.

Loth, Myrna, and H. Close Hesseltine. "Therapeutic Abortion at the Chicago Lying-In Hospital." *American Journal of Obstetrics and Gynecology* 72 (August 1956): 304–311.

Loudris, Manuel D. *Diary of an Unborn Child: An Unborn Baby Speaks to Its Mother.* New York: Gill & Macmillan, 1993.

Ludmerer, Kenneth M. *Genetics and American Society: A Historical Approach.* Baltimore: Johns Hopkins University Press, 1972.

Lukas, J. Anthony. *Common Ground: A Turbulent Decade in the Lives of Three American Families.* New York: Vintage Books, 1986.

Luker, Kristen. *Abortion and the Politics of Motherhood.* Berkeley: University of California Press, 1984, 1998.

Lunbeck, Elizabeth. *The Psychiatric Persuasion: Knowledge, Gender and Power in Modern America.* Princeton: Princeton University Press, 1994.

Lundberg, Ferdinand, and Marynia F. Farnham. *Modern Woman: The Lost Sex.* New York: Harpers & Brothers, 1947.

Lupo, Alan. *Liberty's Chosen Home: The Politics of Violence in Boston.* Boston: Little, Brown, 1977.

MacKinnon, Catherine. "Difference and Dominance." In *Feminism Unmodified: Discourses on Life and Law.* Cambridge: Harvard University Press, 1987.

Macklin, Ruth. "Consent, Coercion, and Conflicts of Rights." *Perspectives in Biology and Medicine* 20, no. 3 (Spring 1977): 360–371.

Maienschein, Jane. *Whose View of Life? Embryos, Cloning, and Stem Cells.* Cambridge: Harvard University Press, 2003.

"Make Electric Recordings of Unborn Baby's Heart." *Science News Letter* 41 (February 7, 1942): 92.

Mall, Franklin. "A Human Embryo, Twenty-Six Days Old." *Journal of Morphology* 5 (1891): 459–480.

———. "A Contribution to the Study of the Pathology of Early Human Embryos." *John Hopkins Hospital Reporter* 1 (1900): 1–68.

———. "A List of Normal Human Embryos Which Have Been Cut into Serial Sections." *Anatomical Record* 4, no. 10 (1910): 355–367.

———. "Methods of Preserving Human Embryos." *American Naturalist* 25 (1891): 1144–1146.

———. "A Plea for an Institute of Human Embryology." *Journal of American Medical Association* 60 (1913): 1599–1601.

———. "Report upon the Collection of Human Embryos at the Johns Hopkins University." *Anatomical Record* 5:7 (1911): 343–357.

"Man Tells Us What We Must Do." *Ladies Home Journal* (February 1946): 25.

Manning, Frank A. *Fetal Medicine: Principles and Practice.* Norwalk: Appleton & Lange, 1995.

Marcus, Seymour. "Torts: Prenatal Injury: Right of Injury in Non-Viable Fetus." *Cornell Law Quarterly* 39 (1954): 542–547.

Marcy, Henry. "Education as a Factor in the Prevention of Criminal Abortion and Illegitimacy." *Journal of the American Medical Association* 47 (1906): 1889.

Margulies, Martin M. "Dying after Edelin." *Columbia Forum* 4, no. 2 (spring 1975): 48–50.

Markowitz, Gerald, and David Rosner. *Deceit and Denial: The Deadly Politics of Industrial Pollution.* Berkeley: University of California Press, 2002.

Marsh, Carole. *Nine Months in My Mommy! Autobiography of an Unborn Baby.* New York: Gallopade, 1994.

Marsh, Margaret, and Wanda Ronner. *The Empty Cradle: Infertility in America from Colonial Times to the Present.* Baltimore: Johns Hopkins University Press, 1990.

———. *The Fertility Doctor: John Rock and the Reproductive Revolution.* Baltimore: Johns Hopkins University Press, 2008.

Martin, Anne. "Everywoman's Chance to Benefit Humanity: An Everlasting Benefit You Can Win in a Week." *Good Housekeeping* 17 (January 1920): 20.

Martin, Emily. "The Egg and the Sperm." *Signs* 16, no. 3 (1991): 485–501.

———. "The Fetus as Intruder: Mother's Bodies and Medical Metaphors," In Robbie Davis-Floyd and Joe Dumit, eds., *Cyborg Babies: From Techno-Sexto Techno-Tots.* New York: Routledge, 1998.

———. *The Woman in the Body: A Cultural Analysis of Reproduction.* Beacon Press, 1987.

Mason, Carol. *Killing for Life: The Apocalyptic Narrative of Pro-Life Politics.* Ithaca, N.Y.: Cornell University Press, 2002.

———. "Minority Unborn." In *Fetal Subjects and Feminist Positions,* edited by Lynn M. Morgan and Meredith W. Michaels. Philadelphia: University of Pennsylvania Press, 1999.

Mathieu, Deborah. *Preventing Prenatal Harm: Should the State Intervene?* Washington, D.C.: Georgetown University Press, 1996.

Maxwell, Carol J. C. *Pro-Life Activists in American: Meaning, Motivation, and Direct Action.* Cambridge: Cambridge University Press, 2002.

May, Elaine Tyler. *Homeward Bound: American Families in the Cold War Era*. New York: Basic Books, 1988.

————. *Barren in the Promised Land: Childless Americans and the Pursuit of Happiness*. Cambridge: Harvard University Press, 1995.

Mayes, Linda C., et al. "The Problem of Prenatal Cocaine Exposure: A Rush to Judgment." *Journal of American Medical Association* 267 (1992): 406–408.

Maynard-Moody, Steven. *The Dilemma of the Fetus: Fetal Research, Medical Progress, and Moral Politics*. New York: St. Martin's Press, 1995.

Mayor's Committee on Drug Addiction. "Report of Study on Drug Addiction among Teenagers." New York: City of New York, December 11, 1950.

McClay, Wilfred M. *The Masterless: Self and Society in Modern America*. Chapel Hill: University of North Carolina Press, 1994.

McGee, Glenn. *The Perfect Baby: Parenthood in the New World of Cloning and Genetics*. New York: Rowman & Littlefield, 2000.

McGirr, Lisa. *Suburban Warriors: The Origins of the New American Right*. Princeton: Princeton University Press, 2002.

McKay, H. T., and A. P. McKay. "Abortion Training in the United States." *Family Planning Perspectives* 27 (1995): 112–115.

McLaren, Anne. "Why Study Early Human Development." *New Scientist* 24 (April 1986): 49–52.

McLaughlin, Loretta. *The Pill, John Rock, and the Church*. New York: Little, Brown, 1982.

McNamara, Eileen. "Factory and Fertility." *Boston Globe* (October 17, 1989), 1.

McNulty, Molly. "Pregnancy Police: The Health Policy and Legal Implications of Punishing Pregnant Women for Harm to Their Fetuses." *New York University Review of Law and Social Change* 26 (1987): 277–303.

Meckel, Richard A. *Save the Babies: American Public Health Reform and the Prevention of Infant Mortality, 1950–1929*. Baltimore: Johns Hopkins University Press, 1990.

Melbye, Mads. "Induced Abortion and the Risk of Breast Cancer." *New England Journal of Medicine* 336 no. 2 (January 9, 1997): 81–85.

Melnick, R. Shep. *Between the Lines: Interpreting Welfare Rights*. Washington, D.C.: Brookings Institute, 1994.

Melzack, Ronald. *The Puzzle of Pain*. New York: Basic Books, 1973.

Menand, Louis. *The Metaphysical Club: A Story of Ideas in America*. New York: Farrar, Strauss, and Giroux, 2001.

Menon, Elizabeth K. "Anatomy of a Motif: The Fetus in Late 19th-Century Graphic Art," *Nineteenth Century Art Worldwide: A Journal of 19th-Century Visual Culture* 3, no. 1 (2004), http://19thc-artworldwide.org/index.php/spring04/283-anatomy-of-a-motif-the-fetus-in-late-19th-century-graphic-art (accessed June 8, 2010).

Merewood, Anne. "Studies Reveal Men's Role in Producing Healthy Babies." *Chicago Tribune*, January 12, 1991, 8.

Merrick, Janna. "Caring for the Fetus to Protect the Born Child? Ethical and Legal Dilemmas in Coerced Obstetrical Intervention." *Women & Politics* 13 nos. 3–4 (1993): 63–81.

Metler, Suzanne. *Divided Citizens: Gender and Federalism in New Deal Public Policy*. Ithaca, N.Y.: Cornell University Press, 1998.

Meyer, Arthur. *The Rise of Embryology*. London: Oxford University Press, 1939.

Meyerowitz, Joanne, ed. *Not June Cleaver: Women and Gender in Postwar America, 1945–1960*. Philadelphia: Temple University Press, 1994.

Meyr, Berl Ben. *Your Own True Story*. Idaho: Caxton, 1940.

Miller, Donald M. "The White City." *American Heritage* 44 (July/August 1993): 84.

Mink, Gwendolyn. *Whose Welfare*. Ithaca, N.Y.: Cornell University Press, 1999.

Minkoff, Howard, and Lynn M. Paltrow. "The Rights of 'Unborn Children' and the Value of Pregnant Women." *Hastings Center Report* 36, no. 2 (March 1, 2006): 26–28.

Minow, Martha. *Making All the Difference: Inclusion, Exclusion, and American Law*. Ithaca, N.Y.: Cornell University Press, 1990.

Mitchell, Mary. "Infanticide: Its Moral and Legal Aspects." MD thesis, Women's Medical College of Pennsylvania, 1884.

Mitchell, William J. *The Reconfigured Eye: Visual Truth in the Post-Photographic Era*. Cambridge: Massachusetts Institute of Technology, 1992.

Mitford, Jessica. *The American Way of Death*. New York: Simon and Schuster, 1963.

Mohr, James C. *Abortion in America: The Origins and Evolution of National Policy, 1800–1900*. New York: Oxford University Press, 1978.

——. *Doctors and the Law: Medical Jurisprudence in Nineteenth Century America*. New York: Oxford University Press, 1993.

Montagu, Ashley. *Life before Birth*. New York: New American Library, 1962.

Montagu, Ashley, and Joseph Shalit. "New Light on Life before Birth." *Science Digest*, October 1950, 63–67.

Mooney, Chris. "Research and Destroy: How the Religious Right Promotes Its Own 'Experts' to Combat Mainstream Science," *Washington Monthly*, October 2004, http://www.washingtonmonthly.com/features/2004/0410.mooney.html (accessed June 10, 2010).

Moore, Robert Laurence, and David S. Moore. *In Search of White Crows: Spiritualism, Parapsychology in American Culture*. New York: Oxford University Press, 1993.

Morantz-Sanchez, Regina. *Sympathy and Science: Women Physicians in American Science*. New York: Oxford University Press, 1985.

Morello-Frosch, Rachel. "The Politics of Reproductive Hazards in the Workplace: Class, Gender, and the History of Occupational Lead Exposure." *International Journal of Health Services* 27, no. 3 (1997): 501–521.

Morgan, Ann Haven. "Zoology at Mount Holyoke," *Mount Holyoke Alumnae Quarterly* 5, no. 1 (1921): 17–23.

Morgan, Lynn. "The Embryography of Alice B. Toklas," *Comparative Studies in Society and History*. 50, nos. 1 (2008): 304–325.

——. *Icons of Life: A Cultural History of Human Embryos*. Berkeley: University of California Press, 2009.

——. "Imagining the Unborn in the Ecuadoran Andes." *Feminist Studies* 23, no. 2 (1997): 323–350.

―――. "Materializing the Fetal Body." In *Fetal Subjects and Feminist Positions*, edited by Lynn M. Morgan and Meredith W. Michaels. Philadelphia: University of Pennsylvania Press, 1999.

―――. "'Properly Disposed Of': A History of Embryo Disposal and the Changing Claims on Fetal Remains." *Medical Anthropology* 21, nos. 3–4 (2002): 247–274.

―――. "The Rise and Demise of a Collection of Human Fetuses at Mount Holyoke College." *Perspectives in Biology and Medicine* 49, no. 3 (2006): 435–451.

―――. "Trafficking in Fetal Remains." *College Street Journal* 13, no. 12 (November 19, 1999).

Morgan, Lynn M., and Meredith W. Michaels, eds. *Fetal Subjects and Feminist Positions*. Philadelphia: University of Pennsylvania Press, 1999.

Morowitz, Harold J., and James S. Trefil. *The Facts of Life: Science and the Abortion Controversy*. New York: Oxford University Press, 1992.

Morris, David. *The Culture of Pain*. Berkeley: University of California Press, 1993.

Moskowitz, Mark. *The Haunting Fetus: Abortion, Sexuality, and the Spirit World in Taiwan*. Honolulu: University of Hawaii Press, 2001.

Moynihan, Daniel Patrick. *The Negro Family: The Case for National Action*. Washington, D.C.: Government Printing Office, March 1965.

Mohammed, Khalil. "Islamic Tradition and Reproductive Choice." Religious Coalition for Reproductive Choice, Educational Series No. 15, n.d..

Graham-Mulhall, Sara. *Opium: The Demon Flower*. New York: Howard Vinal, 1926.

Mulkay, Michael. *The Embryo Research Debate: Science and the Politics of Reproduction*. Cambridge: Cambridge University Press, 1997.

Mullen, William. "A Work in (and of) Progress: The Museum of Science and Industry, in the Middle of an 11-year Philosophy of Hands-on Education." *Chicago Tribune*, June 19, 2008, 1.

Munstermann, Richard. "Torts: A Right of Viable Child to Maintain a Tort Action for Negligent Prenatal Injury." *Nebraska Law Review* 26 (1947): 431–436.

Murchison, Carl. "Origin and Prenatal Growth of Behavior." *Handbook of Childhood Psychology*. Worcester, Mass.: Clark University Press, 1933.

Musgrave, Kate. *Womb with Views: A Contradictionary of the English Language*. Racine, Wis.: Mother Courage Press, 1989.

NARAL Pro-Choice America Foundation. "Factsheet: Anti-Choice Violence and Intimidation," 2006, http://www.prochoiceamerica.org/issues/abortion/access-to-abortion/clinic-violence/ (accessed June 8, 2010).

Nathanson, Bernard. *Aborting America*. New York: Pinnacle Books, 1981.

―――. "Ambulatory Abortion Experience with 26,000 Cases, July 1, 1970 to August 1, 1971." *New England Journal of Medicine* 286 (1972): 403–407.

―――. *The Hand of God: A Journey from Death to Life by the Abortion Doctor Who Changed His Mind*. Washington, DC: Regency, 2001.

National Cancer Institute. "Fact Sheet: Abortion, Miscarriage, and Breast Cancer." May 30, 2003, http://www.cancer.gov/cancertopics/factsheet/Risk/abortion-miscarriage (accessed July 15, 2008).

Nebinger, Andrew. *Criminal Abortion: Its Extent and Prevention*. Philadelphia: Collins, 1870.

Needham, Joseph. *A History of Embryology*. Cambridge: Cambridge University Press, 1934.

Nelson, Hilde Lindemann. "Dethroning Choice: Analogy, Personhood, and the New Reproductive Technologies." *Journal of Law, Medicine & Ethics* 23, no. 2 (1995): 129–135.

———. "Paternal-Fetal Conflict." *Hastings Center Report* 22, no. 3 (March/April 1992): 3.

Nelson, Jennifer. "From Abortion Rights to Reproductive Freedom: Feminism, Nationalism, and Identity Politics." PhD diss., Rutgers University, 1999.

Nesmith, Jeff. "Studies Link Agent Orange to Birth Defects in Children of Vietnam Vets." *Atlanta Constitution*, March 15, 1996, A14.

"New Attack on Abortion." *Time*, May 27, 1974, 84.

"New Test for Pregnancy." *Newsweek*, November 21, 1938, 26.

"A New Theory in Prenatal Injuries: The Biological Approach." *Fordham Law Review* 26 (Winter 1957/1958): 687.

Newman, Karen. *Fetal Positions: Individualism, Science, Visuality*. Stanford, Calif.: Stanford University Press, 1996.

"NIH Bans Research on Live Fetuses." *Science News*, April 21, 1973, 253–254.

Nilsson, Lennart. "Drama of Life before Birth." *Life*, April 30, 1965, 54–70.

Niswander, Kenneth J. "Medical Abortion Practices in the United States." In *Abortion and the Law*, edited by David Smith. Cleveland: Case Western Reserve University Press, 1967.

Nix, Joseph T.. *The Unborn: Medical, Legal, and Moral Aspects of Abortion*. New Orleans: J. T. Nix Clinic, 1924.

Nolan, "The Use of the Embryo or Fetus in Transplantation: What Is There to Lose?" *Transplant Proclamation* 22 (1990): 1028.

Nolen, William A. *The Baby in the Bottle: An Investigative Review of the Edelin Case and Its Larger Meaning for the Controversy over Abortion Reform*. New York: Coward, McCann & Geoghegan, 1978.

Noonan, John T., Jr. "The Experience of Pain by the Unborn." In *New York Perspectives on Human Abortion*, edited by Thomas W. Hilgers, Dennis Horan, and David Mall. Frederick, Md.: University Publications of America, 1981.

———. *The Morality of Abortion: Legal and Historical Perspectives*. Cambridge: Harvard University Press, 1970.

Noyes, John Humphrey. "Essay on Scientific Propagation with an Appendix Containing a Health Report on the Oneida Community by Theodore R. Noyes, M.D." Oneida, N.Y.: Oneida Community, 1872.

Oaks, Laury. "Fetal Spirithood and Fetal Personhood: The Cultural Construction of Abortion in Japan." *Women's Studies International Forum* 17, no. 5 (1994): 511–523.

———. "Irish Trans/national Politics and Locating Fetuses," In *Fetal Subjects and Feminist Positions*, edited by Lynn M. Morgan and Meredith W. Michaels. Philadelphia: University of Pennsylvania Press, 1999.

Oakley, Ann. *The Captured Womb: A History of the Medical Care of Pregnant Women*. Oxford: Basil Blackwell, 1984.

O'Connor, John J. "TV: Heroin Addiction in the Newborn." *New York Times*, January 10, 1973, 82.

O'Connor, Thomas H. *South Boston, My Hometown: The History of an Ethnic Neighborhood*. Boston: Northeastern University Press, 1994.

Okin, Susan Moller. *Justice, Gender, and the Family*. New York: Basic Books, 1991.

Olasky, Martin. *Compassionate Conservatism: What It Is, What It Does, and How It Can Transform America*. New York: Free Press, 2000.

———. *Renewing American Compassion*. Washington, D.C.: Regnery, 1997.

Oldfield, Josiah. *The Mystery of Birth*. New York: Rider, 1948.

Olsham, Andrew F., et al. "Birth Defects among Offspring of Firemen." *American Journal of Epidemiology* 131 (1990): 313–321.

O'Neill, Nena, and George O'Neill. *Shifting Gears: Finding Security in a Changing World*. New York: M. Evans, 1974.

O'Rahilly, Ronan, and Fabiola Muller. *Development Stages in Human Embryos: Including a Revision of Streeter's "Horizons" and a Survey of the Carnegie Collection*. Washington, D.C.: Carnegie Institution of Washington, 1987.

Ortiz, Ann Teresa. "'Bare-Handed' Medicine and Its Elusive Patients: The Unstable Construction of Pregnant Women and Fetuses in Dominican Obstetrics Discourse." *Feminist Studies* 23:2 (1997): 263–288.

Overall, Christine. "Frozen Embryos and 'Father's Rights': Parenthood and Decision-Making in the Copreservation of Embryos." In *Reproduction, Ethics and the Law: Feminist Perspectives*, edited by Joan C. Callahan. Bloomington: Indiana University Press, 1995.

Packer, Herbert L., and Ralph L. Gambell. "Therapeutic Abortion: A Problem in Law and Medicine." *Stanford Law Review* 11 (May 1959): 417–455.

Padgett, Faye M., and Mazo, Earl., eds. *The Presidential Campaign, 1976*, vol. 1. Washington, D.C.: U.S. Government Print Office, 1978.

Page, Connie. "Dr. Edelin and Dr. Sabath: They've Never Met: Indicted Doctors Talk on Abortion Issue." *Boston Phoenix*, May 21, 1974, 1.

Paige, Carole. *The Right-to-Lifers: Who They Are, How They Operate, Where They Get Their Money*. New York: Summit Books, 1983.

Paltrow, Lynn. "Criminal Prosecution against Pregnant Women: National Update and Overview." *Annual Report for the Center for Reproductive Law and Policy*. New York City, 1992.

———. "Our Common Struggle." *Harm Reduction Coalition Newsletter*, Spring 1999.

———. "Pregnant Drug Users, Fetal Persons, and the Threat to *Roe v. Wade*." *Albany Law Review* 999 (1999): 62.

———. "Punishing Women for Their Behavior during Pregnancy: An Approach That Undermines Women's Health and Children's Interests." *Annual Report for the Center for Reproductive Law & Policy*. New York: Center for Reproductive Law & Policy, 1996.

"Panel Says Caesarians Are Used Too Often." *New York Times*, November 3, 1987, C5.

Parsons, Talcott. "The Science Legislation and the Role of the Social Sciences." *American Sociological Review* 11, no. 6 (December 1946): 653–666.

Pascoe, Peggy. "Miscegenation Law, Court Cases, and Ideologies of 'Race' in Twentieth-Century America." *Journal of American History* 83, no. 1 (June 1996): 44–69.

Pateman, Carole. *The Sexual Contract.* Stanford: Stanford University Press, 1988.

"The Patient within the Patient: Problems in Perinatal Medicine." Special issue of *Birth Defects* 21 (1985).

Patterson, James T. *Grand Expectations: The United States, 1946–1974.* New York: Oxford University Press, 1996.

Paul, Annie Murphy. "The First Ache." *New York Times Magazine*, February 19, 2008, 45–59.

Paul, Diane. *Controlling Human Heredity: 1865 to the Present.* Amherst, N.Y.: Humanity Books, 1998.

Paul, John R. *A History of Poliomyelitis.* New Haven: Yale University Press, 1971.

Paul, Maureen, Cynthia Daniels, and Robert Rosofsky. "Corporate Response to Reproductive Hazards in the Workplace: Results of the Family, Work, and Health Survey." *American Journal of Industrial Medicine* 16 (1989): 279–289.

Pauley, Philip J. "How Did the Effects of Alcohol on Reproduction Become Uninteresting?" *Journal of the History of Biology* 29 (1996): 1–28.

Pear, Robert. "Abortion Proposal Sets Condition on Aid." *New York Times*, July 15, 2008, A17.

Pearse, Harry A., and Harold A. Ott. "Hospital Control of Sterilization and Therapeutic Abortion." *American Journal of Obstetrics and Gynecology* 60 (August 1950): 285.

Peiss, Kathy. *Cheap Amusements: Working Women and Leisure in Turn-of-the-Century New York.* Philadelphia: Temple University Press, 1986.

Pence, Gregory. "Abortion: Kenneth Edelin." In *Classic Cases in Medical Ethics: Accounts of Cases that Have Shaped Medical Ethics with Philosophical, Legal and Historical Backgrounds.* New York: McGraw Hill. 1990.

Perl, Rebecca. "Cocaine May Travel to Egg through Sperm, Study Says." *Atlanta Constitution*, October 9, 1991, 16.

Perlstein, M. A. "Congenital Morphinism: Rare Cause of Convulsions in the Newborn." *Journal of American Medical Association* 135 (November 8, 1947): 633.

Perlstein, Rick. *Nixonland: The Rise of a President and the Fracturing of America.* New York: Scribner, 2008.

Pernick, Martin S. *The Black Stork: Eugenics and the Death of "Defective" Babies in American Medicine and Motion Pictures since 1915.* New York: Oxford University Press, 1996.

———. *A Calculus of Suffering: Pain, Professionalism and Anesthesia in Nineteenth-Century America.* New York: Columbia University Press, 1985.

Perone, Nicole. "In Vitro Fertilization and Embryo Transfer: A Historical Perspective." *Journal of Reproductive Medicine* 39 (1994): 698–720.

Petchesky, Rosalind. *Abortion and Woman's Choice: The State, Sexuality, & Reproductive Freedom.* Boston: Northeastern University Press, 1984, 1991.

———. "Fetal Images: The Power of Visual Culture in the Politics of Reproduction." *Feminist Studies* 13 (summer 1987): 263–292.

————, ed. "Workers, Reproductive Hazards, and the Politics of Protection." Special issue, *Feminist Studies* 5, no. 2 (Summer 1979).

Peterfy, Agota. "Fetal Viability as a Threshold to Personhood: A Legal Analysis." *Journal of Legal Medicine* 16, no. 4 (1995): 607.

Peurala, Alice. "People in the Plant Looked on Me as a Fighter." In *Rocking the Boat: Union Women's Voices, 1915–1975*, edited by Brigid O'Farrell and Joyce L. Kornbluh. New Brunswick, N.J.: Rutgers University Press, 1996.

Philipson, Agneta, et al. "Transplacental Passage of Erythromycin and Clyndamycin." *New England Journal of Medicine* 288, no. 23 (June 7, 1973): 1219–1221.

Pilati, Joseph. "Edelin Was Not the Only One Who Was on Trial, Pilot Says." *Boston Globe*, February 21, 1975, 8.

Pinto-Correia, Clara. *The Ovary of Eve: Egg and Sperm and Preformation*. Chicago: University of Chicago Press, 1997.

"Place of Science in Society Today." *Science Monthly*, December 1954, 365–367.

Planned Parenthood Federation of America. *The Facts Speak Louder: Planned Parenthood's Critique of "The Silent Scream"* (1985 pamphlet).

Pollard, Edward B. *The Rights of the Unborn Race*. Philadelphia: American Baptist Publication Society, 1914.

Pollitt, Katha. "'Fetal Rights': A New Assault on Feminism." *Nation* 26 (March 1990): 409–418.

Poovey, Mary. "The Abortion Question and the Death of Man." In *Feminists Theorize the Political*, edited by Judith Butler and Joan Scott. New York: Routledge, 1992.

Porter, Roy. *The Greatest Benefit to Mankind: A Medical History of Humanity*. New York: W. W. Norton, 1997.

"Pre-Birth Sex Determination." *Science News Letter*, September 22, 1956, 182.

"Prenatal Diagnosis of Sex Using Cells from the Amniotic Fluid." *Science* (March 30, 1956), 548.

Prescott, James. W. "'The Abortion of 'The Silent Scream': A False and Wrongful Cry for Human Pain, Suffering and Violence." *Humanist* (September/October 1986): 10–17.

Pressley, Sue Anne. "S.C. Verdict Fuels Debate over Rights of the Unborn." *Washington Post*, May 27, 2001, A3.

Price, Janet, and Margrit Shildrich, eds. *Feminist Theory and the Body: A Reader*. New York: Routledge, 1999.

Prince, Michael K. *Rally 'Round the Flag, Boys! South Carolina and the Confederate Flag*. Columbia: University of South Carolina Press, 2004.

Pritchard, Jack A., and Louis M. Hellman, eds. *Williams Obstetrics*, 14th ed. New York: Appleton-Century-Crofts, 1971.

"Procuring Abortions," Editorial, *Boston Medical and Surgical Journal* 51, no. 10 (1855): 205.

Purdy, Laura Martha. *Reproducing Persons: Issues in Feminist Bioethics*. Ithaca, N.Y.: Cornell University Press, 1996.

Quindlen, Anna. "In the Name of the Father." *Newsweek*, July 16, 2001, 62.

Rachels, James. *The End of Life*. Oxford: Oxford University Press, 1986.

Ramsey, Paul. *Ethics at the Edges of Life: Medical and Legal Intersections.* New Haven: Yale University Press, 1980.

Randall, Donna M., and James F. Short, Jr. "Women in Toxic Work Environments: A Case Study of Social Problem Development." *Social Problems* 30, no. 3 (April 1983): 410–423.

Randall, Vernellia R. "Slavery, Segregation and Racism: Trusting the Health Care System Ain't Always Easy! An African American Perspective on Bioethics." *Saint Louis University Public Law Review* 15 (1996): 191–223.

Rapp, Rayna. *Testing Women, Testing the Fetus: The Social Impact of Amniocentesis in America.* New York: Routledge, 1999.

Rapson, Richard L. *Individualism and Conformity in the American Character.* Boston: Heath, 1967.

Rawls, John. *Political Liberalism.* New York: Columbia University Press, 1993.

————. *A Theory of Justice.* Cambridge: Harvard University Press, 1971.

Reagan, Leslie. *When Abortion Was a Crime: Women, Medicine, and Law in the United States, 1867–1973.* Berkeley: California University Press, 1997.

Reagan, Ronald. "Remarks at the National Religious Broadcasters Convention." Washington, D.C., January 30, 1984. Transcript available online at Ronald Reagan Presidential Library, University of Texas, http://www.reagan.utexas.edu/archives/speeches/1984/13084b.htm (accessed July 14, 2008).

Reardon, David. *Aborted Women: Silent No More.* Westchester, Ill.: Crossway Books, 1987.

————. *Making Abortion Rare: A Healing Strategy for a Divided Nation.* Springfield, Ill.: Acorn Books, 1996.

————. "Their Deepest Wound: An Analysis." *Post-Abortion Review* 4, nos. 2–3 (spring and summer 1996): 2–3.

Reardon, David, and Theresa Burke. *Forbidden Grief: The Unspoken Pain of Abortion.* Springfield, Ill.: Acorn Books, 2002.

Reardon, David, et al. "Deaths Associated with Abortion Compared to Childbirth—A Review of New and Old Data and the Medical and Legal Implications." *Journal of Contemporary Health Law and Policy* 20 (2003–2004): 280–283.

Reed, Charles B. "Therapeutic and Criminal Abortion." *Illinois Medical Journal* 7, (January 1905): 27.

Reich, Warren T., ed. *Encyclopedia of Bioethics,* vol. 2. New York: Free Press, 1978.

Reinhold, Robert. "Boston Indicts Doctors in Fetus Case." *New York Times,* April 12, 1974, 1.

————. "Boston vs. the Doctors: Strange Case." *New York Times,* April 21, 1974, 223.

————. "3 Boston Doctors Are Reinstated." *New York Times,* April 19, 1974, 42.

Remnick, David. "Whose Life Is It Anyway? Angie Carder Lived a Very Simple Life…and Died a Very Complicated Death." *Washington Post,* February 21, 1988, 276.

Rentoul, Robert Reid. *Race Culture; or, Race Suicide? A Plea for the Unborn.* New York: Walter Scott, 1906.

"Reproductive Health and Rights of Workers." American Public Health Association Policy Statement reprinted at www.apha.org (November 7, 1979). Available at http://ethics.iit.edu/indexOfCodes-2.php?key=24_594_1339 (Accessed on June 8, 2010).

Reverby, Susan M., ed. *Tuskegee's Truths: Rethinking the Tuskegee Syphilis Experiment.* Chapel Hill: University of North Carolina Press, 2000.

Rey, Roselyn. *The History of Pain.* Cambridge: Cambridge University Press, 1995.

Reynolds, Barbara. "How Soon the Cheering Stops When Veterans Become Ill." *USA Today*, November 11, 1994, 1.

Rhode, Deborah. *Justice and Gender: Sex Discrimination and the Law.* Cambridge: Harvard University Press, 1990.

Rhoden, Nancy K. "Caesarians and Samaritans," *Law, Medicine & Health Care* 15, no. 3 (Fall 1987): 118.

———. "The Judge in the Delivery Room: The Emergence of Court-Ordered Caesarians." *California Law Review* 74 (December 1986): 1959.

Richards, Ellen H. Swallow. *Euthenics: The Science of Controllable Environment, a Plea for Better Conditions as a First Step towards Higher Efficiency.* Boston: Whitcomb & Barrods, 1910.

Richards, Robert. *Darwin and the Emergence of Evolutionary Theories of Mind and Behavior.* Chicago, IL: University of Chicago Press, 1989.

Richardson, Ruth. *Death, Dissection, and the Destitute.* Chicago: University of Chicago Press, 1987.

Rieder, Jonathan. *Canarsie: The Jews and Italians against Liberalism.* Cambridge: Harvard University Press, 1987.

"The Rights of the Unborn." *Good Housekeeping*, October 1912, 32.

"The Rights of Unborn Children." *Harvard Law Review* 12 (1901): 209–210.

"Right-to-Life: Two Crusaders." *Newsweek*, March 3, 1975, 29.

"Rise of Scientific Understanding." *Science*, September 3, 1948, 241.

Risen, James, and Thomas, Judy L. *Wrath of Angels: The American Abortion War.* New York: Basic Books, 1998.

"Risk to Fetus Ruled as Barring Women from Jobs." *New York Times*, October 3, 1989, A16.

Rivera, Geraldo (producer). *The Littlest Junkie: A Children's Story.* New York City: ABC-TV, January 10, 1973.

R.M.L. "Torts: Prenatal Injuries: Rights of an Infant to Sue." *Brooklyn Law Review* 15 (1949): 322–325.

Roberts, Dorothy. *Killing the Black Baby: Race: Reproduction and the Meaning of Liberty.* New York: Pantheon, 1997.

———. "Punishing Drug Addicts Who Have Babies: Women of Color, Equality, and the Right of Privacy." *Harvard Law Review* 104 (1991): 1419–1482.

Roberts, S. S. "Potential Cure, Ethical Questions." *Diabetes Forecast* 48, no. 8 (1995): 42.

Robertson, John. "Procreative Liberty and the Control of Conception, Pregnancy, and Childbirth." *Virginia Law Review* 405 (1983): 405–464.

———. "The Right to Procreate and *In Utero* Fetal Therapy." *Journal of Legal Medicine* 63 (1982): 333.

Robinson, James C. *Toil and Toxics: Workplace Struggles and Political Strategies for Occupational Health.* Los Angeles: University of California Press, 1991.

Robinson, Walter, and Nick King. "Jurors Say 'Negligence' Was Basis." *Boston Globe*, February 16, 1975, 1.

Robinson, William J. *Birth Control, or the Limitations of Offspring by Prevenception.* New York: Eugenics, 1929.

———. *Fewer and Better Babies, or the Limitations of Offspring.* New York: Critic and Guide, 1915.

Rock, John, and Menkin, Miriam F. "In Vitro Fertilization and Cleavage of Human Ovarian Eggs." *Science* 100, no. 2588 (August 4, 1944): 105–107.

Rodgers, Daniel T. *Atlantic Crossings: Social Politics in a Progressive Age.* Cambridge: Belknap Press of Harvard University Press, 1998.

———. "In Search of Progressivism." *Reviews in American History* 10 (1982): 113–132.

Rodrique, Jessie. "The Black Community and the Birth Control Movement." In *Unequal Sisters: A Multicultural Reader in U.S. Women's History*, edited by Ellen DuBois and Vicki Ruiz. New York: Routledge, 1990.

Roe, Shirley. *Matter, Life, and Generation: Eighteenth-Century Embryology and the Haller-Wolf Debate.* Cambridge: Cambridge University Press, 1981.

Rom, William. "Effects of Lead on the Female and Reproduction: A Review." *Mount Sinai Journal of Medicine* 43 (1976): 542–552.

Roosevelt, Theodore. "A Letter from President Roosevelt on Race Suicide," *American Monthly Review of Books* 35, no. 5 (1907): 550–551.

Rorty, Amélie Oksenberg. *The Identities of Persons.* Berkeley: University of California Press, 1976.

Rosen, Harold. "The Psychiatric Implications of Abortion: A Case Study in Hypocrisy." In *Abortion and the Law*, edited by David Smith. Cleveland: Case Western Reserve University Press, 1967.

Rosen, Howard, ed. *Therapeutic Abortion: Medical, Psychiatric, Legal, Anthropological, and Religious Considerations.* New York: Julian Press, 1954.

Rosenberg, Charles. "The Bitter Fruit: Heredity, Disease, and Social Thought in Nineteenth Century America." *Perspectives in American History* 8 (1974): 189–235.

———. *No Other Gods: On Science and American Social Thought.* Baltimore: Johns Hopkins University, 1961.

Rosenberg, Harriet G. "From Trash to Treasure: Housewife Activists and the Environmental Justice Movement." In *Articulating Hidden Resistance: Exploring the Influence of Eric Wolf.* Berkeley: University of California Press, 1993.

Rosenberg, Rosalind. *Beyond Separate Spheres: Intellectual Roots of Modern Feminism.* New Haven: Yale University Press, 1982.

Rosenthal, Theodore, Sherman W. Patrick, and Donald C. Krug. "Congenital Neonatal Narcotics Addiction: A Natural History." *American Journal of Public Health.* 54, no. 8 (August 1964): 1252–1262.

Rosner, David, and Gerald Markowitz. *Deadly Dust: Silicosis and the Politics of Occupational Disease in Twentieth-Century America.* Princeton: Princeton University Press, 1994.

———. *Dying for Work: Workers' Safety and Health in Twentieth Century America.* Bloomington: Indiana University Press, 1987.

Rosof, Libby. "Embryo Use or Abuse Taints Groundbreaking Study." *Compass* 43, no. 30 (April 15, 1997): 8–9.

Ross, Loretta J. "African-American Women and Abortion." In *Abortion Wars: A Half Century of Struggle, 1950–2000*, edited by Rickie Solinger. Berkeley: University of California Press, 1998.

———. "African American Women and Abortion, 1800–1970." In *Mothers & Motherhood: Readings in American History*, edited by Rima D. Apple and Janet Golden. Columbus: Ohio State University Press, 1997.

Rostand Jean. *Adventures before Birth*. Trans. Joseph Needham. London: Victor Gollancz, 1936.

Roth, Rachel. "At Women's Expense: The Cost of Fetal Rights." In *The Politics of Pregnancy*, edited by Janna C. Merrick and Robert H. Blank. London: Haworth Press, 1993.

———. *Making Women Pay: The Hidden Costs of Fetal Rights*. Ithaca, N.Y.: Cornell University Press, 2000.

Rothman, Barbara Katz. *The Tentative Pregnancy: Prenatal Diagnosis and the Future of Motherhood*. New York: W. W. Norton, 1986.

Rothman, David J. "Human Experimentation and the Origins of Bioethics in the United States." In *Social Science Perspectives on the Medical Ethics*, edited by George Weisz. Dordrecht, The Netherlands: Kluwer Academic, 1990.

———. *Strangers at the Bedside: A History of How Law and Bioethics Transformed Medical Decision Making*. New York: Basic Books, 1991.

Rothman, David J., and Sheila M. Rothman. *The Willowbrook Wars*. New York: Harper & Row, 1984.

Rudd, Jim. "Fetal Pain Legislation Is Bogus." *CovenantNews.com*, January 31, 2005, http://www.covenantnews.com/rudd050131.htm (accessed July 14, 2008).

Rudder, Lynn Baker. *Persons and Bodies: A Constitutional View*. Cambridge: Cambridge University Press, 2000.

Rushton, Alan. *Genetics and Medicine in the United States, 1800–1922*. Baltimore: Johns Hopkins University Press, 1994.

Russell, Keith P. "Changing Indications for Therapeutic Abortions: Twenty Years' Experience at Los Angeles Community Hospital." *Journal of the American Medical Association* 151 (January 10, 1953): 108.

Rutherford, Charlotte. "Reproductive Freedoms and African American Women." *Yale Law Journal of Law and Feminism* 4 (1992): 255–275.

Ryan, Joseph G. "Wrestling with the Angel: The Struggle of Roman Catholic Clergy, Physicians, and Believers with the Rise of Medical Practice, 1807–1940." PhD diss., American University, 1997.

Rydell, Robert W. *All the World's a Fair: Visions of Empire at America's International Expositions, 1876–1916*. Chicago: University of Chicago Press, 1884.

Rymph, Catherine. *Republican Women: Feminism and Conservatism from Suffrage through the Rise of the New Right*. Chapel Hill: University of North Carolina Press, 2006.

Sabin, Alfred B. "Oral Poliovirus Vaccine." *Journal of the American Medical Association* 194, no. 8 (1965): 872–876.

Sabin, Florence. *Franklin Paine Mall: The Story of a Mind*. Baltimore: Johns Hopkins Press, 1934.

Safire, William. "What's with Boston?" *New York Times*, March 10, 1975, 29.

Saletin, Williams. *Bearing Right: How Conservatives Won the Abortion War*. Berkeley: University of California Press, 2004.

———. "I Feel Your Fetus' Pain: Compassionate Conservatism Enters the Womb." Human Nature, *Slate*, August 31, 2005, http://www.slate.com/id/2125299 (accessed July 11, 2008).

Salk, Jonas E. "Studies in Human Subjects on Active Immunization against Poliomyelitis." *Journal of the American Medical Association* 151, no. 13 (1953): 1081–1098.

Samuels, Suzanne Uttaro. *Fetal Rights, Women's Rights: Gender Equality in the Workplace*. Madison: University of Wisconsin Press, 1995.

Sandel, Michael. *Liberalism and the Limits of Justice*. Cambridge: Harvard University Press, 1982.

Sandroff, Ronni. "Invasion of the Body Snatchers: Fetal Rights vs. Mother's Rights." *Vogue*, October 1988, 330.

Sappol, Michael. *A Traffic of Dead Bodies: Anatomy and Embodied Social Identity in Nineteenth-Century America*. Princeton: Princeton University Press, 2002.

Sarbin, Theodore R., and John I. Kitsue, eds. *Constructing the Social*. London: Sage, 1994.

Sarkos, Chrysso Barbara. "The Fetal Tissue Transplant Debate in the United States: Where Is King Solomon When You Need Him?" *Journal of Law and Politics* 7, no. 2 (1991): 379–416.

Sasson, Vanessa R., and Law, Marie Jane, eds. *Imagining the Fetus: The Unborn in Myth, Religion, and Culture*. New York: Oxford University Press, 2009.

Satter, Beryl E. *Each Mind a Kingdom: American Women, Sexual Purity, and the New Thought Movement, 1875–1920*. Berkeley: University of California Press, 2001.

Sauer, R. "Attitudes to Abortion in America, 1870–1973." *Population Studies* 28, no. 1 (March 1974): 58.

"Save Lives of Unborn." *Science News Letter*, March 27, 1954, 194.

Savitz, David A., and Jianjua Chen. "Paternal Occupation and Childhood Cancer: Review of Epidemiological Studies," *Environmental Health Perspectives* 88 (1990): 325–337.

Savitz, David, Nancy Sonnefeld, and Andrew Olshan. "Review of Epidemiologic Studies of Paternal Occupational Exposure and Spontaneous Abortion." *American Journal of Industrial Medicine* 25 (1994): 361–383.

Saxton, Marsha. "Prenatal Screening and Discriminatory Attitudes about Disability." In *Embryos, Ethics, and Women's Rights: Exploring the New Reproductive Technologies*, edited by Elaine Hoffman Baruch, Amadeo F. D'Adamo, and Joni Seager. New York: Haworth Press, 1988.

Scarry, Elaine. *The Body in Pain: The Making and Unmaking of the World*. New York: Oxford University Press, 1985.

Scheinfeld, Amram. *Why Are You You?* New York: Abelard-Schuman, 1958.

Schlafly, Phyllis. "American Citizenship Is Precious." Phyllis Schlafly Columns, Eagle Forum website, October 12, 2005, http://www.eagleforum.org/column/2005/oct05/05–10–12.html (accessed July 14, 2008).

Schlictmann, Laura. "Accommodation of Pregnancy-Related Disabilities on the Job." *Berkeley Journal of Employment and Labor Law* 15 (1994): 335–361.

Schmidt, William E. "Risk to Fetus Ruled as Barring Women from Jobs." *New York Times*, October 3, 1989, A16.

Schoenwald, Jonathan M. *A Time for Choosing.* New York: Oxford University Press, 2002.

Schrag, Peter. "The Forgotten American." *Harper's*, August 1969, 27–34.

Schroedel, Jean Reith. *Is the Fetus a Person? A Comparison of Policies across the Fifty States.* Ithaca, N.Y.: Cornell University Press, 2000.

———. "Law, Religion, and Fetal Personhood." Religious Coalition for Reproductive Choice Research Report. N.D.

Schrödinger, Erwin. *What Is Life?: With Mind and Matter, and Autobiographical Sketches.* Cambridge: Cambridge University Press, 1944.

Schuck, Peter H. *Agent Orange on Trial: Mass Toxic Disasters in the Courts.* Cambridge: Harvard University Press, 1986.

Schulman, Bruce J. *The Seventies: The Great Shift in American Culture, Society, and Politics.* Cambridge: Da Capo Press, 2001.

Schulman, Bruce J., and Julian E. Zelizer, eds. *Rightward Bound: Making American Conservative in the 1970s.* Cambridge: Harvard University Press, 2008.

Schultz, Suzanne. *Body Snatching: The Robbing of Graves for the Education of Physicians.* Jefferson, N.C.: McFarland Press, 1992.

Schutte, Anne Jacobson. "'Such Monstrous Births': A Neglected Aspect of the Antinomian Controversy." *Renaissance Quarterly* 38, no. 1 (1985): 85–106.

Schweitzer, Albert. *The Rights of the Unborn & the Peril Today: Annihilation without Representation.* Chicago: Albert Schweitzer Education Foundation, 1958.

"Science and the Citizen." *Scientific American*, May 1947, 223.

"Science and the Citizen." *Science*, December 13, 1957, 1225–1229.

"Science and Human Values." *Nation*, December 29, 1956, 550–556.

"Science and the Public." *Science*, July 11, 1947, 23–25.

"Scientific Thought in the Coming Decades." *Harpers*, November 1948, 44–48.

"Scientists: A Moral Obligation to be Intelligible." *Science Monthly*, February 1950, 17.

"Scientists Succumb to Public Role." *Business Week*, March 22, 1958, 133.

Scott, Douglas R. "Unborn Child Pain Awareness Act Could Backfire," *Christian Newswire*, December 5, 2006, http://www.christiannewswire.com/index.php?module=releases&task=view&releaseID=1664 (accessed July 14, 2008).

Scott, James Foster. "Criminal Abortion." *American Journal for Obstetrics and Diseases for Women* 33 (January 1896): 72–86, 128–132.

Scott, Janny. "Study Finds Cocaine Can Bind Sperm." *Los Angeles Times*, October 9, 1991, A1.

Scott, Joan. "The Evidence of Experience." *Critical Inquiry* 17 (Summer 1991): 773–797.

Scott, Judith A. "Keeping Women in Their Place: Exclusionary Policies and Reproduction." In *Double Exposure: Women's Health Hazards on the Job and at Home,* edited by Wendy Chavkin. New York: Monthly Review Press, 1984.

Seld, Arthur. "Torts: Prenatal Injuries: Rights of an Infant to Sue." *Cornell Law Review* 32 (1947): 609.

Selden, Steven. *Inheriting Shame: The Story of Eugenics and Racism in America*. New York: Teachers College Press, 1999.

Selle, Raymond M. "Before a Baby Is Born." *Parents Magazine* (May 1939), 29.

Sellers, Christopher. *Hazards of the Job: From Industrial Disease to Environmental Health*. Chapel Hill: University of North Carolina, 1999.

Serrano, Richard. "Birth Defects in Gulf Vets' Babies Stir Fear, Debate." *Los Angeles Times*, November 14, 1994, 1.

"Setback for Abortion." *Time*, February 24, 1975, 67.

Shain, Barry Alan. *The Myth of American Individualism: The Protestant Origins of American Thought*. Princeton: Princeton University Press, 1994.

Shanley, Mary L. "Fathers' Rights, Mothers' Wrongs? Reflections on Unwed Fathers' Rights, Patriarchy, and Sex Equality." In *Reproduction, Ethics and the Law: Feminist Perspectives*, edited by Joan C. Callahan. Bloomington: Indiana University Press, 1995.

Shannon, Christopher. *Conspicuous Criticism: Tradition, the Individual, and Culture in American Social Thought from Veblen to Mills*. Baltimore: Johns Hopkins University Press, 1996.

Shannon, T. W. *Nature's Secrets Revealed: Scientific Knowledge of the Laws of Sex Life and Heredity, or Eugenics*. Marietta, Ohio: S. A. Mullikin, 1916.

Shaw, Lucien. "Recognition of New Interests in the Law of Torts." *California Law Review* 10 (1922): 469.

Shaw, Marjorie. "Conditional Prospective Rights of the Fetus." *Journal of Legal Medicine* 5 (1984): 63.

Sheehan, Alan H. "BCH Fetus Case: Research at Stake." *Boston Sunday Globe*, June 2, 1974, 1.

———. "BCH Officials Say Doctor Can Return to Work." *Boston Globe*, February 19, 1975, 1.

———. "Edelin Returns to Work at City Hospital." *Boston Globe*, February 20, 1975, 1.

———. "Edelin Sentenced to Year's Probation." *Boston Globe*, February 19, 1975, 1.

———. "Manslaughter Is Charged in BCH Abortion." *Boston Globe*, April 12, 1974, 1.

Sherman, Rorie. "Keeping Baby Safe from Mom." *National Law Journal* (October 3, 1988): 24.

Shriner, Thomas L. "Maternal versus Fetal Rights: A Clinical Dilemma." *Obstetrics and Gynecology* 53, no. 4 (April 1979): 518–519.

Sicherman, Barbara. *Alice Hamilton: A Life in Letters*. Cambridge: Harvard University Press, 1987.

Siegal, Reva B. "Abortion as Sex Equality: Its Basis in Feminist Theory." In *Mothers in Law: Feminist Theory and the Legal Regulation of Motherhood*, edited by Martha Albertson Fineman and Isabel Karpin. New York: Columbia University Press, 1995.

———. "The New Politics of Abortion: An Equality Analysis of Women-Protective Abortion Restrictions." 2006 Baum Lecture. *University of Illinois Law Review* 991 (2007): 991–1053.

———. "The Right's Reasons: Constitutional Conflict and the Spread of Woman-Protective Antiabortion Argument." 2008 Brainerd Curie Lecture. *Duke Law Journal* 57 (2008): 1641–1692.

The Silent Scream, film produced by Donald S. Smith. American Portrait Films, 1984.

Silverman, Kenneth, comp. *Selected Letters of Cotton Mather*. Baton Rouge: Louisiana State University Press, 1971.

Sinclair, Brevard. *The Crowing Sin of the Age*. Boston: H. L. Hastings, 1991.

Sinclair, Upton. *The Brass Check: A Study of American Journalism*. Urbana: University of Illinois Press, 2003.

Singer, Peter, and Deanne Wells. *Making Babies: The New Science and Ethics of Conception*. New York: Scribner's Sons, 1985.

"Sins of the Father." *Economist*, February 23, 1991, 87.

Sitaraman, Bhavani. *The Middleground: The American Public and the Abortion Debate*. New York: Garland, 1994.

"60-Minute Pregnancy. " *Science Digest*, November 1951, 51.

Sjostrom, Henning, and Robert Nilsson. *Thalidomide and the Power of Drug Companies*. New York: Penguin, 1972.

Slaughter, M. M. "The Legal Construction of 'Mother.'" In *Mothers in Law: Feminist Theory and the Legal Regulation of Motherhood*, edited by Martha Albertson Fineman and Isabel Karpin. New York: Columbia University Press, 1995.

Slevin, Peter. "Ruling Gives South Dakota Doctors a Script to Read." *Washington Post*, July 20, 2008, A3.

Slezas, Roman V. (producer-director). *Crisis to Crisis. Voices of a Divided City*. U.S. Corporation for Public Broadcasting, CEBA Award Collection for the World Institute of Black Communications, 1982.

Smith, Arthur. "Prenatal Education." *Arena*, August 1907, 149–154.

Smith, Henry Craven. *A Plea for the Unborn: An Argument that Children Could and Therefore Should Be Born with a Sound Mind in a Sound Body, and that Man May Become Perfect by Means of Selection and Stirpiculture*. London: Watts, 1897.

Smith, William Benjamin. *The Color Line: Brief for the Unborn*. New York: McClure, Philips, 1905.

Smith-Rosenberg, Carroll. "The Abortion Movement and the AMA, 1850–1880." In *Disorderly Conduct: Visions of Gender in Victorian America*. New York: Oxford University Press, 1986.

———. *Disorderly Conduct: Visions of Gender in Victorian America*. New York: Oxford University Press, 1986.

———. "The Female World of Love and Ritual." *Signs* 1, no. 1 (autumn 1975): 1–29.

Sobran, Joseph. "The Averted Gaze: Liberalism and Fetal Pain." *Human Life Review* 10, no. 2 (spring 1984): 5–15.

Solinger, Ricki. *The Abortionist: A Woman against the Law*. New York: Free Press, 1994.

———, ed. *Abortion Wars: A Half Century of Struggle, 1950–2000*. Berkeley: University of California Press, 1998.

———. *Wake Up Little Susie: Single Pregnancy and Race Before Roe v. Wade*. New York: Routledge, 1992.

"Some Causes of Congenital Deformities." *Quarterly Journal of Inebriety* 21 (1899): 201–204.

Sontag, Lester W. *Annual Report of the Samuel S. Fels Research Institute for the Study of Prenatal and Postnatal Environment*. Yellow Springs, Ohio: Antioch College, February 1938.

Sontag, Susan. *Regarding the Pain of Others*. New York: Picador, 2003.

Speckhard, Anne. *Psycho-Social Stress following Abortion*. Kansas City: Sheed & War, 1987.

Speert, Harold. *Illustrated History of Gynecology and Obstetrics* (Paris: Roger Dacosta, 1973).

———. *Obstetric and Gynecological Milestones*. New York: Informa Healthcare, 1996.

Spock, Benjamin. *Pocket Book of Baby and Child Care*. New York: Pocket Books, 1946.

Squier, Susan Merrill. *Babies in Bottles: Twentieth-Century Visions of Reproductive Technologies*. New Brunswick, N.J.: Rutgers University Press, 1994.

Stabile, Carol. "Shooting the Mother: Fetal Photography and the Politics of Disappearance." *Camera Obscura* (January 28, 1992): 178–205.

Stafford, Barbara Maria. *Body Criticism: Imagine the Unseen in Enlightenment Art and Medicine*. Cambridge: Harvard University of Press, 1991.

Stage, Sarah. "Ellen Richards and the Social Significance of the Home Economics Movement." In *Rethinking Home Economics*, edited by Sarah Stage and Virginia B. Vincenti. Ithaca, N.Y.: Cornell University Press, 1997.

Stander, Henricus J. *Williams Obstetrics: A Textbook for the Use of Students and Practitioners*, 9th ed. New York: Appleton-Century-Crofts, 1945.

Stason, E. Blythe, and Samuel D. Estep, and William J. Pierce. *Atoms and the Law*. Ann Arbor: University of Michigan Press, 1959.

Steinbock, Bonnie. *Life before Birth: The Moral and Legal Status of Embryos and Fetuses*. New York: Oxford University Press, 1992.

Stellman, Jeanne. *Women's Work, Women's Health: Myths and Realities*. New York: Pantheon Books, 1977.

Stern, Roy. "The Pregnant Addict: A Study of 66 Case Histories, 1950–1959." *American Journal of Obstetrics and Gynecology* (January 15, 1966): 253–257.

Stevens, Leonard. "When Is Death?" *Reader's Digest* 94 (1969): 225–226.

Stevens, Tina. *Bioethics in America: Origins and Cultural Politics*. Baltimore: Johns Hopkins University Press, 2000.

———. "Redefining Death in America, 1968." *Caduceus: A Humanities Journal for Medicine and Health Sciences* 11, no. 3 (Winter 1995): 207–209.

Stock, Gregory. *Engineering the Human Germline: An Exploration of the Science and Ethics of Altering the Genes We Pass to Our Children*. New York: Oxford University Press, 2000.

Stocking, George W. *Race, Culture, and Evolution: Essays in the History of Anthropology*. Chicago: University of Chicago Press, 1982.

Storer, Horatio Robinson. *On Criminal Abortion: Its Nature, Its Evidence, Its Law*. Cambridge: John Wilson & Son, 1868.

———. *Why Not? A Book Intended for Every Woman*. Boston: Lee and Shepard, 1868.

Stormer, Nathan. *Articulating Life's Memory: U.S. Medical Rhetoric about Abortion in the Nineteenth Century*. Oxford: Lexington Books, 2002.

Stotland, Nada. "The Myth of the Abortion Trauma Syndrome." *Journal of the American Medical Association* 268, no. 15, 1992, 2078–2079.

Strain, Bruce Francis. *Being Born*. New York: D. Appleton-Century Co., 1937.

Stratton, Ethel. "X-Rays and Pregnancy." *Today's Health*, June 1954, 27.

Strecker, Edward A. *Their Mother's Sons: The Psychiatrist Examines an American Problem*. New York: J. B. Lippincott, 1946.

Stuart, Asch S. "Psychiatric Complications: Mental and Emotional Problems." In *Rovinsky & Guttmacher's Medical, Surgical, and Gynecological Complications of Pregnancy*, 3rd ed. Baltimore: Williams and Wilkins, 1985.

Sungard, Arnold. *The Miracle of Growth*. Urbana: University of Illinois Press, 1950.

Sussman, Warren. *Culture as History: The Transformation of the American Society in the Twentieth Century*. New York: Pantheon, 1984.

Swerdlow, Amy. *Women Strike for Peace: Traditional Motherhood and the Radical Politics of the 1960s*. Chicago: University of Chicago Press, 1993.

Tabor, Nathan. "Believe It or Not: Abortion Causes Illegal Immigration." *RenewAmerica.us*, August 24, 2005, http://www.renewamerica.us/columns/tabor/050824 (accessed July 14, 2008).

Tager, Jack. *Boston Riots: Three Centuries of Social Violence*. Boston: Northeastern University Press, 2000.

Tallack, Douglas. *Twentieth-Century America: The Intellectual and Cultural Context*. London: Longman Group, 1991.

Tanner, Lindsey. "Crack Is the Major Peril to Infants, but Not the Only Danger." *Chicago Sun Times*, March 28, 2001, 1.

Tate, Cassandra. "American Dilemma of Jobs, Health in an Idaho Town." *Smithsonian* 12, no. 6 (1981), 74–83.

———. "Women Shifted From Bunker Hill Smelter Jobs." *Morning Tribune* (Lewiston, Idaho) April 17, 1975, 1.

Taussig, Frederick. *Abortion Spontaneous and Induced: Medical and Social Aspects*. St. Louis: C. V. Mosby, 1936.

———. *The Prevention and Treatment of Abortion*. St. Louis: C. V. Mosby, 1910.

Taylor, Charles. *Human Agency and Language*. Cambridge: Cambridge University Press, 1985.

Taylor, James. "Ward Hall: King of the Sideshows," *Shocked and Amazed! On and Off the Runway*. Baltimore, Md.: Dolphin-Moon Press/Atomic Books: 2000.

Taylor, Janelle. "Images of Contradiction: Obstetrical Ultrasound in American Culture." In *Reproducing Reproduction: Kinship, Power and Technological Innovation*, edited by Sarah Franklin and Helena Ragone. Philadelphia: University of Pennsylvania Press, 1998.

———. "The Public Fetus and the Family Car: From Abortion Politics to a Volvo Advertisement." *Public Culture* 4, no. 2 (1992): 47–59.

"Tell Child's Sex before Baby Born." *Science News Letter*, February 11, 1956.

Terry, Charles E., and Mildred Pellens. *The Opium Problem*. New York: Bureau of Social Hygiene, 1928. Reprinted Montclair, N.J.: Patterson Smith, 1970.

Terry, Jane. "Conflict of Interest: Protection of Women from Reproductive Hazards in the Workplace." *Industrial and Labor Relations Forum* 15 (1981): 43–45.

Terry, Jennifer. "The Body Invaded: Medical Surveillance of Women as Reproducers." *Socialist Review* 89, no. 3 (1988): 13–44.

"Test-Tube Babies." *Newsweek*, December 27, 1954, 48–49.

"Test-Tube Babies." *Time*, December 27, 1954, 16.

Thelberg, Elizabeth B. "Instruction of College Students in Regard to Reproduction and Maternity." *New York Medical Journal* 95 (1912): 1269–1270.

Theriot, N. M. "Women's Voices in Nineteenth-Century Medical Discourse: A Step toward Reconstructing Science," *Signs* 19, no. 1 (1993): 1–31.

"Thirty Moved from Smelter." *Spokane Daily Chronicle*, April 17, 1975, 5.

Thomas, Kenneth R. *Anti-abortion Protests and Medical Clinic Blockades: Statutory and Constitutional Implications.* Major Studies and Issue Briefs of the Congressional Research Service. Washington, D.C.: Congressional Research Service, 1993.

Thomson, Judith Jarvis. "A Defense of Abortion." *Philosophy and Public Affairs* 1, no. 1 (1971): 47–66.

Thurow, Lester. *The Zero-Sum Society: Distribution and the Possibilities for Economic Change.* New York: Basic Books, 1980.

Tingley, Katherine. *The Gods Await.* Point Loma, California: Women's International Theosophical League, 1926.

Tomasi, Timothy B. and Jess A. Velona. "All the President's Men? A Study of Ronald Reagan's Appointments to the U.S. Court of Appeals." *Columbia Law Review* vol. 87, no. 4 (May 1987): 766–793.

Tone, Andrea. *Controlling Reproduction: An American History.* Wilmington, Del.: Scholarly Resources, 1997.

Tong, Rosemarie. "The Personhood Debate in Abortion." *The World & I* no. 5 (1992).

Tordjman, Dan. "Nine-Year-Old Girl and Mother Killed in House Fire, Family Visits Crime Scene." *WIS News* 10, June 5, 2007.

Torres, Aida, et al. "Public Benefits and Costs of Government Funding for Abortion," *Family Planning Perspectives* 18, no. 3 (1986): 111, 117.

"Torts: Child's Right of Action for Prenatal Injuries." *Indiana Law Journal* (December 1949): 91–95.

"Torts—Right of Parent to Recover for Prenatal Injuries Causing Death of a Child." *Texas Law Review* 11 (1933): 396–397.

Toumey, Christopher. *Conjuring Science: Scientific Symbols and Cultural Meanings in American Life.* New Brunswick, N.J.: Rutgers University Press, 1996.

Toufexis, Anastasia. "Innocent Victims," *Time*, May 13, 1991, 56–60.

Treub, Hector. *The Right to Life of the Unborn Child.* New York: Joseph F. Wagner, 1903.

Tribe, Lawrence. *Abortion: The Clash of Absolutes.* New York: W. W. Norton, 1990.

———. *American Constitutional Law*, 2nd ed. New York: Foundation Press, 1988.

Trussell, James., et al. "The Impact of Restricting Medicaid Financing for Abortion." *Family Planning Perspectives* 12 (1986): 120, 127.

Tuana, Nancy. "The History of Embryology." In *The Encyclopedia of Reproductive Technologies.* New York: Garland, 1996.

Tucker, Cora. *Women Make It Happen*. In *Empowering Ourselves: Women and Toxics Organizing*, edited Robbin Lee Zeff, Marsha Love, and Karen Stults. Falls Church, Va.: Citizens Clearinghouse for Hazardous Waste, 1987.

Turner, Frederick Jackson. "The Significance of the Frontier in American History." Delivered at the meeting of the American History Association in Chicago, July 12, 1893. Published in the *Proceedings of the State Historical Society of Wisconsin* 14 (1893).

Turner, McRae, Jr. "Torts: Recovery for Prenatal Injuries." *Mississippi Law Journal* 21 (1949): 174–175.

Ulrich, Laurel Thatcher. "The Living Mother of a Living Child: Midwifery and Mortality in Eighteenth-Century New England." *William and Mary Quarterly* 3rd series 66 (1989): 27–48.

"The Unborn Child." *University of Toronto Law Review* 4 (1941–1942): 278–295.

"Unborn Heartbeats." *Newsweek* (November 30, 1942): 74.

"University Presses and the Polarization of Science." *Science Monthly* (July 11, 1947): 28.

UPI. "Doctor, Convicted in Abortion, Charges Prejudice Barred Fair Trial in Boston." *New York Times*, February 17, 1975, 41.

———. "Medical Implications of Edelin Verdict Studied." *Boston Globe*, February 23, 1975, 1.

"U.S. District Judge Blocks Pregnant Women's Deportation, says Fetus is U.S. Citizen," *Washington Times*, May 29, 2004, 1.

Van Blarcom, Carolyn Conant. *Getting Ready to Be a Mother: A Little Book of Information and Advice for the Young Women Who is Looking Forward to Motherhood*. New York: Macmillan, 1922.

Van De Carr, F. Rene, et al. *While You Are Expecting: Creating Your Own Prenatal Classroom*. Humanics Ltd. Partners, 1996.

Varigny, Henry M. de. "The Experimental Psychology Laboratory of the University of Wisconsin of Madison." *Revue Scientifique* 1 (1894): 624–629.

Vawter, Dorothy, Warren Kearney, Karen G. Gervais, Arthur L. Caplan, Daniel Garry, and Carol Tauer. *The Use of Human Fetal Tissue: Scientific, Ethical, and Policy Concerns, a Report of Phase I of an Interdisciplinary Research Project Conducted by the Center for Biomedical Ethics*. Minneapolis: University of Minnesota, January 1990.

Veith, Gene Edward. "Worldview Warehouse." *World Magazine*, July 17, 1999, http://www.worldmag.com/articles/3007 (accessed June 8, 2010).

Verney, Thomas. *The Secret Life of the Unborn Child*. New York: Dell, 1981.

Vietor, Richard. *Energy Policy in America since 1945: A Study of Business-Government Relations*. New York: Cambridge University Press, 1984.

"Violence Continues in Boston: Kennedy Is Jostled by Crowd." *Worcester Telegram*, April 14, 1975, 1.

Von Raffler-Engel, Walburga. *The Perception of the Unborn Across the Cultures of the World*. Seattle, Wash.: Hogrefe & Huber, 1994.

Vrazo, Fawn. "Causing an Outcry with a 'Silent Scream.'" *Philadelphia Inquirer*, March 5, 1985, 8E.

Wall, Patrick. *Pain: The Science of Suffering*. New York: Columbia University Press, 2001.

Wall, Patrick, and Ronald Melzack, ed. *The Textbook of Pain*. Edinburgh: Churchill Livingston, 1994.

Walsh, Mary Roth. *"Doctors Wanted: No Women Need Apply": Sexual Barriers in the Medical Profession, 1835–1975*. New Haven: Yale University Press, 1977.

Walters, L. "Ethical Issues in Fetal Research: A Look Back and a Look Forward." *Clinical Research* 36 (1988): 209–214.

Wampler, F. J. *Industrial Medicine*. Baltimore: Williams and Wilkins, 1943.

Warren, Rosalind. *Women's Glibber: State of the Art Women's Humor*. Freedom, Calif.: Crossing Press, 1992.

Washington, Peter. *Madame Blavatsky's Baboon: A History of the Mystics, Mediums, and Misfits Who Brought Spiritualism to America*. New York: Schocken Books, 1993.

Weddington, Sarah. *A Question of Choice*. New York: Grosset/Putnam, 1992.

Weisman, Jonathan. "House to Consider Abortion Anesthesia Bill: Conservatives Vow More Tests for Democrats on Social Issues When Congress Returns." *Washington Post*, December 5, 2006, A6.

Weiss, Gail. *Body Images: Embodiment as Intercorporeality*. New York: Routledge, 1999.

Weiss, Gail, and Honi Fern Haber, eds. *Perspectives on Embodiment: The Intersections of Nature and Culture*. New York: Routledge Press, 1998.

Weiss, Nancy Pottishman. "Mother: The Invention of Necessity: Dr. Benjamin Spock's *Baby and Child Care*," *American Quarterly* 29 (Winter 1977): 519–546.

Weiss, Rick. "New Status for Embryos in Research," *Washington Post*, October 30, 2002, A01.

Welsome, Eileen. *The Plutonium Files: America's Secret Medical Experiments in the Cold War*. New York: Dell Books, 2000.

Welter, Barbara. "The Cult of True Womanhood, 1830–1960." *American Quarterly* 16 (1966): 151–174.

Welton, Donn, ed. *Body & Flesh: A Philosophical Reader*. London: Blackwell, 1998.

Westberg, Jenny. "Grim Technology for Abortion's Older Victims." *Life Advocate*, http://www.lifeadvocate.org/arc/dx.htm (accessed 15 July 2008).

Weyrich, Paul. "Unborn Pain." RenewAmerica.us, June 25, 2004, http://www.renewamerica.us/columns/weyrich/040625 (accessed July 14, 2008).

Whitcover, Jules. *Marathon: The Pursuit of Presidency, 1972–1976*. New York: Viking Press, 1997.

White, Diane. "Abortion Procedure Explained." *Boston Globe*, January 15, 1975, 1.

———. "Acquittal Motion Denied in Edelin Trial." *Boston Globe*, January 31, 1975, 1.

———. "Curtis Testifies Fetus Can Inhale Intrauterine Fluids." *Boston Globe*, January 24, 1975.

———. "Curtis Testifies Fetus Can Inhale Intrauterine Fluids. *Boston Globe*, January 25, 1975, 1.

———. "Duty to Mother, Not Fetus, Edelin Says." *Boston Globe*, February 4, 1975.

———. "Edelin Colleague Supports Contention of Prosecutor." *Boston Globe*, January 17, 1975, 1.

———. "Edelin Defense Asks Dismissal after New U.S. Ruling on Juries." *Boston Globe*, January 28, 1975, 1.

———. "Edelin Delay in Taking Fetus Proper Practice, Expert Says." *Boston Globe* February 7, 1975, 1.

———. "Edelin Jury: Their Faces Told Nothing." *Boston Globe*, January 13, 1975, 8.

———. "Edelin's Judgement Sound, Says Expert." *Boston Globe*, February 11, 1975, 1.

———. "Edelin Trial Arguments Conclude, Jury May Get Case Today." *Boston Globe*, February 14, 1975, 9.

———. "Fetus Never Breathed, Says Pathologist." *Boston Globe*, February 7, 1975, 1.

———. "Jury Convicts Edelin of Manslaughter." *Boston Globe*, February 16, 1975, 1.

———. "Medical Examiner Tell Court Fetus Has 'Respiratory Activity.'" *Boston Globe*, January 24, 1975, 1.

———. "Pathologist Say Fetus in Edelin Case Breathed." *Boston Globe*, January 29, 1975, 1.

———. "Survival 'Rare' at 1½ Pounds, Edelin Tells Jury." *Boston Globe*, February 6, 1975, 1.

———. "2 BCH Nurses Say No Clock on Wall When Edelin Operated." *Boston Globe*, February 5, 1975, 1.

———. "Witness Says Fetus 'Very Likely' Dead before Abortion." *Boston Globe*, February 12, 1975, 1.

White, Margaret. *Whence in Power of Ann Hite*. Boston: Christopher, 1937.

Whiting, Ellis W. *The Story of Life*. Chicago: Wilcox & Follett, 1933.

Whitner, Cornelia. "Letter to the Governor of South Carolina," National Advocates for Pregnant Women, November 10, 1999, http://advocatesforpregnantwomen.org/issues/corneliatr.htm.

Whyte, William H. *The Organization Man*. New York: Simon & Schuster, 1956.

Wiebe, Robert. *The Search for Order, 1877–1920*. New York: Hill and Wang, 1967.

Wikander, Ulla, Jane Lewis, and Alice Kessler-Harris, eds. *Protecting Women: Labor Legislation in Europe, The United States, and Australia, 1880–1920*. Urbana: University of Illinois, 1995.

Wilcox, Ella Wheeler. *The Heart of the New Thought*. Chicago: Psychic Research, 1902.

———. "Splendid Amazons and Pygmy Men." In *Today Then: America's Best Minds Look 100 Years into the Future on the Occasion of the 1893 World's Columbian Exposition*. Compiled and introduced by Dave Walter. Helena, Mont.: American & World Geographic, 1992.

Wilcox, Fred. *Waiting for an Army to Die: The Tragedy of Agent Orange*. New York: Vintage, 1983.

Wilde, Melissa J. *Vatican II: A Sociological Analysis of Religious Change*. Princeton: Princeton University Press, 2007.

Wilkinson, Signe. *Abortion (On Demand) Cartoons*. Broad Street Books: Philadelphia, 1992.

Williams, Alaine. "American Cyanamid: The Fight against Exclusionary Policies." Speech prepared for the PHILAPOSH Reproductive Hazards Workshop, February 21, 1987.

Williams, Glanville. *The Sanctity of Life and Criminal Law*. New York: Knopf, 1957.

Williams, John W. *Obstetrics: A Textbook for the Use of Students and Practitioners*, 9th ed. New York: Appleton, 1903.

Williams, S. J. "Modern Medicine and the 'Uncertain Body': From Corporeality to Hyperreality?" *Social Science & Medicine* 45, no. 7 (1997).

Williams, Wendy. "Firing the Woman to Protect the Fetus: The Reconciliation of Fetal Protection with Employment Opportunity Goals under Title VII." *Georgetown Law Journal* 69 (1980–1981): 641–704.

Willis, Claudia. "Silent Scream." *Time*, March 25, 1985, 54.

Willke, J. C. "Twenty Five Years of Loving Them Both." *Life Issues Connector*, July 1997, http://www.abortionfacts.com/dr_willke/connector_july_97.asp (accessed July 14, 2008).

Wilson, Sloan. *The Man in the Gray Flannel Suit*. New York: Da Capo Press, 1955.

Witcover, Jules. *Marathon: The Pursuit of the Presidency, 1972–1976*. New York: Viking Press, 1977.

Witt, Doris. "What (N)ever Happened to Aunt Jemima: Eating Disorders, Fetal Rights, and Black Female Appetite in Contemporary American Culture." *Discourse* 17, no. 2 (1994): 98–122.

Wolfe, Alan. *Impasse: The Rise and Fall of the Politics of Growth*. New York: Pantheon Books, 1981.

"Women for ROAR vs. Edelin Supporters." *Boston Phoenix*. Photograph caption, May 5, 1975, 1.

Woman's Needs and Necessities ~ or ~ A Plea for the Unborn and Infancy. Willimantic, Conn.: Hall and Rice, 1894.

Wong, Kenneth K., and Anna C. Nicotera. "Brown v. Board of Education and the Coleman Report: Social Science Research and the Debate on Educational Equality." *Peabody Journal of Education* 79, no. 2 (March 2004): 122–135.

Wood, Thomas. "Can One Influence an Unborn Child?" *Parents Magazine*5 (September 1930), 19.

World's Columbian Exposition: Chicago, Official Catalogue Exhibition of the German Empire., Berlin: Reichsdruckerei, 1893.

"World-Wide: Fathers Who Smoke." *Wall Street Journal*, January 24, 1991, 3.

Wright, Brett. "Smokers' Sperm Spell Trouble for Future Generations." *New Scientists*, March 6, 1993, 10.

Wright, Michael. "Reproductive Hazards and 'Protective' Discrimination." *Feminist Studies* 5, no. 2 (Summer 1979): 303–352.

Wylie, Philip. *Generation of Vipers*. New York: Pocket Books, 1942.

Yazigi, Ricardo, et al. "Demonstration of Specific Binding of Cocaine to Human Spermatozoa." *Journal of the American Medical Association* 266 (1991): 1596–1959.

Yergin, Daniel. *The Prize: The Epic Quest for Oil, Money, and Power*. New York: Simon & Schuster, 1991.

Yoken, Edward. "Seeing with Sound: A Study of the Development of Medical Images." In *The Social Construction of Technological Systems: New Directions in the Sociology and History of Technology*, edited by W. Bijker, T. Hughes, and T. Pinch. Cambridge: Massachusetts Institute of Technology, 1987.

Young, Iris. *Justice and the Politics of Difference*. Princeton: Princeton University Press, 1990.

Young, Nugent Alice. "Interpreting the Dangerous Trades: Workers' Health in America and the Career of Alice Hamilton, 1910–1935." PhD diss., Brown University, 1982.

Yudkin, Marcia. "Earth, Air, Water, Hearth: The Woman Who Founded Ecology." *Vassar Quarterly* (Spring 1982), 32–34.

Zaitchik, Alexander. "'Christian' Nativism." *Intelligence Report* 124 (Winter 2006): 2, http://www.splcenter.org/intel/intelreport/article.jsp?pid=1313 (accessed July 14, 2008).

Ziegler, Friedrich. *Prospectus Uber Die Zu Unterrichtszwecken hergestellten embrylogischen Wachsmodelle*. Freiberg. 1893.

Zimmerman, David R. *Rh: The Intimate History of a Disease and Its Conquest*. New York: Macmillan, 1973.

Zuckerman, Barry, and Deborah Frank. "Crack Kids: Not Broken." *Pediatrics* 89 (1992): 337–339.

Zwerin, Raymond A., and Shapiro, Richard J. "Abortion: Perspectives from Jewish Traditions." Religious Coalition for Reproductive Choice, Educational Series No. 5, n.d.

Index

abortifacient drugs, 16
abortion, 110, 155
  breast cancer (ABC) link, 162
  criminal, 17–18, 20, 21, 64
  induced, 162
  legalizing, 2, 4, 41, 64, 66, 69, 165
  Provider Refusal Rule and, 184
  restriction on second trimester, 98–99
  surgical, 16
  third trimester, 171
abortion boards, 64
abortion reform law, 65
Advisory Committee on Human
    Research Protections, 1
Aid to Families with Dependent
    Children (AFDC), 62–63, 165
Alito, Samuel, 154, 180
Allaire v. St. Luke's Hospital
    (1900), 23, 62
American Bar Association, 66
American Civil Liberties Union
    (ACLU), 31, 127, 129, 133, 141, 146
  Reproductive Freedom Project, 119,
    137, 150
American College of Obstetricians and
    Gynecologists, 65, 99, 113, 150, 157
American Cyanamid, 126–29
American History of Natural
    History, 36
American Law Institute (ALI), 64
  Model Penal Code (1962), 204n132
American Medical Association
    (AMA), 20, 21, 40, 48, 64, 149, 150
  Committee on Criminal Abortion, 16
American Pediatrics Association, 149
American Psychological Association,
    47, 163
American Public Health
    Association, 130, 150
Americans for Democratic Action, 75

Americans United for Life (AUL), 155,
    158, 168, 231n33
American Theosophical Society, 25
amniocentesis, 5, 68, 70, 93, 174
antenatal diagnosis, 71
antiabortion movement, 2, 5, 16, 17, 19,
    154–55, 157–58, 161–66, 169, 175–77,
    178, 229n10
Antioch College, Ohio, 200n43
Application of Donald L. Clarke, for a
    Writ of Habeas Corpus (1957), 62
Aristotle, 12
Army of God, 154
Arney William, 114
artificial insemination, 43
Asch, Stuart, 116
AT&T, 126
Atkins, Thomas, 104, 106
atomic and fetal culture, linking, 52
atomic energy, legal implications of, 59
Atoms and the Law, 59

Ballantyne, John William, 11
Barnum, P. T., 28
Bauer, Gary, 157
Bertin, Joan, 141
Besant, Annie, 25, 28
beta-thalassemia, 70
Beth Israel Hospital, 99, 109
Biography of the Unborn, The, 50
Blackmun, Harry, 66, 135
Boas, Franz, 28
Bobbitt, Lorena, 161
Boggs, Justice, 23
Bonbrest v. Katz (1946), 4, 52, 54, 55, 56,
    57, 62, 202n76
Bork, Robert, 128, 129
Borstelmann, Thomas, 57
Boston busing crisis, 8, 67–68, 72, 73, 83,
    104, 106–8, 109

Boston City Hospital (BCH), 8, 67,
74–75, 98, 101, 111
Committee on Human
Experimentation, 72
conscience clause, 69
Department of Obstetrics and
Gynecology, 69
Thorndike Memorial Laboratory, 68
Boston City Morgue, 79
Boston Globe, 84, 91, 98
Boston Medical and Surgical Journal, 19
Boston Phoenix, 80, 108
Boston School Committee, 106
Boston University, 86, 106, 150
Law School, 83
Medical School, 111, 216*n*233
Boston Women's Health Book
Collective, 75
Bradwell v. Illinois (1873), 182
Breast Cancer Prevention Institute, 162
Breyer, Stephen, 182
Brigham and Women's Hospital, 70
Brind, Joel, 162, 163
Brodie, Janet Farrell, 16
Broken Justice, 80
Brookline Free Hospital for Women, 42
Brownback, Sam, 178
Brown v. Board of Education (1954), 54
Buchanan, Patrick J., 147, 157, 185
Buckley, James, 78, 100
Buckley, William, 105
Buck v. Bell (1927), 36, 197*n*129
Bunker Hill Mining Company, 123–25
Bunning, Jim, 172
Burns v. Alcala (1975), 63
Bush, George W., 154, 165, 176, 184,
233*n*70
Button, Helen L., 39–40, 41
Byrne, Garrett, 74, 79, 104

Calderone, Mary S., 64
California Appellate Court, 62
Campbell, Nancy, 142–43
Canady, Charles, 169

Cangemi, Gary, 187, 188
Carder, Angela, 119
Carey, Eban James, 38, 39, 40
Carnegie Institute, 30, 36, 41, 47, 56
Department of Embryology,
15, 42, 70
Carter, Jimmy, 109, 128, 143
Casper, Monica, 201*n*4, 202*n*18,
216*n*6, 227*n*8
Catholic Charities Appeal and the
United Way, 83
Catholic Church, 72
Catholics for a Free Choice, 165
Catholic University, 83
Catholic University of America, 231*n*28
Center for Reproductive Law and
Policy (CLRP), 148
Center for Reproductive Rights, 178
Century of Progress World's Fair, 38, 43
Charles, David, 69, 75
Charleston County, South Carolina, 145
Charles v. Carey (1980), 167
Chasnoff, Ira, 137
Chavkin, Wendy, 140
Chessick, Robert J., 138
Chicago-Kent Law Review, 54
Chicago Medical Society, 21, 22
child development and democracy,
relationship between, 58
child neglect, 146
Children's Bureau, 31, 35
Children's Hospital, 70
Christian Coalition, 154
Christian Science, 26
Church, Louisa Randall, 51
Civil Liberties Union of
Massachusetts, 75
Civil Rights Act (1964), 5, 121, 122
Clement, Paul, 179, 180
Clinton, Bill, 143, 144, 149, 173, 175, 176
clyndamycin, 68, 69
Coalition for the Reproductive Rights of
Workers (CRROW), 130, 133
Coalition of Labor Union Women, 130

Coalition on Abortion/Breast
    Cancer, 162
Cobb, Matthew, 11
Coburn, Tom, 163
cocaine, 2, 140, 141, 145–48, 150, 151–52
Collins, Vincent J., 158
Color Line, The, 24
Columbia Presbyterian Hospital, 114
Columbia University, 80
Combahee River Collective, 99
Commonwealth of Massachusetts v.
    Kenneth Edelin (1976), 214n183
Commonwealth v. Gricus (1944), 101
compassion, 164–65
compassionate conservatism, 165
Compassionate Pain Relief Act, 165
Concerned Women for America
    (CWA), 155
Condon, Charles, 145, 147, 148, 151
Conference on Women and Health, 99
Connelly, Thomas, 69, 70, 72, 73
Contract with America, 144
Conyers, John, 176
Cook County Hospital, 39, 40
Corea, Gena, 187
Cornell Law Quarterly, 54, 58
Cornell Medical Center, New York
    Hospital, 160
Corner, George Washington, 41, 42, 43,
    44, 49–50
Coronet magazine, 47
Costello, Coreen, 174, 175
Council of Vienne, 19
Cox, Ruth, 92
crack babies, 2, 142, 144, 146
crack mothers, 137
Crick, Francis, 13
criminal abortion, 17–18, 20, 21, 64
Criminal Abortion, 20
Crystal Ferguson et al v. City of Charleston
    (2001), 149, 151
Curley, James Michael, 108
Curran, William J., 110
Curtis, Ellyn, 92, 93

Curtis, George T., 79, 80, 82, 91, 92
Cushing, Richard Cardinal, 73

Daniels, Cynthia, 117, 118
Darrow, Clarence, 31
Darwin, Charles, 28
Davenport, Charles Benedict, 30
Dawes, Rufus, 43
Death of the West, The, 157
DeCamp, James A., 167
Decision Research Corp., 83
Decreten, 19
Degler, Carl, 19
Delahunt, William, 70, 71, 206n23
de Lamarck, Jean Baptiste, 30
delayed ensoulment, 19, 195n59
delayed hominization, 19
Democratic Leadership Council
    (DLC), 143
Democratic Party, 108, 109, 145
Department of Health and Human
    Services (DHHS), 1, 137, 184, 210n88
    Office for Civil Rights (OCR), 148
Department of Human Resources, 117
Department of Justice, 125
Department of Labor, 123, 125
dependent child, 62–63
Depo-Provera, 76
D-HEW report, 124
diethylstilbestrol (DES), 76
Dietrich v. Northampton (1884), 4, 22, 23,
    52, 53, 54, 55, 56, 57
DiGeorge syndrome, 76, 208n66
dilation and evacuation (D&E)
    method, 169, 174
dilation and extraction (D&X)
    procedure, 169, 174, 175, 176
Dilemma of the Fetus, The, 110
disability rights movement, 76
District of Columbia
    Circuit Court, 128
    Court of Appeals, 119
Donald, Ian, 5
Dorland, William A. Newman, 18

Douglas, William O., 139
Dow Chemical, 126
Dudziak, Mary, 57
Dufour, Lew, 38, 39, 40, 43
Dyer, Frederick, 16

Eagle Forum, 154, 156
Eastman Kodak, 126
Edelin, Kenneth, 8, 67, 69, 80, 81, 83, 84,
    91, 92, 93, 94–96, 97, 98, 100, 101, 102,
    103, 107, 110–11, 186, 216*n*233
Edelin, Ramona Hoage, 104, 106
electronic fetal monitoring
    (EFM), 116
Elliot Institute for Social Science
    Research, 161, 232*n*50
embryo, 1, 3, 7, 10, 12, 13–15, 18, 22, 27, 38,
    40, 42, 44, 46, 52, 194*n*28
embryologists, 13–16, 42–43
embryon, 12
Em-bry-on-ics Learning System, 186
epigenesist, 12, 13
Equal Employment Opportunity
    Commission (EEOC), 124, 125,
    126, 127, 133
Equal Rights Amendment (ERA), 67,
    107, 123
erythromycin, 68
eugenics, 24, 29–30, 31, 36, 37
Eugenics Record Office, 30
euthenics, 24, 30–31, 37
evolutionary model of embryology,
    of Haeckel, 14
Ewalt, Jack, 70
exclusionary policies. *See* fetal protection
    policies
Experimental Negotiating
    Agreement, 125
ex utero life, 93

Fair Labor Standards Act (1938), 123
Falwell, Jerry, 159
Family Research Council, 154, 157
family values ideology, 155, 156

Ferguson, Crystal, 148
Ferguson v. The City of Charleston
    (2001), 5
fertilization, 32–33, 43
    in-vitro, 42
fetal pain, 163–83
    liberalism and, 164–67, 171, 173
Fetal Pain hearings, 166
fetal protect policies, 8, 113, 120, 121, 122,
    124, 126, 127, 128, 129, 130, 131, 132–33,
    134, 135, 220*n*59
fetal psyche, 48
fetal research, 8, 68, 69, 70, 71, 72, 75–76,
    77, 78–79, 82, 86, 100
Fetal Research, 79
Fewer and Better Babies, 23
Finkbine, Sherri, 64, 65
Finney, Charles, 29
Firestone Tire, 126
First National Conference on
    Abortion Laws, 66
Fitzgerald, "Honey Fitz," 108
Flanagan, Newman, 74, 79, 83, 84, 85, 88,
    90, 91–92, 95–96, 97, 102, 103–4, 106,
    205*n*5, 208*n*52
Florida, 140
Flynn, Raymond L., 70, 71, 72, 106,
    207*n*33
Focus on the Family, 154, 155
Food and Drug Administration (FDA), 184
food stamps, 165
Fordham Law Review, 58
Fourteenth Amendment, 148, 156
Fourth Amendment, 149
Frank, Deborah, 150
Freedom of Access to Clinics Entrances
    Act (FACE) (1994), 2
Free Thought, 27
Frist, Bill, 176
From, Al, 143
frontier anxiety, 113

Gallagher, Janet, 114
Galton, Francis, 28

Garrity, W. Arthur, 71, 83, 106
General Motors, 126
Generation of Vipers, 49
genetics, 30
Georgetown University, 209*n*75
   Hospital, 115
Georgia Right to Life Committee, 101
Georgia Supreme Court, 58
Gesell, Arnold, 47, 52
Gestalt school of psychology, 47
Gilbert, Margaret Shea, 50
Gimenez-Jimeno, Enrique, 81, 90, 92, 96,
   103, 212*n*124
Gingrich, Newt, 144
Ginsburg, Ruth Bader, 179, 182, 183
Globe, 102
Gonzales v. Carhart and Gonzales v.
   Planned Parenthood Federation of
   America, Inc., et al. (2007), 8, 153,
   154, 179, 180, 183 237*n*142
Governor's Commission on the Status
   of Women, 107
grave-robbing statute, 67, 205*n*1
Great Depression, 46
Great Society, 8, 108, 165
Gruenberg, Sidonie Matsner, 51

Haeckel, Ernst, 14
Hall, Faneuil, 107
Hall, G. Stanley, 28
Hall, Ward, 40, 41, 67
Hall of Science exhibit, 38, 40
Hamilton, Alice, 122, 131
Handbook of Public Assistance, 63
Harlem's Joint Disease, 141
Harman, Moses, 27
Harrington, Monsignor Paul, 73
Harrison, Michael, 119
Harris Poll, 76, 97
Harris v. McRae (1980), 216*n*230
Hartsoecker, Niklass, 13
Harvard Medical School, 16, 68, 70,
   86, 94, 122
Harvey, William, 12

Haskell, Martin, 169, 180
Hastings Center, 77, 209*n*75
Hatch, Orrin G., 164
Head Start, 165
Healing Hearts, 161
Health and Hospital Committee, 71
heredity, 24, 29, 36, 31, 34–35
Heritage Foundation, 229*n*10
heroin crisis, 135, 138–39
Hertig, Arthur, 5, 42, 43, 70, 93
Hertwig, Oscar, 13
Herzog, Maximillian, 23
Hicks, Louise Day, 72, 74, 106, 107
Hildebrand, Kit, 44
Hippocrates, 12, 17
His, Wilhelm, 14
History of Man, The: Embryology
   exhibit, 38–39, 39*f*, 43
Hodge, Hugh Lenox, 17, 18–19, 21
Holbo, Christine, 31
Hollander, Nicole, 131, 132*f*
Holmes, Oliver Wendell, 22, 36–37, 52
Holmes, Rudolph, 21, 22
Holtrap, Hugh, 81, 88, 210*n*96
Homans, William, 82, 83, 84, 85, 86, 88,
   89, 91, 92, 93, 94–97, 98, 101, 103, 104,
   106, 211*n*107
Hornbuckle v. Plantation Pipe Line
   (1956), 58
House Democratic Caucus, 143
House Judiciary Committee
   Subcommittee on the
   Constitution, 174
House Ways and Means Committee, 63
Hrdlicka, Alex, 36
Hudson v. Michigan (2006),
   233*n*72
Humanae Vitae, 73
Human Life Amendment,
   100, 109, 114
Human Pain Relief Act, 166
"Hyde Amendment," 110
Hygeia magazine, 40
hysterotomy, 82, 88, 90, 94

Idaho Human Rights Commission
    (IHRC), 125, 126
Illinois Right to Life Committee, 101
Indiana Law Journal, 62
infertility, 49
informed consent, 167–68
innate physical and mental abilities,
    measuring, 28–29
In re A.C. (1990), 4, 119
Institute for Learning Innovation, 186
Institute for Pregnancy Loss,
    161, 232n49
"Interagency Policy on Cocaine Abuse
    in Pregnancy," 145
International Music Society for Prenatal
    Development, 186
International Right to Life
    Federation, 156
International Society for Traumatic
    Stress Studies, 232n49
in utero life, 49, 52, 55, 84, 88, 114, 120,
    122, 127, 133, 135, 146, 174, 175, 187
in vitro fertilization, 42
involuntary sterilization law (1907),
    197n129
Irish-Catholic identity, 69, 71, 74, 83, 103,
    104, 105, 107, 108, 145
Istook, Ernest, 171

Japan, 125
Jastrow, Joseph, 28
Jefferson, Jessie Mae, 117, 118
Jefferson, Mildred, 73, 86, 212n124
Johns Hopkins University, 5
    School of Medicine, 10, 11, 14
Johnson, Douglas, 169
Johnson, Lyndon B., 165
Johnson Controls, 133, 134
Jones, Jessie, 115
Jones, Maggie, 120
*Journal of American Physicians and
    Surgeons*, 162
*Journal of the American Medical
    Association* (JAMA), 163, 177–78

Kanner, Leo, 57, 58
Kansas Liberal, 27
Kelly, James E., 20
Kelsey, Frances, 204n134
Kennedy, Anthony, 168, 180, 181, 182, 183
Kennedy, Edward, 144
Kennedy, Jack, 108
Kennedy, Ted, 78, 79
Kennedy Institute, 77
Kenner, Francis, 218–19n32
Kenney, Sally, 129
King, Jr., Martin Luther, 188
Kinsey, Alfred, 64
Klyne, Robert, 126–27
Knights of Columbus, 83, 208n52
"knock-and-announce" rule, 233n72
Kogan, Herman, 45
Koop, C. Everett, 232n49
Kopp, James, 3
Kornberg, Arthur, 76

Ladies Home Journal, 51
Lake County Fair, 40
Lamson, Armenouhie Tashjian, 10, 11,
    31–35, 39
Lathrop, Julia, 31
lead, 121, 122–23, 124, 125–26, 127, 128, 129,
    131, 133–34
Lead Industries Association, 121
League of Women Voters, 75
Lieberman, J. R., 116, 117
Liebling, A. J., 38, 39
Life, 46
Life Advocate, 169, 170
Life Decisions International, 229n10
Life Issues, 156
Liley, William, 5, 113
Lincoln, Abraham, 45
Lippmann, Walter, 11
Littlest Junkie, The, 135
Long Island Coalition for Life, 109
Lowe, Ernest W., 101
Loyola University exhibit, 38, 39, 40, 44
Luckhardt, Albert E., 53

Mall, Franklin Paine, 5, 14, 15
Malpighi, Marcello, 12
Malthus, Thomas, 23
Manifesto for the Saving of the Unborn Child and the Restoration of the Republic, A, 189
manslaughter
  accusation of, 83–84
  interpretation of, 98, 100
Manual of Obstetrics, 18
March of Dimes, 150
Marshall, Thurgood, 154
Massachusetts Association of Hospitals, 105
Massachusetts Citizens for Life (MCL), 69, 71, 72, 75, 100, 104, 106, 212*n*124
Massachusetts Institute of Technology, 30
Massachusetts Organization for the Repeal of Abortion Laws rights, 75
Massachusetts State House, 107
Massachusetts Youth for Life, 72
maternal impressions, 48
Maynard-Moody, Stephen, 110
McDonough, Patrick F., 72, 106
McFall v. Shrimp (1978), 218*n*20
McGuire, James P., 54, 83, 84, 85, 88, 91, 92, 98, 101, 214*n*183
McKnight, Regina, 151, 152
Mecklenburg, Fred E., 212*n*124
Medeiros, Humberto Cardinal, 73
Medicaid, 165
Medical College of Virginia, 160
Medical University of South Carolina (MUSC), 145, 147–48
Meharry Medical College, 80
Melting Pot, The, 24
Menkin, Miriam, 42
metaphor, fetal body as, 11, 33
microscope, 13
Militant, 106
Minnesota Supreme Court, 55

"Miracle of Growth" exhibit, 43–44, 50, 52, 58
Missouri Doctors for Life, 212*n*124
Missouri House of Representatives, 156
Mitchell, Mary, 20
Mitchell v. Couch (1955), 203*n*99
Moakley, Joe, 108
momism, 49
Mondale, Walter, 76
Moral Majority, 154, 159
Morgan, Lynn, 15
Morgan v. Hennigan (1973), 71
Moseley, Kathryn, 167
Mount Sinai Medical Center, Department of Obstetrics and Gynecology, 166
Moynihan, Daniel Patrick, 144
Muller v. Oregon (1908), 121, 122, 123, 182
Museum of Science and Industry, Chicago, 41, 43, 44, 45, 186
Muskie, Ed, 143
My Birth: The Autobiography of an Unborn Infant, 10, 31, 35
Myer, Edwin C., 160

NAACP Legal Defense and Educational Fund, 216*n*233
NARAL Pro-Choice America, 178, 234*n*86
Nassau Medical Center, 109
Nathan, David, 70, 71, 74
Nathanson, Bernard, 8, 153–54, 159, 160–61, 163, 164, 166
National Abortion Federation, 178
  Risk Management Seminar, 169, 180
National Abortion Rights Action League (NARAL), 99
National Association for Prenatal Psychology and Education, 186
National Association for Repeal of Abortion Laws (NARAL), 66, 159
National Black Feminist Organization, 99
National Cancer Institute (NCI), 163

National Child Neurology Society, 160
National Commission for Human Life, 101
National Commission for the Protection of Human Subjects of Biomedical and Behavioral Research, 78, 100
National Health Services Corps, 140
National Institutes of Health (NIH), 69, 77–78, 148
National Organization for Women (NOW), 75
National Religious Broadcasters convention, 157
National Research Act (1974), 78
National Review, 105, 164, 233*n*66
National Right to Life Committee (NRLC), 73, 101, 154, 155, 156, 162, 163, 169, 178, 187
National Right to Life Organization, 100
National Student Conference Against Racism (NSCAR), 106, 107
National Woman's Party, 10, 123
Nebraska Law Review, 54
negative eugenics, 30, 36–37
negligence, 22, 23, 53
    guilty of, 102–3
    imputed, 62
    suing for, 52, 55
    in tort liability cases, 52–55, 59
New Deal, 108, 123
New England Deaconess Hospital, 99
New England Hospital for Women and Children, 16
New England Journal of Medicine (NEJM), 42, 69, 70, 110, 117, 118, 136, 163
New England Telephone Company, 102
Newsweek, 43, 45, 101
New Thought, 25
New Woman, 138
New York City, 140, 141
    Welfare Council report, 224*n*142
New Yorker, 38
New York Medical College, Metropolitan Hospital, 138

New York Times, 18, 74, 75, 98, 108, 120, 142
Nilsson, Lennart, 46, 91, 135, 136*f*
Nix, Joseph, 22
Nixon, Richard, 78, 108
"no-knock" laws, 233*n*72
Noonan, John T., 158, 231*n*28
North Dakota, 185
North General Hospital, 141
Noyes, John Humphrey, 29
Nuremberg Code (1949), 77

Obama, Barack, 184
Obstetricians, 114
Occupational Health and Safety Review Commission (OHSRC), 128
O'Connor, Sandra Day, 154, 168, 233*n*85
Office of Technological Assessment (OTA), 121
Ohio State Law Journal, 56
Oil, Chemical, and Atomic Workers Union (OCAW), 127, 128, 133
Olasky, Marvin, 165
Oneida community, 29
O'Neil, Albert "Dapper," 69, 70, 71, 72, 73, 74, 79, 86, 106
O'Neill, Thomas P. "Tip," 108
Operation Rescue. *See* Operation Save America
Operation Save America, 154, 189, 229*n*10
Opium: The Demon Flower, 138
Oprah Winfrey Show, 112
Osborn, Henry Fairfield, 36
Occupational Health and Safety Administration (OSHA), 124, 127, 128, 129
O'Steen, David, 163
Ourselves Unborn, 49

Paige, Connie, 80, 108, 205*n*5
pain, 231*n*27. *See also individual entries*
Parents magazine, 44
partial-birth abortion, 169–72
Partial Birth Abortion Ban Act, 8, 153, 154, 176, 179, 180, 235*nn*108, 121

Paul, Annie Murphy, 158
Penza, James F., 82, 88, 89
Pernick, Martin, 158
Personal Responsibility and Work
    Opportunity Reconciliation
    Act. *See* Welfare Reform Act
personhood, of fetus, 34
personhood bill, 185
PersonhoodUSA, 184
Person in the Womb, The, 50
Petchesky, Rosalind, 187
Philipson, Agnita, 68, 69, 75
pickled fetus, 40, 41, 67
Pilot, 83, 105
Pincus, Gregory, 42
Pinto-Correia, Clara, 13
Plan B, 184
Planned Parenthood, 64, 99, 109, 111, 160
Planned Parenthood Federation of
    America, 178, 216n233
*Planned Parenthood of Southeastern
    Pennsylvania v. Casey* (1992), 168,
    169, 176, 181, 182, 236n138
Plea for the Unborn, A, 24
Podhoretz, Norman, 233n66
Pope Pius IX, 19
positive eugenics, 30
post-abortion trauma, 161, 163
postwar pronatal culture and
    prenatal culture, 44
preformationists, 12–13
pregnancy, 2, 5, 18, 22, 23, 24, 26, 35,
    116–17, 149 (*see also* abortion)
    and copulation, 11–12
Pregnancy Counseling Service, 75
prenatal care, inadequate, 149
prenatal culture, 24, 25–28, 37, 44
prenatal development, 46–47
prenatal mind, 48
prenatal neglect, 62
prenatal neurosis, 48
prenatal psychology, 47
prenatal torts, 52–55
Prescott, James W., 165, 166

President's Commission on Health
    Science and Society, 76
Prince v. Massachusetts (1944), 218n20
Prisoners of Christ, 154
Pritchard, Jack, 93
Pro-Child Life Score, 165
Progressive Era, 7, 11, 14, 24, 29, 30, 31, 36,
    41, 122, 185, 186
progressivism, 24
pro-life movement, 72, 100, 101, 110,
    229n10
Provider Refusal Rule, 184
Public Interest Research Group, 218n24

Q-test, 43

Race Culture or Race Suicide?, 24
race suicide, 21
Rachel's Vineyard Ministries, 161
Racial Imbalance Act (1965), 71
Rakic, Pasko, 160
Raleigh-Fitkin-Paul Morgan Memorial
    Hospital, 115
Rangel, Charles, 143–44
Reagan, Ronald, 109, 128, 154, 157, 163
Reardon, David, 161, 162, 232n50
Redstockings, 66
reproductive endocrinologists, 43
Republican National Coalition for
    Life, 156
Republican Party, 137, 144, 154, 165
research, on fetus, 77–79
Restore Our Alienated Rights
    (ROAR), 72, 106, 107
Reyes, Margaret, 139
Rhoden, Nancy, 119
Ribicoff, Abe , 76
Richards, Ellen Swallow, 30–31
Richards, Justice, 62
Riggs, Betty, 126, 127
*Right of the Child to Be Well Born,
    The,* 24
Rights of the Unborn Race, The, 24
Rights of Unborn Children, The, 24

Right to Life Committee, 100, 187
Right to Life of the Unborn Child, The, 24
Rivera, Geraldo, 135
Road to H, The, 138
Roberts, Dorothy E., 137
Roberts, John, 180
Robinson, William J., 23
Robinson v. California (1962), 139
Rock, John, 5, 42, 43, 93
Rockefeller, John D., 66
Roe, Alice, 81, 82, 88, 94, 95, 103, 210n96
Roe v. Wade (1973), 2, 4, 41, 64, 66, 67, 68, 69, 71, 72, 78, 79, 92, 100, 105, 109, 110, 113, 135, 153, 154, 167, 168, 182, 185, 208n53
Rogers, Joe, 38, 39, 40, 43
Rogers v. Danforth (1975), 212n124
Roman Catholic Church, 6
Romper Room, 64
Roosevelt, Franklin D., 188
Roosevelt, Theodore, 21
Roth, Rachel, 133, 218n32, 223n117
Rudolph, Eric, 3
Rue, Vincent, 161, 232n49
Ryan, Kenneth, 70, 100

Sabath, Leon, 68, 69
Safe Haven, 161
Safire, William, 108
Salisbury, Lynn, 75
Samuel S. Fels Research Institute, 46, 47, 48, 56, 100, 200n43
Samuelson, Peter, 168
San Diego County, 139–40
Santorum, Rick, 176
Scalia, Antonin, 180
Scarry, Elaine, 158
Schlafly, Phyllis, 156
Schloendorff v. Society of New York Hospital (1914), 218n20
Schultz, A. H., 36
Schweitzer, Albert, 52
Science magazine, 75
Science News Letter, 43
Scopes Trial (1925), 100

Search for the Beloved, The, 48
Second International Congress of Eugenics, 36
Senate Finance Committee, 63
Senate Subcommittee on the Constitution of the Committee of the Judiciary, 164
Sensenbrenner, James, 176
"separate spheres," 155
Seventh Circuit Court of Appeals, 134
sex discrimination, 127, 129–30, 133, 141
Shafer, Brenda P., 174, 180
Shalala, Donna, 148, 149
Sheehan, Alan, 208n53
Sheehan, J. M., 21
Sheila, Sister, 73
Sheppard-Towner Maternity and Infancy Protection Act (1921), 35, 37
Siegel, Reva, 229n5
Silberman, Alan, 81, 89
Silent Scream, The, 8, 153, 159–60, 164
simultaneous animation, 195n59
Sinclair, Upton, 193n6
Slepian, Bernard, 3
Smith, Senator Gordon, 172, 173
Smith, Theresa Joller, 53
Smith v. Luckhardt (1938), 53
Snowflake Embryo Donation and Adoption Awareness Program, 185
Sobran, Joseph, 164–65, 166, 233n66
social Darwinists, 36
Social Science Resource Commission (1946), 202n70
Social Security Act, 63
Social Security Board, 62
Society for the Protection of Unborn Children (SPUC), 114
sonogram images, 3
Sontag, Lester W., 48, 200n43
Souter, David, 168, 182
South Boston High School, 106
South Carolina, 145–46
South Carolina Advocates for Pregnant Women, 147, 150

South Dakota Taskforce to Study
    Abortion, 156
Speckhard, Anne, 161, 232*n*53
Spencer, Herbert, 23
Spock, Benjamin, 57
St. Augustine, 19, 195*n*59
St. Luke's Hospital, 23
St. Thomas Aquinas, 19
State Child Health Insurance Program
    (S-CHIP), 1
state intervention, in immigration and
    reproduction regulation, 36
Stella, Vikki, 171
Stemmer, Pauline, 53
Stenberg v. Carhart (2000), 175, 176
Stern, Roy, 138, 139
Sternberg, Julie, 150
Stevens, John Paul, 149, 179, 180, 182
Stewart, Pamela Rae, 139
Stockbridge School, 80
Storer, Horatio Robinson, 5, 16–17, 20,
    21, 30, 43, 156, 186
Stormer, Nathan, 20
Stotland, Nada, 163
Stowe, Harriet Beecher, 164
Strecker, Edward, 49
Studies in Law and Medicine, 158
Sundgaard, Arnold, 50
Super Baby, 186
Supreme Judicial Court of
    Massachusetts, 101, 110
surgical abortions, 16

Taft, William Howard, 31
Taussig, Frederick, 22
Taylor v. Louisiana (1975), 211*n*107
Tertullian, 19, 195*n*60
thalidomide, 64
Their Mothers' Sons, 49
theosophy, 25
therapeutic abortion, 64, 69
Thomas, Clarence, 154, 180
Tiller, George, 2
Time magazine, 45, 53, 75, 141

Tingley, Katherine, 25
Today's Health magazine, 48
"Treatise on the Soul," 19
Turner, Frederick Jackson, 31
Tuskegee syphilis study, 162

ultrasound technology, 1, 174
Umbert the Unborn, 187
Unborn Child Pain Awareness Act
    (UCPAA) (2006), 153, 154, 178
Unborn Patient, The, 119
Unborn Victim of Violence Act, 157
Unborn Victims of Violence
    Act (2004), i
Uncle Tom's Cabin, 164
Union Carbide, 126
*Union Pacific Railway Company v.
    Botsford* (1891), 218*n*20
United Auto Workers of America
    (UAW), 133, 135
United Auto Workers v. Johnson Controls
    (1991), 5, 135
United States Museum of Natural
    History, 36
United Steelworkers Association of
    America (USWA), 124, 125
University of Auckland, Postgraduate
    School of Obstetrics and
    Gynaecology, 114
University of California, 231*n*28
University of Chicago, 14
University of Colorado Medical
    Center, 218*n*32
University of Illinois Law Forum, 56
University of Illinois Medical School, 48
University of Michigan, 14, 58
University of North Carolina, 94
University of Notre Dame, 231*n*28
University of Pennsylvania Medical
    School, 17
University of South Carolina, 145
University of Washington, Laboratory
    for the Study of Human Embryos
    and Fetuses, 68

University of Wisconsin, 28
U.S. Air Force Hospital, 80
U. S. Department of Health, Education,
    and Welfare, 78, 79, 121
*Using Women: Gender, Drug Policy, and
    Social Justice,* 142
U.S. Public Health Service, 46

Value of Life Committee, 72
VanDerHoef, Kenneth, 101
vasectomy, 134
Verkennes v. Corniea (1949),
    55, 202*n*93
viability, 89, 93
    shift to conception, 58
    transformation from
        separability, 57
Victims of Choice, 161
violation of sepulture, 67
Virginia, 141
von Baer, Karl Ernst, 13
vulnerability, of fetus, 46

Wallace, George, 108
Ward, John, 92, 93
War on Poverty, 165
Washington, George, 188
Washington Post, 77, 98
Watson, James, 13
Webster v. Reproductive Health Services
    (1989), 233*n*85
Weismann, August, 13, 30
Welby, Marcus, 105
Welfare Reform Act (1996), 144
Westberg, Jenny, 169
Weyrich, Paul, 229*n*10
While You're Expecting, 186
White, Diane, 91, 102
White, Leon, 72, 75
Whitner, Cornelia, 2, 145–46
"Why can't we love them both?"
    campaign, 156

*Why Not? A Book Intended for Every
    Woman,* 16
Wilberforce, William, 171
Wilcox, Ella Wheeler, 25, 26
Wilkinson, Signe, 131
Williams Obstetrics, 56, 59
Williams v. Marion Rapid Transit Inc.
    Supreme Court of Ohio (1949),
    55–56, 57
Willke, J. C., 156
Willowbrook State School for
    the Retarded, 76
Wilson, Pete, 142
Wofford, Harris, 144
Woman Citizen, The, 35
Women's Bureau of, 123, 131
Women's Health and Human
    Life Protection Act (2006), 153, 156
women's health movement, 217*n*12
Women Exploited by Abortion
    (WEBA), 161
*Wonderful Story of How You Were Born,
    The,* 51
Woods v. Lancet (1951), 203*n*99
World's Columbian Exposition, Chicago
    (1893), 25, 29, 30
World's Parliament of Religions, 25
World Medical Association, Declaration
    of Helsinki, 77
Wright, Frances, 29
Wright Patterson Air Force Base,
    Ohio, 80
Wylie, Philip, 49

Yale Research Institute for the Study of
    Prenatal and Postnatal
    Environment, 47
Yale University, 50
    School of Medicine, 160, 166

Zero Population Growth, 75
Ziegler, Friedrich, 25, 38

Printed in the USA/Agawam, MA
January 27, 2015

607369.016